Questions and Answers in Small Animal Anesthesia

Questions and Answers in Small Animal Anesthesia

EDITED BY

Lesley J. Smith DVM, DACVAA

Clinical Professor of Anesthesiology, Department of Surgical Sciences
School of Veterinary Medicine, University of Wisconsin
Madison, Wisconsin, USA

WILEY Blackwell

This edition first published 2016 © 2016 by John Wiley & Sons, Inc.

Editorial offices: 1606 Golden Aspen Drive, Suites 103 and 104, Ames, Iowa 50010, USA

The Atrium, Southern Gate, Chichester, West Sussex, PO19 8SQ, UK

9600 Garsington Road, Oxford, OX4 2DQ, UK

For details of our global editorial offices, for customer services and for information about how to apply for permission to reuse the copyright material in this book please see our website at www.wiley.com/wiley-blackwell.

Library of Congress Cataloging-in-Publication Data

Questions and answers in small animal anesthesia / [edited by] Lesley J. Smith.
    p. ; cm.
  Includes bibliographical references and index.
    ISBN 978-1-118-91283-6 (paper)
    I. Smith, Lesley J., 1962- , editor.
    [DNLM: 1. Anesthesia–veterinary–Problems and Exercises. 2. Analgesia–veterinary–Problems and Exercises. 3. Anesthetics–therapeutic use–Problems and Exercises. SF 914]
    SF914.Q47 2015
    636.089'796–dc23

                                                              2015018227

A catalogue record for this book is available from the British Library.

Wiley also publishes its books in a variety of electronic formats. Some content that appears in print may not be available in electronic books.

Typeset in 9.5/13pt MeridienLTStd by SPi Global, Chennai, India.
Printed in Singapore by C.O.S. Printers Pte Ltd

1   2016

This book is dedicated to the many veterinary patients and students that have taught me so much over the years about anesthesia and about how to teach it. It is also dedicated to my husband and companion animals, who remind me on a daily basis why I do what I do, and how important these creatures are in our lives.

Contents

List of Contributors

Richard M. Bednarski, DVM, MSc, DACVAA
Professor, Veterinary Anesthesiology, Department of Veterinary Clinical Sciences, College of Veterinary Medicine, The Ohio State University, USA

Javier Benito, LV, MS
Resident in Veterinary Anesthesiology, Département de Sciences Cliniques, Faculté de Médecine Vétérinaire, Université de Montréal, Canada

Benjamin M. Brainard VMD, DACVAA, DACVECC
Associate Professor, Critical Care, College of Veterinary Medicine, University of Georgia, USA

Andrew Claude DVM, DACVAA
Assistant Professor and Service Chief, Anesthesiology, Mississippi State University College of Veterinary Medicine, USA

Tanya Duke-Novakovski BVetMed, MSc, DVA, DACVAA, DECVAA
Professor of Veterinary Anesthesiology, Department of Small Animal Clinical Sciences, Western College of Veterinary Medicine, University of Saskatchewan, Canada

Berit L. Fischer DVM, DACVAA, CCRP
Anesthesia Director, Animal Medical Center, New York City, USA

Stephen A. Greene DVM, MS, DACVAA
Professor of Anesthesia & Analgesia, Department of Veterinary Clinical Sciences, College of Veterinary Medicine, Washington State University, USA

Tamara Grubb DVM, PhD, DACVAA
Assistant Clinical Professor of Anesthesia & Analgesia, Department of Veterinary Clinical Sciences, College of Veterinary Medicine, Washington State University, USA

Rebecca A. Johnson DVM, PhD, DACVAA
Clinical Associate Professor of Anesthesia and Pain Management, Department of Surgical Sciences, School of Veterinary Medicine, University of Wisconsin, USA

Martin J. Kennedy DVM
Anesthesiologist, MedVet Animal Medical and Cancer Center for Pets, Ohio, USA

Carolyn Kerr DVM, DVSc, PhD, DACVAA
Professor of Anesthesiology and Department Chair Department of Clinical Studies,
Ontario Veterinary College, University of Guelph, Canada

Katrina Lafferty BFA, CVT, VTS (Anesthesia)
Senior Technician, Section of Anesthesia and Pain Management, Director, Veterinary
Technician Student Internship Program, University of Wisconsin-Madison, USA

Lydia Love DVM, DACVAA
Anesthesia Director, Animal Emergency & Referral Associates, USA

Beatriz Monteiro DVM
Département de Biomédecine Vétérinaire, Faculté de Médecine Vétérinaire,
Université de Montréal, Canada

Jo Murrell BVSc, PhD, DECVAA
School of Veterinary Sciences, University of Bristol, UK

Odette O DVM, DACVAA
Assistant Professor of Anesthesiology, Ross University School of Veterinary Medicine,
St. Kitts

Lysa Pam Posner DVM, DACVAA
North Carolina State University, USA

Jane Quandt DVM, MS, DACVAA, DACVECC
Associate Professor Comparative Anesthesiology, College of Veterinary Medicine,
University of Georgia, USA

Gregg S. Rapoport DVM, DACVIM (Cardiology)
Assistant Professor, Cardiology College of Veterinary Medicine, University of
Georgia, USA

Carrie Schroeder DVM, DACVAA
Clinical Instructor, Department of Surgical Science University of Wisconsin School of
Veterinary Medicine, USA

Andre C. Shih DVM DACVAA
Associate Professor Anesthesia, University of Florida, College Veterinary Medicine, USA

Lesley J. Smith DVM, DACVAA
Clinical Professor of Anesthesiology, Department of Surgical Sciences, School of
Veterinary Medicine, University of Wisconsin, USA

Jason W. Soukup, DVM, DAVDC
Clinical Associate Professor, Dentistry and Oral Surgery Department of Surgical Sciences, School of Veterinary Medicine, University of Wisconsin, USA

Paulo Steagall MV, Ms, PhD, DACVAA
Assistant Professor in Veterinary Anesthesiology Département de Sciences Cliniques, Faculté de Médecine Vétérinaire, Université de Montréal, Canada

Ann B. Weil MS, DVM, DACVAA
Clinical Professor of Anesthesiology, Department of Veterinary Clinical Sciences, College of Veterinary Medicine, Purdue University, USA

Erin Wendt-Hornickle DVM, DACVAA
Assistant Clinical Professor, Department of Veterinary Clinical Sciences, College of Veterinary Medicine, University of Minnesota, USA

Preface

This book is intended to be a practical tool to guide veterinary practitioners, technicians, and veterinary students in the anesthetic management of small animal patients. It is constructed as a step-by-step text that starts at patient evaluation, and then takes the reader through preparation for anesthesia, premedication, induction, maintenance, monitoring and troubleshooting, recovery, and pain management. The book finishes by addressing anesthetic management for specific disease conditions in dogs and cats, breed considerations in dogs, anesthetic specifics in cats, and anesthetic management of small pocket pets and birds. My hope is that it will be a go-to source for anesthesia and analgesia questions that arise on an everyday basis.

1 Patient Evaluation

Prevention is the Best Medicine!

Lesley J. Smith

Department of Surgical Sciences, School of Veterinary Medicine, University of Wisconsin, USA

KEY POINTS:

- A thorough physical exam should be performed on all patients unless it causes undue stress to the patient or is dangerous to the anesthetist.

- An overall impression of health, temperament, and body condition score are important to assess in every patient in order to plan drug protocols and doses.

- The physical exam should focus on the cardiovascular and respiratory systems, most importantly.

- Basic blood work for every patient should include a PCV and TP

- Many other additional tests may be indicated depending on the patient's health status and reasons for anesthesia.

Q. Why is it important to perform a complete patient evaluation?

A. Almost without exception, all anesthetic and analgesic drugs have potential toxic effects on organ systems. For example, the inhalant anesthetics significantly decrease blood pressure and organ perfusion such that an animal with pre-existing renal compromise may suffer irreversible renal damage if inhalants are used without monitoring and support of blood pressure. This damage may be even worse if nonsteroidal anti-inflammatory drugs (NSAIDs) are used prior to or during anesthesia.

A complete patient evaluation allows the veterinarian to identify potential health concerns and temperament issues that will affect how that animal responds to the various anesthetic drugs that may be used. In some cases, it may be important to avoid certain anesthetic or analgesic drugs because of identified health concerns. Often many, if not most, anesthetic drugs can be used in patients with significant health problems, but the dose of those drugs may need to be adjusted to minimize known side effects that may be harmful to that particular patient. To continue with the example provided above, in a patient with renal disease inhalants can still be used to maintain anesthesia,

---

Questions and Answers in Small Animal Anesthesia, First Edition. Edited by Lesley J. Smith.
© 2016 John Wiley & Sons, Inc. Published 2016 by John Wiley & Sons, Inc.

but the dose of those inhalants should be kept as low as possible to minimize their negative effects on blood pressure and renal perfusion. Keeping the inhalant dose very low can be achieved by adding other anesthetic or analgesic drugs to the anesthetic protocol, as will be covered in depth in later chapters.

Q. Under what circumstances may patient evaluation be less than complete?

A. Occasionally a patient may be simply too aggressive or unhandled to allow for any physical examination to be conducted safely. Some animals, for example birds, may undergo significant stress from excessive handling and will benefit from a more limited physical examination. Even under these circumstances, however, careful observation "from a distance" can provide important information such as body condition (obese, thin, or just right?), haircoat and general appearance of health, posture and gait (normal or abnormal?), respiratory pattern and effort.

Q. What important questions should I ask the owner when taking a history?

A. The owner may volunteer a lot of information in the history that is or isn't relevant to anesthesia. Some questions that should be asked include:

✓ Has your pet had anesthesia previously and how was his/her recovery at home? – This may alert you to risks of prolonged effects of sedative or other drugs used in the anesthetic protocol.

✓ Are you aware of any problems that your pet had with anesthesia in the past? – Often owners will not know, or will be unsure of, which anesthetic drugs were used previously, but if they recall a specific event (e.g., the vet said he/she had a rough recovery) this can alert you to potential drugs to avoid or to use (e.g., perhaps the rough recovery was because the dog experienced emergence delirium, so this time a longer acting sedative may be indicated).

✓ Are you aware of any relatives of your pet that have experienced complications with anesthesia? – For example, herding breeds of dogs may experience prolonged and profound sedation from certain sedatives and opioids.

✓ Is your pet allergic to any foods or medications that you know of? – Clearly, known allergies to certain medications would indicate that those medications, or ones that are in the same class, should be avoided. Rarely, dogs will have an allergy to eggs, which would make propofol contra-indicated, as propofol contains egg lecithin.

✓ How is your pet's general energy level? Does he/she tire easily or get out of breath quickly during exercise? – Exercise intolerance is a red flag to be on the lookout for cardiovascular or respiratory disease, anemia, or endocrine disease!

✓ Are there any recent changes in drinking or urination habits? – Increases in frequency of water intake should put you on the medical hunt for diseases that cause PU/PD, such as renal disease or diabetes.

✓ Has there been any weight loss or gain that you've noticed recently? – Again if these cannot be explained by a diet change or lifestyle change, then you should be on the hunt for underlying medical issues that could lead to weight gain or loss (e.g., thyroid disorders).

✓ What medications is your pet currently taking? What about nutraceuticals or herbal remedies? – Some medications can directly and significantly impact how the animal responds to anesthetics. For example, ACE inhibitors (e.g., enalapril) can lead to low blood pressure under anesthesia that is unresponsive to most normal interventions.

Q. What are important considerations to look for on initial patient evaluation?

A. The initial patient assessment, before beginning the physical exam, can give you a lot of information. Make a note of the breed, as some breeds warrant special management considerations. Make a note of the animal's temperament: are they quiet, calm, lethargic? If so, then sedative drug doses may need to be reduced. Conversely, are they anxious? Then sedative drugs that provide anxiolysis may be indicated (e.g., acepromazine, midazolam). Are they aggressive and/or dangerous to handle? Then you may need to plan for heavy premedication with drugs that render the animal extremely sedate if not lightly anesthetized. If the dog is athletic and "works for a living" then it may have a normally low resting heart rate, which will be reflected in their heart rate under anesthesia. If that heart rate is normal for them, then you may not need to treat it, even if you consider it bradycardic by most standards.

Also make note of the animal's general appearance of wellbeing. Is their hair coat glossy and clean, or does it have a rough, dry, unkempt, or ungroomed appearance, which may indicate underlying disease, poor nutrition, or lack of self-grooming secondary to disease, stress, or pain.

Lastly, but importantly, assess the animal's body condition. Ideally you will obtain an accurate body weight during your physical, but prior to that, get an impression of whether the animal is close to an ideal weight or not. Obese patients will not breathe well under anesthesia because abdominal and thoracic fat increase the work of breathing and limit thoracic compliance. You should plan to assist ventilation in these patients. Also, drug dose calculations should be adjusted for ideal or lean body weight, otherwise you will be giving a relative overdose of anesthetic drugs. All anesthetic drugs circulate first to organs that receive a high percentage of cardiac output, and because adipose tissue receives very little blood flow, the relative concentration of drugs in the more vascular tissues will be too high if the drug dose is administered based on the obese body weight.

If an animal is too thin, drug doses should be calculated based on the actual body weight. A thin animal, however, may get colder sooner during anesthesia because of the lack of insulating fat.

Q. How should I estimate the patient's ideal weight?

A. Recent studies have reported that ~40% of dogs in the USA and other countries are overweight and between 5–20% are obese [1, 2]. A commonly used
body condition scoring system uses a subjective 9-point scale, where 1 is a
morbidly thin animal and 9 is a morbidly obese animal, with a spectrum of
body conditions ranked on the scale between these extremes [3]. This system
is validated for dogs with < 45% body fat, so may not accurately identify dogs
that are extremely obese, which is becoming a more common finding.

A subjective but common-sense approach to estimating ideal weight is to consider the species, breed, and age of the animal and assign a body weight that
would be typical for that animal *if* it had a body condition score of 5–6 (ideal).
For example, a typical adult yellow Labrador of average size *should* weigh
approximately 30–33 kg.

Q. What are general considerations for very young or geriatric patients?

A. Very young patients (i.e., less than 5 months of age) have immature liver
function [4]. This means that they are slower to metabolize many drugs and
are not very efficient at gluconeogenesis, so glucose should be checked and
monitored during anesthesia, with supplementation if needed. When glucose falls below 60 g/dl, adding enough dextrose to make a 2.5% (25 mg/ml)
solution of dextrose in a balance electrolyte fluid, for example plasmalyte-R,
with fluids run at normal anesthetic maintenance rates (see Chapter 9: Fluid
Therapy), will maintain normal glucose levels.

Geriatric patients should be carefully screened for diseases common to older
animals, such as cardiac, renal, hepatic, CNS, and neoplastic disease. As a general rule, doses of sedative drugs should be tapered down in geriatric animals
because of delayed clearance. Anesthetic monitoring should also be vigilant in
order to quickly address complications that may compromise organ function,
such as hypoxemia, hypotension, hypercapnia, and hypothermia. Underlying
arthritis should be considered when positioning the patient for procedures,
with attention to padding and positioning joints carefully to minimize patient
discomfort or stiffness after recovery from anesthesia.

Q. What are the key organ systems to focus on during my physical examination
that are relevant to anesthetic planning?

A. The most important organ systems with respect to anesthesia are the cardiovascular and respiratory systems. This is because so many of the negative
effects of anesthetic drugs are cardiac and respiratory. A good grasp of abnormalities in these two systems in any given patient will allow for pre-emptive
planning in advance in order to minimize anesthetic risk.

The chapters on anesthetic management for cardiovascular and respiratory
disease will provide guidelines for how to plan anesthesia for patients where
abnormalities in these organ systems exist. With respect to physical examination, the following checklist may help:

✓ Mucous membrane color should be pink.

✓ Mucous membranes should be wet/moist with a capillary refill time of <2 s.

✓ Hydration status should appear normal.

✓ Heart rate should be "normal" for this species and breed.

✓ Are there any murmurs heard? Any arrhythmias?

✓ Are there strong peripheral pulses and are they synchronous with the heart beats?

✓ Is respiratory effort minimal? Does the animal "work to breathe"?

✓ Is there good airflow through both nostrils when the mouth is held shut?

✓ Are normal breath sounds heard in all four lung fields?

Q. Are there any other organ systems I should examine?

A. The abdomen should be gently palpated to search for organomegaly or effusion, both of which can signal neoplastic, hepatic, or cardiac disease. A basic evaluation of CNS function should check that the patient has normal mentation, normal visual reflexes, and responds to voice. Check that the mouth can be easily opened so that intubation will be easy. If not (e.g., mandibular myopathy), you may need to be prepared with an endoscope to visualize the larynx or, worst case, for a tracheostomy.

Q. What bloodwork is important for a young, healthy animal?

A. A suggested minimum data base for a healthy animal should be packed cell volume (PCV) and total protein concentration. These tests are inexpensive and easy to perform and provide a lot of information. PCV will alert you to dehydration (if high) or to anemia (if low), which compromises oxygen carrying capacity and oxygen delivery to tissues. A PCV < 25%, if an acute decrease, should be addressed prior to anesthesia with blood products (packed RBCs, whole blood). Total protein concentration also can indicate dehydration (if high) or a chronic inflammatory disease (if high, because of increases in gamma globulins). Low total protein concentration can indicate poor liver function (e.g., portosytemic shunt) and makes the animal more at risk for hypotension because of low plasma oncotic pressure (fluids will not stay in the vascular space). Coagulation factors may also be low if liver function is poor, so the animal will be at a higher risk for surgical blood loss, even in routine procedures such ovariohysterectomy. Low total protein concentration may also indicate protein loss, for example, from protein-losing nephropathy or GI losses.

In young animals, a baseline blood glucose concentration can be important for making decisions about fluid therapy and glucose support. A reagent test strip, for example Azostix, can provide a rough indication of normal or high blood urea nitrogen concentration, which can clue you in to pre-renal dehydration or renal dysfunction. If high, obtaining a urine specific gravity, also easy to perform, will help determine the animal's concentrating ability and distinguish between pre-renal and renal azotemia.

Q. When should I consider performing more blood work? What tests are most important for anesthesia?

A. A retrospective evaluation of canine patient pre-anesthetic records was performed in order to determine the necessity of pre-anesthetic blood screening. Pre-anesthetic blood work was deemed to be unnecessary in 84% of these patients, as it did not alter the anesthetic plan. Less than 1% of patients required alterations of the anesthetic plan based upon blood work [5]. It is important to note that the majority of these patients were classified as ASA I or II. In a separate study evaluating geriatric canine patients (>7 years), pre-anesthetic blood work resulted in a new diagnosis of subclinical disease in roughly 30% of patients [6]. The results of these studies suggest that pre-anesthetic hematologic and biochemical screening is of value in detecting subclinical disease, especially among geriatric patients, but may not be necessary in all patients. Any patient with significant uncompensated or compensated systemic disease, a history of trauma, urinary obstruction, sepsis, and so on, should have a full CBC and serum biochemical profile with electrolytes. Again, this helps in stabilizing the patient prior to anesthesia and in making decisions regarding fluid therapy, as well as interpreting and managing complications that may arise under anesthesia (e.g., arrhythmias associated with K^+ disorders).

Q. Are there other diagnostic tests that should be considered?

A. Thoracic radiographs should probably be taken in any patient in which a previously undiagnosed heart murmur is heard or in a patient with a history of heart disease that is/is not being treated with medications, in order to assess heart size and the possible presence of heart failure. Patients with a history of trauma often have abnormalities on thoracic radiographs (e.g., pulmonary contusions, pneumothorax). Any patient in which lower respiratory abnormalities are ausculted on physical exam should have thoracic radiographs.

Echocardiography can be useful in identifying the significance of murmurs and assessing cardiac contractility in patients with cardiac disease. Abdominal radiographs, computed tomography, and ultrasound, while not necessarily pertinent to anesthetic planning, can help identify co-morbidities (e.g., metastases) that can change the overall patient plan.

Patients that are suspected to have clotting disorders based on breed (e.g., von Willebrand disease [vWD] in Dobermans), history of disease, or physical exam (e.g., petechiae) should have a platelet count (part of the CBC), buccal mucosal bleeding time (to check platelet function in an animal with a normal platelet count), or PT/aPTT tests, depending on the signs and signalment, to rule out/rule in a bleeding disorder that may increase surgical bleeding and risk. If vWD is suspected, a von Willebrand factor antigen assay should be obtained from a reference laboratory.

Q. What is ASA status and how do I rank a patient?

Table 1.1 ASA status categories with descriptions and clinical examples.

Category	Physical status	Examples
I	normal healthy patient	no signs of obvious disease
II	patient with mild systemic disease	compensated cardiac disease, fracture with no shock
III	patient with severe systemic disease	anemia, moderate dehydration, renal or hepatic disease
IV	patient with severe disease that is life-threatening	uncompensated cardiac disease, renal or hepatic failure, sepsis
V	patient that is not expected to live with or without surgery	profound shock, severe multi-organ failure, severe sepsis, severe trauma

WJ Tranquilli, JC Benson, KA Grimm (eds) *Lumb and Jones' Veterinary Anesthesia and Analgesia*, 4th edn. Blackwell Publishing: Ames IA, 2007:Table 2.7.

A. The American Society of Anesthesiologists (ASA) recommends categorizing patients into one of five possible statuses after the patient evaluation has been completed (www.asahq.org) [7]. Table 1.1 summarizes the five categories. Any patient that presents as an emergency is ranked at its appropriate status followed by an E. For example, a dachshund with thoracolumbar disc herniation that is otherwise completely healthy, but that requires an emergency hemi-laminectomy would be an ASA 2E.

References

1 McGreevy PD, Thomson RM, Mellor DJ, *et al*. Prevalence of obesity in dogs examined by Australian veterinary practices and the risk factors involved. *Veterinary Record* 2005; **156**:695–702.

2 Lund EM, Armstrong PJ, Kirk CA, *et al*. Prevalence and risk factors for obesity in adult dogs from private US veterinary practices. *International Journal Applied Research Veterinary Medicine* 2006; **4**:177–186.

3 LaFlamme D. Development and validation of a body condition score system for dogs. *Canine Practice* 1997; **22(4)**:10–15.

4 Root-Kustritz MV. What are normal physical exam findings at various ages in puppies and kittens? In: Root-Kustritz MV (ed.) *Clinical Canine and Feline Reproduction: Evidence-based Answers*, 1st edn. Wiley-Blackwell Publishers: Ames, IA, 2010:278.

5 Alef M, von Praun, F, and Oechtering G. Is routine pre-anaesthetic haematological and biochemical screening justified in dogs? *Veterinary Anaesthesia and Analgesia* 2008; **35**:132–140.

6 Joubert KE. Pre-anesthetic screening of geriatric dogs. *Journal South African Veterinary Association* 2007; **78**:31–35.

7 American Society of Anesthesiologists. *ASA Physical Status Classification System*. https://www.asahq.org/For-Members/Clinical-Information/ASA-Physical-Status-Classification-System.aspx (accessed June 1, 2014).

2 Owner Concerns

Be prepared with answers

Lesley J. Smith

Department of Surgical Sciences, School of Veterinary Medicine, University of Wisconsin, USA

> **KEY POINTS:**
>
> - Trained personnel dedicated to anesthetic monitoring will address many owner concerns about anesthetic risk.
> - Good monitoring (hands-on, temperature, pulse oximetry, blood pressure, ECG, and capnography) will address owner concerns about anesthetic risk.
> - Owners should be prepared that their pet may not be "normal" for several days after anesthesia, even if everything goes exactly according to plan.

The following are questions that a pet owner may ask, with possible scenarios or answers that you may provide, depending on your practice. Some questions are taken from the American College of Veterinary Dentistry website [1].

Q. Who monitors the anesthesia at your practice?

A. Responses here could vary from (i) A board certified veterinary anesthesiologist (i.e., a diplomate of the American College of Veterinary Anesthesia and Analgesia). (ii) A veterinarian with some additional training in anesthesia but who is not a diplomate of the ACVAA. (iii) A veterinarian with no additional training in anesthesia post-graduation. (iv) A dedicated veterinary technician with special training in anesthesia (i.e., a veterinary technician with a certificate of Veterinary Technician Specialist – Anesthesia). (v) A dedicated veterinary technician without special training in anesthesia. (vi) A veterinary technician who also helps with the procedure at the same time. (vii) Kennel staff, office staff, volunteer.

A veterinarian should always be involved in choosing anesthetic drug protocols and doses, even if those are standard protocols that have been established by the practice. The American Animal Hospital Association (AAHA) recommends that all animal anesthetics be monitored by a dedicated individual [2]. Clearly, owners who ask this question will be reassured if they know that their pet's anesthesia will be monitored closely, minute to minute, by a trained individual.

Q. What things do you monitor as standard protocol for your anesthesia?

A. This again can run the gamut of possibilities based on the practice type. Minimal monitoring should be hands-on assessment of depth, membrane color, heart rate and breathing, and temperature. AAHA guidelines indicate that minimal anesthetic monitoring include heart rate and rhythm, membrane color, respiratory rate, pulse oximetry, blood pressure, and temperature [3].

Q. Do you keep an anesthetic record?

A. The anesthetic record should be considered a legal document, because if there are any complications related to that pet and the owner pursues it either legally or via the state licensing office, the absence of an anesthetic record will make defense of any actions taken during the anesthetic period very difficult.

Q. What blood work will you perform on my pet?

A. Answers will depend on what is indicated based on the pet's medical condition, reason for anesthesia, age, overall health status, history, and physical exam findings. A minimum amount of blood work for any animal should be a PCV and TP, even if it is obtained after anesthetic induction to reduce patient stress. See Chapter 1 for other guidelines on pre-anesthetic blood work.

Q. What are the risks of anesthesia?

A. Owners should understand that anesthesia is a risk, for any animal, under any circumstances. Risk can be reduced by careful patient evaluation and anesthetic planning, dedicated anesthesia personnel who monitor the patient on a continuous basis through recovery, and good knowledge of trouble-shooting. Some potential, but hopefully rare, anesthetic risks that should be shared with owners include: anesthetic death, aspiration and pneumonia, regurgitation with subsequent esophageal ulceration or stricture, delayed/prolonged recovery, post-operative pain/discomfort, CNS abnormalities (blindness, confusion), renal failure, worsening of chronic disease such as cardiac or renal disease.

Q. How will you manage my pet's pain?

A. Many owners do not ask this question, as they assume that their pet's pain will be managed much like their own would be in a hospital setting. They should understand that pain medications may cause some sedation lasting into the time the pet arrives home (e.g., opioids) or may cause other abnormalities in behavior if they are prescribed for at-home administration (e.g., sedation from a fentanyl patch, tremors/agitation from tramadol). The NSAIDs are commonly prescribed for post-operative at-home administration and owners should know that some of these drugs have been associated with (rare) hepatotoxicity (e.g., carprofen) and can worsen renal function in geriatric dogs and, particularly, in cats when they are given for prolonged periods or at high doses. These drugs also can cause GI upset, nausea, melena, diarrhea, and GI ulcers, so owners should be advised of these risks as well.

Q. Why does my pet need an IV catheter? I don't want him shaved!

A. An IV catheter is vital for safe anesthetic induction, administration of IV fluids which help to maintain water balance and blood pressure during anesthesia, and for quick delivery of any emergency or pain drugs we might have to use. Only a small square of hair needs to be shaved in order to place a clean IV catheter. The medial saphenous vein can often be used and is relatively "hidden" compared to the cephalic or lateral saphenous locations.

Q. Why does my pet need anesthesia when I don't need it for the same sort of procedure?

A. Pets will not voluntarily hold still for many relatively non-invasive routine preventative procedures such as dental cleanings. Physical restraint for any length of time is stressful to the pet and potentially painful as well. General anesthesia allows us to complete the procedure more efficiently without the pet feeling any pain or stress during the procedure.

References

1 American College of Veterinary Dentistry. *Questions to ask your veterinarian about your pet's dental cleaning.* www.acvd.org (accessed November 12, 2014)
2 American Animal Hospital Association. *AAHA accreditation standards require anesthesia monitoring equipment for your pet's safety.* www.aahanet.org/Accreditation/aspx (accessed November 12, 2014)
3 Bednarski R, Grimm K, Harvey R, *et al.* AAHA Anesthesia guidelines for dogs and cats. *Journal of the American Animal Hospital Association* 2011; **47**:377–385.

3 Patient Preparation

They should be prepared too!

Carrie Schroeder

Department of Surgical Science, University of Wisconsin School of Veterinary Medicine, USA

KEY POINTS:

- Healthy adult patients should be fasted 8–12 h prior to anesthesia, although water may be offered until the time of sedation.
- Fasting time may need to be modified in patients that cannot maintain normoglycemia.
- Fasting should not be for more than a few hours in neonates.
- Depending on the patient's history, physical examination, and anticipated surgical procedure, pre-anesthetic medications or fluids may be indicated.
- Most medications may be administered until the time of anesthesia. However, certain medications may interfere with anesthetic management or may interact adversely with anesthetic agents.
- For patients receiving medications prior to anesthesia, it is important to verify potential adverse effects or adverse interactions of those medications with anesthetics that may be used.

Q. For how long should a patient be fasted prior to anesthesia?

A. Pre-anesthetic fasting is important in order to decrease the volume of gastric contents as well as decrease the risk of peri-operative regurgitation. It is generally recommended that adult patients be fasted for 8–12 h prior to the administration of anesthetic medications. Most patients will have adequate glycogen stores and can maintain blood glucose throughout this fasting period. Water may be offered until the time any anesthetic or sedative agents are administered.

Q. Are there exceptions to this rule of thumb in patients with diseases like diabetes or portosystemic shunts?

A. There are certain disease states in which an animal's blood glucose cannot be maintained during fasting. Patients with a diminished capacity to maintain normoglycemia, such as those with portosystemic shunt, should be fasted for a shorter period of time based upon their blood glucose. Generally, these patients should be able to tolerate 4–6 h of fasting. Blood glucose should

Questions and Answers in Small Animal Anesthesia, First Edition. Edited by Lesley J. Smith.
© 2016 John Wiley & Sons, Inc. Published 2016 by John Wiley & Sons, Inc.

be checked to verify normoglycemia at the time of induction, sooner if the patient has historically been unable to maintain blood glucose within a normal range. Intravenous glucose supplementation (2.5–5% dextrose) should be performed as necessary.

In patients with diabetes, pre-anesthetic fasting should be undertaken with caution as the patient's insulin dose is typically administered along with food to prevent hypoglycemic episodes. Ideally, surgical procedures should be performed first thing in the morning so that post-operative patients may be monitored closely for the duration of the day and restarted on a regular feeding schedule. Opinions vary on the ideal way to manage blood glucose in diabetic patients, but a common approach is an overnight fast, roughly 6–8 h, followed by administration of one-half the usual insulin dose in the morning. Blood glucose should be monitored every hour following administration of insulin until the time of anesthetic induction, with intravenous glucose supplementation administered as necessary.

Q. For how long should a young animal be fasted?

A. Young animals (< 12 weeks) or species with a high metabolism, such as small birds, rodents, and rabbits, should not have food withheld for more than 2–4 h. These patients may become significantly hypoglycemic if fasted for prolonged periods of time. Neonatal patients (< 4 weeks) should be allowed to nurse from the mother until the time of anesthesia.

Q. What medications should be given prior to anesthesia or anesthetic premedication?

A. There is no standard recommendation regarding the timing and type of medications that should be administered prior to sedation or anesthetic induction. Common pharmacologic agents administered prior to anesthesia include antibiotics, nonsteroidal anti-inflammatory drugs (NSAIDs), anticholinergics, and antihistamines.

Pre-operative antibiotics such as cefazolin are often administered prior to major orthopedic or soft tissue surgeries. As a general rule, prophylactic antimicrobials should be administered approximately 30–60 min prior to the initial surgical incision [1,2].

Nonsteroidal anti-inflammatory drugs (NSAIDs) are a highly effective component of a multimodal analgesic plan and are most effective when administered prior to the surgical insult [3,4]. For maximum analgesic effect, NSAIDs should be given at least 30 min prior to surgery. One must use caution in administering these agents in patients with pre-existing hepatic, gastrointestinal, or renal disease or in patients where peri-operative hypotension is anticipated, as hypotension under anesthesia combined with an NSAID "on board" can lead to renal failure [5].

Antihistamines, such as diphenhydramine, and H2-blockers, such as famotidine, are indicated in patients with mast cell tumors to attenuate the negative effects associated with histamine release that may occur with tumor manipulation. It is important that these agents be administered prior to anesthesia in case of mast cell degranulation. These agents should be given roughly 20 min prior to anesthetic induction and can be administered at the time of intramuscular sedation.

Q. What are indications for the administration of pre-anesthetic fluids?

A. While intra-operative fluids are recommended in nearly all patients, the administration of pre-anesthetic intravenous fluids is recommended in selective cases. Patients presenting with renal disease, dehydration, electrolyte abnormalities, and hypovolemic shock are candidates for the administration of pre-anesthetic fluids.

Patients with renal disease, discussed in Chapter 35, should ideally be admitted for intravenous fluid therapy roughly 12–24 h prior to induction of anesthesia. This will allow for stabilization of any possible electrolyte imbalances, correction of dehydration, and optimization of intravenous fluid volume, improving the glomerular filtration rate under anesthesia. Fluid rate should be tailored to each individual patient, based upon the level of dehydration and any concurrent conditions, such as cardiac disease. Patients with renal disease who present on an emergency basis should, at minimum, be administered fluids to replace fluid deficits.

Patients presenting with hypovolemic shock (e.g., gastric dilatation/volvulus), should have fluids administered prior to anesthesia in order to improve cardiac output and tissue perfusion. Ideally, fluid administration rate and amount should be guided by measurement of the patient's central venous pressure (CVP) in order to prevent fluid overload. In the absence of CVP measurement, patient response to fluid administration can be gauged by pulse rate and quality, capillary refill time, auscultation of lung sounds, and respiratory rate and effort.

Q. How can I calculate the rate of administration of pre-anesthetic fluids?

A. The rate of fluid administration for patients with dehydration can be calculated based upon maintenance fluid need (40–60 ml/kg/day or 1.7–2.5 ml/kg/h) plus replacement of any fluid deficit, in addition to fluids to account for ongoing losses such as vomiting, if present. This can be estimated by assessing the patient's level of dehydration and replacing the deficit over 4–6 h or longer if time allows.

For example, a 5 kg patient presenting with 7% dehydration should have an initial fluid rate calculated as:

$$(5 \text{ kg} \times 2.5 \text{ ml/kg/h}) + (5 \text{ kg} \times 1000 \text{ g/kg} \times 7\%)/6 \text{ h}$$

$$= 12.5 \text{ ml (maintenance rate)} + 58\text{ml (dehydration correction)}$$

$$= 70.5 \text{ ml over 6 h}$$

Following correction of dehydration, the rate of administration should be at least the maintenance fluid rate until the time of anesthesia.

Q. I have a patient with heart disease who is on a lot of medications. Should I continue those up to the time of anesthesia? All of them or just some?

A. It is common for patients with cardiovascular disease to require a number of medications, including beta blockers (e.g., atenolol), calcium channel blockers (e.g., amlodipine), angiotensin-converting enzyme inhibitors (ACEIs) (e.g., enalapril), and the phosphodiesterase inhibitor pimobendan. Patients presenting with chronic therapy of these medications often have a finely tuned regimen and it is important to avoid disruption of the homeostasis of therapy. However, refractory hypotension can occur upon concurrent administration of anesthetic agents such as propofol and volatile anesthetics with ACEIs [6–8]. Therefore, it is important that ACEI therapy be temporarily discontinued for 24 h prior to anesthetic induction, unless the ACEI is administered to treat hypertension. All other cardiac medications may be continued as usual. It is important, however, to be aware that patients treated with beta-blockers may be bradycardic and require anticholinergic therapy.

Q. What other types of diseases and/or medications should be continued up to the time of anesthesia?

A. Most medications may be continued until the time of anesthesia, especially those administered to treat chronic conditions. This includes treatments for mast cell tumor, epilepsy, hyper- and hypothyroidism, hyper- and hypo-adrenocorticism, and most cardiac medications, as described previously. It is, however, very important to check for possible reactions with anesthetic agents prior to formulating an anesthetic plan. Fortunately, cross-reactions with anesthetics and other pharmacologic agents are relatively rare but untoward reactions have been known to occur. It is far more common to have additive pharmacologic effects, such as hypotension or excessive sedation.

Q. When should ongoing medications be discontinued prior to anesthesia and for how long?

A. There is no general rule for discontinuing medications prior to anesthesia; the administration guidelines should be based upon the individual patient, disease condition, anesthetic plan, and therapeutic regimen. As stated previously, it is important to know any potential cross-reactions and adverse effects of any therapeutic agent prior to administration of any anesthetic agent. For example, antidepressants such as selective serotonin reuptake inhibitors (SSRIs) or monoamine oxidase inhibitors (MAOIs) may interact with opioids such as meperidine to cause a relatively rare disorder called serotonin syndrome. More commonly, therapeutic agents may compound the known effects of anesthetic agents such as hypotension or sedation.

Insulin and angiotensin-converting enzyme inhibitors (ACEIs) are important examples of pharmacologic agents that need to be adjusted in the peri-anesthetic period. Insulin should be administered at one-half the regular morning dose prior to surgery. Full doses should not be given until the animal is alert enough to eat normally. Blood glucose should be monitored every 2–4 h following anesthesia for 24 h after anesthetic emergence.

References

1 Weese JS, Halling KB. Perioperative administration of antimicrobials associated with elective surgery for cranial cruciate ligament rupture in dogs: 83 cases (2003-2005). *Journal of the American Veterinary Medical Association* 2006; **229**:92–95.

2 Whittem TL, Johnson AL, Smith CW, *et al*. Effect of perioperative prophylactic antimicrobial treatment in dogs undergoing elective orthopedic surgery. *Journal of the American Veterinary Medical Association* 1999; **215**:212–216.

3 Lascelles BD, Cripps PJ, Jones A, *et al*. Efficacy and kinetics of carprofen, administered preoperatively or postoperatively, for the prevention of pain in dogs undergoing ovariohysterectomy. *Veterinary Surgery* 1998; **27**:568–582.

4 Crandell DE, Mathews KA, Dyson DH. Effect of meloxicam and carprofen on renal function when administered to healthy dogs prior to anesthesia and painful stimulation. *American Journal of Veterinary Research* 2004; **65**:1384–1390.

5 Curry SL, Cogar DM, Cook JL. Nonsteroidal antiinflammatory drugs: a review. *Journal of the American Animal Hospital Association* 2005; **41**:298–309.

6 Coriat P, Richer C, Douraki T, *et al*. Influence of chronic angiotensin-converting enzyme inhibition of anesthetic induction. *Anesthesiology* 1994; **81**(**2**):299–307.

7 Ishikawa Y, Uechi M, Ishikawa R, *et al*. Effect of isoflurane anesthesia on hemodynamics following the administration of an angiotensin-converting enzyme inhibitor in cats. *Journal of Veterinary Medical Science* 2007; **69**:869–871.

8 Malinowska-Zaprzalka M, Wojewodzka M, Dryl D, *et al*. Hemodynamic effect of propofol in enalapril-treated hypertensive patients during induction of general anesthesia. *Pharmacology Reports* 2005; **57**(**5**):675–678.

4 Anesthetic Machine and Equipment Check

No one likes surprises!

Richard M. Bednarski

Department of Veterinary Clinical Sciences, College of Veterinary Medicine, The Ohio State University, USA

KEY POINTS:

- Every monitoring device and piece of anesthesia equipment that you plan to use for a case should be checked prior to starting anesthesia.

- Many of the routine equipment and monitoring checks need to be done only once each day while others should be done prior to each case.

- A check-list posted in the anesthesia/surgery area can be useful to verify a systematic equipment and monitoring check has been performed.

Q. What anesthetic equipment should be checked prior to use?

A. Any anesthetic equipment used or anticipated to be used must be inspected and its proper function verified before use. Immediately after anesthetic induction you must be able to deliver oxygen and anesthetic gas, provide assisted ventilation, and have the capability of effectively using all of your monitors. A pre-anesthetic check of equipment prevents a potentially dangerous delay in providing oxygen and inhalant, as well as in monitoring vital signs. Typically the anesthetic machine, breathing system, airway device(s) including endotracheal tube or mask, and any monitoring equipment should be checked.

There is no prescribed standard for verifying the correct function of anesthetic machines, breathing systems, airway devices, or anesthetic monitoring equipment. Because of the wide variety of anesthetic machines, vaporizers, and monitoring equipment available, the user must become familiar with the correct operation of their particular equipment. Although a sales representative should be able to provide a functional overview for the correct operation, there is no substitute for thoroughly reviewing the accompanying manufacturer's owner's manual.

Questions and Answers in Small Animal Anesthesia, First Edition. Edited by Lesley J. Smith.
© 2016 John Wiley & Sons, Inc. Published 2016 by John Wiley & Sons, Inc.

Leaks in the anesthetic machine, breathing system, endotracheal tube, and anesthetic ventilator can contribute to unnecessary exposure of personnel to anesthetic vapors. Although there are no federally mandated restrictions relative to anesthetic gas exposure, the Occupational Safety and Health Administration (OSHA) general duty clause requires that an employer provide a hazard-free working environment even in the absence of a relevant standard. A leak-free anesthetic gas delivery system is an important part of controlling waste anesthetic gas exposure.

Q. Who should perform the check?

A. Ideally the person responsible for anesthesia delivery and monitoring should verify proper equipment function. This person can be an appropriately trained technician or veterinarian. Most importantly, it must be a person familiar with proper use of all of the anesthetic and monitoring equipment.

Q. How often should the equipment be checked?

A. Many checks can be performed periodically, while others (e.g., monitoring equipment) should be performed daily prior to each day's procedures. The oxygen source and associated supply line need to be checked only when problems are suspected, tanks are switched, or when new connections are made to the anesthetic machine. Items that are changed or removed and cleaned between cases, such as endotracheal tubes and breathing system components, should be checked prior to each use.

Q. Is there a good way to ensure the equipment is appropriately checked?

A. Although experienced users can rely on a mental checklist, a written checklist of tasks posted in the anesthetic induction area promotes consistency. Such a task list helps ensure that all anesthesia providers do not overlook anything and adhere to that facility's standard of care (see Box 4.1). The checklist can be posted in the anesthetic induction area to verify that the appropriate anesthetic related supplies needed for each case are ready for use. A more detailed task list should be made available to verify proper anesthetic machine and monitoring equipment function (see Table 4.1). It is convenient to divide your pre-anesthetic equipment check into that associated with the: (i) gas supply; (ii) anesthetic machine; (iii) breathing system; (iv) ventilator; (v) airway supplies; (vi) monitoring equipment; and (vii) emergency equipment.

Q. What are the components of a typical anesthesia machine?

A. See Figure 4.1. A hospital-wide oxygen source (high pressure cylinder(s), liquid oxygen storage tank, or oxygen concentrator and storage tank) is connected to a pressure regulator. Oxygen leaves the regulator at a pressure of 50–55 psi and enters the hospital supply line(s) to be directed to various locations within the facility. The anesthesia machine is connected to a hospital supply line. Alternatively or additionally a transport E cylinder of oxygen is attached directly to the anesthesia machine and pressure regulator. Oxygen from either source is routed to the oxygen flush valve and an oxygen flowmeter. Oxygen exits the flowmeter and is directed through an

Box 4.1 Pre-anesthetic task list: A simple task list can be developed and posted in the anesthetic induction area to ensure that necessary supplies are readily available prior to each anesthetic episode.

SUGGESTED LIST OF SUPPLIES WHEN SETTING UP FOR ANESTHESIA
Clippers with clean blade
Skin disinfectant for catheter site
IV catheter(s)
Tape for catheter(s)
Fluid administration set and IV fluids
Anesthetic induction drugs and adjunctive analgesics/anesthetics
Endotracheal tubes of various sizes, ties, sterile lube, inflation syringe for cuff
Laryngoscope with good light source
Eye ointment
Properly checked anesthetic machine and breathing circuit
Anesthetic record and pen

anesthetic vaporizer. A nitrous oxide E tank can be connected to a nitrous oxide-specific pressure regulator from which point it is routed to a nitrous oxide flowmeter. After leaving its flowmeter nitrous oxide joins the oxygen exiting from the oxygen flowmeter. Gas exits the vaporizer or the oxygen flush valve and is directed through a common gas outlet. In some machines a check valve preventing back-flow into the vaporizer and flowmeter(s) is located within the common gas outlet. Gas from the common gas outlet is directed into a non-rebreathing system or into a circle rebreathing system (Figures 4.2 and 4.3).

Q. How do I check the oxygen and nitrous oxide supply?

A. The facility's central oxygen supply is turned on and the pressure regulator adjusted if necessary to ensure a working pressure of 50–55 psi in the hospital supply lines. The source of any audible leaks should be identified and corrected if possible. Next determine if the volume of gas remaining in the hospital supply is adequate for that day's anesthetic procedures. The required daily volume depends on whether the oxygen supply will be used in other areas of the facility, such as for delivery in ICU or to power an anesthetic ventilator. The user must be familiar with the oxygen source in the facility, whether it is from an oxygen generator and storage tank, a liquid oxygen cylinder, or a manifold of H-size compressed oxygen cylinders. Regardless of the hospital source a transport (E-size) cylinder should be attached to the anesthetic machine for use if the hospital supply becomes unexpectedly depleted. In smaller hospital settings, an E cylinder attached to each anesthesia machine may be adequate to meet all of the oxygen demands for that clinic.

Table 4.1 Pre-anesthesia equipment check procedure: These procedures should be performed prior to the first anesthetic delivery of the day. *Not all procedures need to be performed prior to each subsequent anesthetic delivery.

Equipment	Notes
Gas supply*	Open hospital supply oxygen cylinder valves or turn on oxygen concentrator.
	Ensure adequate tank pressure/volume for day's use.
	Ensure pipeline pressure between 50–55 psi.
	Ensure portable E cylinder (backup) is connected to the anesthesia machine and contains a pressure at least 500 psi.
	Perform high pressure system leak check periodically (refer to text).
Anesthesia machine*	Fill vaporizer(s) and close fill cap(s).
	Rotate vaporizer dial throughout its settings and shut off.
	Verify adequacy of CO_2 absorbent material.
	Connect machine to oxygen source and verify correct flowmeter operation.
	Perform negative-pressure or positive-pressure low-pressure system leak check (refer to text).
Waste gas scavenging system*	Switch on active waste gas scavenging system and confirm its connection to the scavenging interface.
	Ensure waste gas scavenging system interface is properly connected to pop-off valve via transfer hose.
	Test and if necessary adjust waste gas scavenging vacuum.
	If using activated charcoal passive scavenging check the weight of the activated charcoal canister and change if necessary.
Breathing system	Connect appropriate breathing system and rebreathing bag to machine:
	Non-rebreathing <3 kg body weight
	Circle rebreathing >3 kg body weight
	Pressure check the breathing system: Begin with flowmeter off and pop-off valve open →
	– Non-rebreathing: Close pop-off valve. Occlude patient connection using hand or thumb. Activate oxygen flush valve to tightly distend rebreathing bag (30 cm H_2O if pressure gauge present). System should retain pressure for minimum of 10 s. Fully open pop-off to confirm pressure release.
	– Circle rebreathing: Close pop-off valve. Occlude patient connection (Y piece or patient end of coaxial circuit) using hand or thumb. Activate oxygen flush valve to fully distend rebreathing bag (30 cm H_2O). System should retain pressure for minimum of 10 s. Fully open pop-off to confirm pressure release.
Mechanical Ventilator	Plug in electrical power cord and connect ventilator to compressed gas source.
	Connect ventilator transfer hose to rebreathing bag port of anesthesia machine.
	Insert pressure sensor (if present) between inspiratory valve and hose.
	Connect waste gas scavenging port of ventilator to waste gas scavenging system.
	Close pop-off valve.
	Turn flowmeters off.
	Occlude Y-piece.
	Activate oxygen flush valve to fully distend the ventilator bellows.
	Bellows should remain distended for at least 10 s.

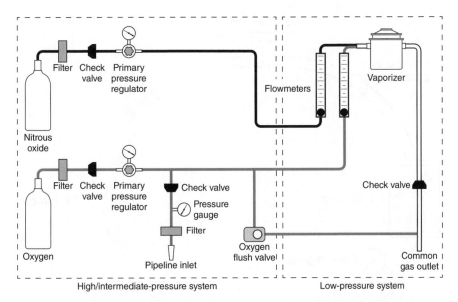

Figure 4.1 Anesthesia machine components: oxygen is delivered to the machine from the hospital bulk supply (pipeline inlet) or the transport cylinders attached to the machine. An anesthetic breathing system connects to the common gas outlet.

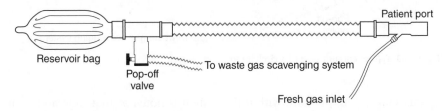

Figure 4.2 Typical components of a non-rebreathing system.

A full E cylinder (2200 psi) contains approximately 650 l of oxygen and, with use, the pressure within the cylinder decreases proportionally to the volume of oxygen used. For example, if the cylinder pressure is equal to 550 psi the cylinder contains approximately 160 l of oxygen. That cylinder would supply oxygen for roughly 160 min at an oxygen flow of 1 l/min. A similar calculation can be made for each H cylinder of oxygen. An H oxygen cylinder contains approximately 6900 l when full and like an E oxygen cylinder its pressure drops proportionally to the volume of oxygen remaining in the cylinder. A full E cylinder of nitrous oxide contains approximately 1600 l. Its pressure is 750 psi, regardless of the volume remaining, until approximately 250 l remains at which time the pressure begins to drop.

Q. How do I check the hospital gas distribution system for leaks?

A. Periodically the piped gas hospital distribution system should be checked for leaks by disconnecting all equipment connected to the pipeline, turning on the gas source to pressurize the lines, and then immediately turning off the

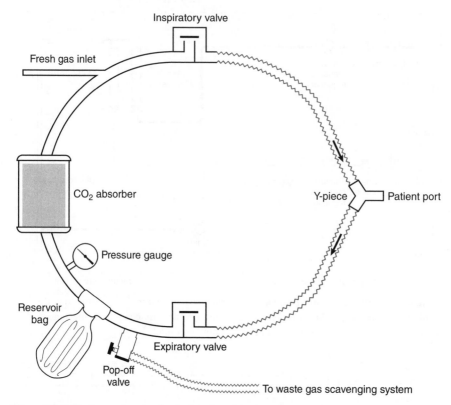

Figure 4.3 Typical components of a circle rebreathing system.

gas source. The pressure within the system is noted at that time and then several hours later. A drop in line pressure indicates a leak. Sources of leaks include a loose connection of the gas source to the supply lines, a leaky regulator, a leak between an oxygen generator and associated holding tank, or leaks within the distribution lines and terminal gas connections.

Q. How do I prepare my anesthesia machine for use?

A. Check the amount of oxygen (and nitrous oxide, if you are using it) at the source, the liquid anesthetic level in the vaporizer(s), and the CO_2 absorbent material. Check for leaks in the anesthetic machine and breathing system, and proper waste-gas scavenger system function.

Q. How should I prepare the anesthetic vaporizer(s) for use?

A. Each vaporizer should be filled at the beginning of the day when a minimum number of personnel are in the area. The fill cap is securely tightened after filling. Check the vaporizer window to make sure you can see a meniscus of liquid that is well above the minimum fill line. The vaporizer dial is rotated to ensure its proper function and then turned off. Prior to each use the vaporizer to be used in that particular instance is put into service by activating the appropriate vaporizer selector mechanism if present.

Q. How do I check the CO_2 absorbent canister?

A. The absorbent material should be changed at the beginning of the day when filling the vaporizer. Typically the canister is filled to within approximately 2 cm of the top. The canister should be gently tapped while filling to ensure that it is uniformly filled. The gasket(s) designed to seal the canister are inspected for dry rot and to ensure that no absorbent granules or absorbent dust is lodged between the canister and the gasket, resulting in a leak.

It can be difficult to determine if an adequate amount of functioning absorbent remains and therefore when it should be replaced. This will depend on the hours of use, the size and number of animals anesthetized since it was last changed, the capacity of the canister and the degree to which it is filled, the type of absorbent material, and the fresh gas flow rates typically used. In some facilities the absorbent is replaced at regular intervals based on historical use (e.g., once per week) whether or not it is needed. A rule of thumb is to change the absorbent material when the color change indicating exhaustion appears 2/3 down the canister. However, color change can be misleading because the color can temporarily revert while the machine is not in use. With some absorbent material the color also changes when the absorbent material becomes desiccated but can still absorb CO_2. An increase in inspired CO_2 concentration seen on a capnograph waveform can indicate absorbent is exhausted. However, erratic patterns of ventilation or relatively large equipment dead space can result in an elevated inspired CO_2 even if the absorbent material is functional.

Q. How do I check my anesthetic machine for leaks?

A. Different parts of the machine are checked differently. Machine leaks can occur in: (i) the high/intermediate pressure portion of the system which includes the gas cylinder connection(s) to the machine, and the pressure regulator(s); (ii) the low-pressure system which includes the flowmeter(s), vaporizers, and the connections to the breathing circuit; and (3) the breathing system, including bag, hoses, absorbent system, and ventilator. Most veterinarians are familiar with procedures for checking the breathing system for leaks but are less familiar with checking the high and low pressure systems of the anesthetic machine for leaks.

In general, larger leaks can be detected by passing your hand over and near the suspected leak sites. Smaller leaks can be detected by applying a solution of soapy water to the suspect areas. A leak will be indicated by bubble formation at the leak site.

Q. How do I check the high-pressure system of my anesthetic machine for leaks?

A. This check needs to be performed only periodically but regularly. It is good practice to check the high-pressure system for leaks whenever tanks are changed. The machine should be disconnected from the central hospital oxygen supply when performing this leak check. Leaks in the gas cylinder connections, if large, are audible as a loud hissing noise. Non-audible leaks within the machine are detected by turning off the flowmeter(s) and then turning on the cylinder valve(s). Next the cylinder valves are turned off. A drop in pressure of more than 50 psi within 2–5 min as indicated on the high-pressure gauge indicates a significant leak. Smaller leaks can be detected by following the same procedure, marking the position of the gauge indicator-needle with a piece of tape and then several hours later checking to see if the pressure on the gauge dropped. No movement confirms a leak-free high-pressure system. A leak in the oxygen supply is wasteful. A leak in the nitrous oxide supply is wasteful and contributes to unnecessary exposure of personnel to nitrous oxide.

Easily corrected sources of leaks in the high pressure system include cross-threaded or loose connections between H cylinders and their connection to the machine or a worn or missing plastic washer between an E cylinder and its connection to the anesthetic machine. Leaking pressure regulators will produce a loud hiss and must immediately be taken out of service and replaced by a qualified service person.

Q. How and when do I check the low-pressure system for leaks?

A. This leak check should be done whenever a vaporizer or flowmeter is replaced or serviced, or whenever a leak in the breathing system is suspected but can't be isolated to the breathing system. Some anesthetic machines contain a check valve in their outflow just downstream from the vaporizer (Figure 4.1). The function of this check valve is to prevent positive pressure within the breathing circuit (such as that generated from squeezing the rebreathing bag or generated from a ventilator) from being transmitted back through the vaporizer. Presence of a check valve will prevent the commonly used positive pressure leak check of the breathing system from detecting a leak in the vaporizer or flowmeters. For this reason a negative pressure leak test of the low-pressure system is considered universal.

To perform this test, negative pressure is exerted at the vaporizer outlet or common gas outlet with the oxygen cylinder turned on and the flowmeter(s) and vaporizer(s) turned off. The test is repeated with each vaporizer in the on position. To perform this test a hand-held suction bulb is squeezed and inserted into the flexible hose leading from the vaporizer(s) and oxygen flush valve (Figure 4.4). The bulb is then released. The bulb should remain empty for a minimum of 10 s indicating a negligible leak.

For machines and vaporizers without a check valve, a positive pressure check of the breathing system can detect a leak within the low-pressure system. When pressure checking the breathing system the oxygen and nitrous oxide flowmeters must be turned off and each vaporizer opened to allow pressurized gas from the breathing circuit to back-flow into the vaporizer.

Sources of low-pressure system leaks include the vaporizer, vaporizer connections, the flowmeter and associated connections, or any conducting tube or hose between the flowmeter, vaporizer, and breathing circuit. A vaporizer

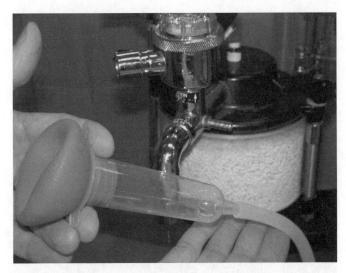

Figure 4.4 Negative pressure leak check: the fresh gas outlet tubing has been disconnected from its attachment to the circle system. A surgical suction bulb is compressed, inserted into the tube, and released. The bulb should remain depressed for at least 10 s indicating a negligible leak (see text for further explanation).

can leak from the fill valve if it was not properly closed and tightened. Other sources of vaporizer leaks must be professionally identified and serviced.

Q. How do I check the circle rebreathing system for leaks?

A. The corrugated breathing hoses/Y-piece or coaxial system (Unilimb, Universal F system) and the rebreathing bag should be attached to the circle absorber unit and the waste gas scavenging transfer hose connected to the pop-off valve. When using a coaxial system the outer corrugated hose is connected to the exhalation port of the circle absorber unit of the anesthetic machine. The hoses and bag should be snugly attached by pushing and twisting them onto the mountings. The machine is connected to the facility bulk oxygen supply or the E oxygen cylinder is turned on. The oxygen flowmeter should be turned off. The patient connection of the breathing system is occluded with the thumb or palm of hand. The pop-off valve is closed and the oxygen flush valve activated to fill the bag and pressurize the system to 30 cm H_2O (Figure 4.5). The system should hold this pressure for at least 10 s. If the pressure begins to drop the leak rate can be quantitated by slowly turning on the flowmeter until the pressure within the system stabilizes. The indicated flow is equal to the leak rate. A leak rate less than 350 ml/min is acceptable. The final step in checking the system for leaks is to open the pop-off valve and observe the pressure drop back to zero.

Common and easily correctable sources of leaks include forgetting to completely close the pop-off valve or not fully occluding the Y-piece. Other correctable causes are tears or holes in the bag and leaks associated with the CO_2 absorbent canister. Canisters can leak if cracked or if absorbent granules

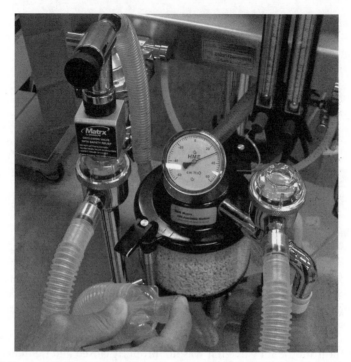

Figure 4.5 Pressure check of a circle rebreathing system. The pop-off valve is closed, the Y-piece occluded, and the O_2 flush valve is activated to distend the bag and develop a pressure equal to 30 cm H_2O.

become lodged between the gasket and canister. The absorbent canister can be inserted improperly and might not seal completely when closed with the cam- or screw-operated closure mechanism. If a leaking canister is identified it should be removed and the gaskets cleaned of absorbent material. The canister should be carefully aligned while activating the closure mechanism.

Q. How do I check a non-rebreathing system (e.g., Jackson – Reese, T – piece, Bain) for leaks?

A. The non-rebreathing system should be connected to the fresh gas outlet of the anesthetic machine. The bag should be attached and the pop-off valve connected to the waste gas scavenging system via a corrugated transfer hose. If using a Bain circuit the inner gas delivery hose should be inspected to determine if it is properly attached to its mounting near the endotracheal tube connection. The machine flowmeter is turned completely off and the pop-off valve of the non-rebreathing system closed. The patient end of the non-rebreathing system is occluded and the system pressurized using the oxygen flush valve. Systems without a pressure gauge should be pressurized until the bag is full and tight. Systems with a pressure gauge should be pressurized to 30 cm H_2O. The system should retain pressure for at least 10 s. The pop-off valve should be opened to verify its proper function.

Q. How do I prepare an anesthetic ventilator for use?

A. The instruction manual supplied with the ventilator should be read thoroughly because different ventilators vary in their details of operation. Most modern anesthetic ventilators contain a ventilator bellows attached at the base and surrounded by a plastic canister. The bellows is designed to fill (ascend) during exhalation and compress (descend) while delivering a breath. These ventilators need to be connected to the electric power and to a compressed gas source, typically the facility's oxygen supply. The 22 mm diameter corrugated hose that connects the ventilator to the anesthesia machine is pushed and twisted on to the bag mount of the circle absorber or the bag mount of the non-rebreathing system. The pressure detection sleeve of the ventilator, if present, is inserted between the inhalation side of the absorber and its connection to the corrugated breathing system hose of the circle rebreathing system. The pop-off valve of the breathing system is closed. The maximum pressure control/alarm located on the face of the ventilator control panel, if present, is set to the desired maximum pressure. The anesthetic machine flowmeter is turned off. The patient end of the breathing hoses is occluded. The oxygen flush valve is activated to completely fill the bellows. The bellows should stay inflated if no leak is present. If the bellows descend a leak is present. The leak rate can be quantified by turning on the flowmeter until the bellows no longer descends. The flow indicated on the flowmeter is equal to the leak rate. A leak rate less than 350 ml/min is acceptable. If the breathing system was determined to be leak free before attaching the ventilator then any leak detected with the ventilator connected must be in the ventilator circuit. Leaks can result from a loosely connected or leaky ventilator transfer hose or a misconnection in the bellows to the housing or hole in the ventilator bellows. Alternatively the ventilator can be leak-checked before attaching it to the breathing system. To do so the operator blows into the ventilator bellows through the hose that attaches the ventilator to the anesthesia machine. That hose is then occluded. If the ventilator is leak free the bellows will not descend.

Q. How do I determine if the waste gas scavenging system is functioning properly?

A. A waste gas scavenging system consists of a 19 or 30 mm diameter corrugated "transfer" hose connected to the scavenging port of the pop-off valve. Waste gas removal is either passive or active. In a passive system the distal end of the transfer hose is directed into an activated charcoal canister or it is directed out of the room via a connection to a through-the-wall opening or to the exhaust vent of a non-recirculating room ventilation system. Periodically the transfer hose should be inspected for leaks. This is done by completing the breathing system leak check as previously described, but instead of closing the pop-off valve it is left open and the distal end of the transfer hose occluded until 30 cm H_2O pressure develops within the breathing system and is sustained for 10 s. The pressure within the system should return to zero when the transfer hose is no longer occluded. The distal end of the transfer hose should then be reconnected to its point of destination. Any "through-the-wall" pipe should be periodically inspected for patency. Insects or other foreign material can clog the opening causing backpressure on the transfer tubing that can result in positive pressure within the breathing system. If an activated charcoal canister is used it should be weighed periodically and discarded when its weight increases by the amount specified in the accompanying manual. A fresh canister should be reconnected to the distal end of the transfer hose.

Active scavenging systems are those that use a vacuum system or a dedicated exhaust fan to remove waste gas from the transfer tubing. These systems ultimately are vented to the outdoors. Typically an adjustable interface mounted on the anesthetic machine is inserted between the distal end of the transfer tubing and the vacuum source. Proper scavenging system function is tested daily when performing a breathing system leak check. To verify proper function, the vacuum source or the fans should be turned on and the transfer tubing leading from the pop-off valve connected to the vacuum interface. At the conclusion of the breathing system leak check the pop-off valve is opened to release the pressure from the breathing system. The waste gas scavenging system should be capable of removing the volume of gas released from the system resulting in complete emptying of the rebreathing bag. Next the system is checked for excessive negative pressure. The Y-piece or patient port of the breathing system is occluded, the flowmeters turned off, and the pop-off valve left open. The pressure gauge within the breathing system should indicate a maximum negative pressure of 2 cm H_2O. If the pressure gauge indicates a more negative pressure than that the vacuum should be adjusted (decreased).

Q. How do I prepare my anesthetic monitoring equipment for use?

A. Refer to the owner's manual supplied with each monitoring device to determine how to appropriately configure the monitor for patient use. Monitors with rechargeable batteries should be plugged in when not in use so that a fully charged monitor is ready for the next patient. Depending on the monitor, it can be turned on prior to the first case of the day and shut down when all cases for that day are complete. Typically alarm limits, the order of traces and their colors on the monitoring screen are set at the time the monitor is first put into service and do not need to be reset. Refer to the owner's manual for any suggested calibration schedule and procedure. Most manuals contain a trouble-shooting section for reference should a particular monitor fail to provide meaningful data.

Q. What are some good references if I want more detail on this material?

A. Both Dorsch and Dorsch [1] and the American Society of Anesthesiologists website [2] provide excellent detailed information on machine and equipment.

References

1 Dorsch JA, Dorsch SE. Equipment Checkout and Maintenance. In: Dorsch JA, Dorsch SE (eds) *Understanding Anesthesia Equipment*, 5th edn. Lippincott Williams & Wilkins: Philadelphia, 2008:931–954.
2 American Society of Anesthesiologists. *Guidelines for Pre-Anesthesia Checkout Procedures.* https://www.asahq.org/For-Members/Clinical-Information/2008-ASA-Recommendations-for-PreAnesthesia-Checkout.aspx/ (accessed December 10, 2014).

5 Pre-Anesthetic Sedative Drugs

Let's make the patient more relaxed and comfortable!

Lesley J. Smith[1] and Jo Murrell[2]

[1] Department of Surgical Sciences, School of Veterinary Medicine, University of Wisconsin, USA
[2] School of Veterinary Sciences, University of Bristol, UK

KEY POINTS:

- Pre-anesthetic sedation reduces patient and personnel stress and reduces the required doses of induction and inhalant drugs, leading to less cardiopulmonary depression overall.

- Acepromazine provides moderate, dose-dependent sedation but reduces blood pressure because of vasodilation.

- Benzodiazapines have few significant side effects but also provide minimal sedation by themselves in healthy patients. They are mostly used to enhance muscle relaxation.

- Alpha-2 agonists provide moderate to profound sedation but also cause significant depression of cardiac output. Required doses of injectable and inhalant anesthestics are significantly reduced.

- Dissociatives are not sedatives, but can provide chemical restraint in very fractious patients.

Q. What is the purpose of pre-anesthetic sedation?

A. Pre-anesthetic sedation has many potential benefits. Among them are reduced patient stress and anxiety, and easier patient handling resulting in less stress to personnel. Because patients are easier to handle there is reduced risk of injury to veterinary staff or to the patient from excessive or aggressive restraint. Perhaps most importantly, pre-anesthetic sedation, depending on the drugs chosen, significantly reduces the required dose of induction agent and of anesthetic inhalant. Reducing doses of induction and inhalant drugs results in less overall cardiovascular and respiratory depression, which are the main players with respect to anesthetic morbidity and mortality. Finally, pre-anesthetic sedation will smooth the recovery process because there is less risk of emergence delirium or dysphoria on recovery.

Q. What drugs are used in small animal medicine for pre-anesthetic sedation or restraint?

Questions and Answers in Small Animal Anesthesia, First Edition. Edited by Lesley J. Smith.
© 2016 John Wiley & Sons, Inc. Published 2016 by John Wiley & Sons, Inc.

A. Most commonly the following drugs are used for sedation/restraint in the pre-anesthetic period.
   ✓ The phenothiazine tranquilizer: acepromazine.
   ✓ The benzodiazepine anxiolytics: midazolam and diazepam.
   ✓ Telazol: A proprietary combination of the dissociative tiletamine and the benzodiazepine zolazepam.
   ✓ The dissociative: ketamine.
   ✓ The alpha-2 agonists: medetomidine, dexmedetomidine.
   Chapter 6 will cover opioids and NSAIDs, which are generally used for their analgesic effects. Opioids can provide sedation in dogs and cats, but not reliably so, and NSAIDs provide no sedation.

Q. What should I know about acepromazine in dogs and cats?

A. Acepromazine is a relatively long-acting sedative that is metabolized by the liver. Depending on the dose used, this drug may have residual sedative effects and prolong the time to extubation [1]. Acepromazine is a relatively reliable sedative drug, but aggressive or fractious animals will override its effects, particularly if it is used alone. The long duration of acepromazine may be an advantage in excitable or anxious patients because it can help to smooth recovery. However, animals that are scheduled to go home the same day, geriatric patients, any patient with compromised hepatic function, and any patient with depressed mentation will exhibit undesirably prolonged sedation from acepromazine.

The most important negative side effect of acepromazine is a decrease in blood pressure secondary to vascular smooth muscle relaxation and vasodilation [2]. This decrease in blood pressure is dose-dependent, so low doses of acepromazine (see Table 5.1) will cause only modest decreases in blood pressure in *healthy* patients. It is also important to keep in mind that hypotension secondary to acepromazine will be additive when inhalants are administered, particularly at higher vaporizer settings.

Q. So when should I think about using acepromazine for sedation and when should I avoid it?

A. Acepromazine is an excellent sedative choice, particularly in combination with opioids (see Chapters 6 and 8) in young, healthy non-fractious dogs. In this population, sedation is generally reliable, blood pressure decreases are modest, and the long-ish duration of acepromazine helps in the recovery phase. In cats, acepromazine combined with an opioid does not always provide adequate sedation, so often a dissociative is added to the combination (see below on Dissociatives).

Acepromazine should probably be avoided, or used at the very lowest end of the dose range, in geriatric patients or those with significant systemic disease (ASA 3–5). It should be avoided in any patient with dehydration or blood loss from hemorrhage because negative effects on blood pressure can be anticipated. It should perhaps be avoided in patients with coagulopathies, because surgical blood loss will contribute to hypotension. Historically, acepromazine was reported to "lower the seizure threshold," but there is no convincing evidence that acepromazine administration is associated with an increase in seizure frequency, even in dogs with a seizure history [3].

Q. When is it useful to consider the benzodiazepine drugs, midazolam or diazepam? How do they work?

A. Benzodiazapine drugs work by enhancing Cl⁻ conductance at the GABA receptor, producing mild sedation and reduced anxiety in animals. The sedative effects are *minimal* in young, healthy dogs and cats. Often, these patients will become excitable and more difficult to restrain, particularly if the benzodiazepine is used alone. Most often, in order to achieve some degree of sedation, the benzodiazapines are combined with opioids in dogs and cats (see Chapters 6 and 8). The duration of effect of the benzodiazapines is short; in dogs an IM dose of midazolam results in sub-therapeutic plasma concentrations within an hour, with similar results via the IV route [4].

Benzodiazapines, combined with an opioid, are good choices for pre-anesthetic sedation in patients with significant systemic disease (ASA 3–5) and in geriatric patients who cannot tolerate low blood pressure during anesthesia because of reduced organ "reserve." Even combined with opioids, the benzodiazapines will not provide reliable sedation in fractious patients.

The benzodiazapines are extremely safe, however, as they cause virtually no change in cardiovascular or respiratory function in dogs and cats. There is some debate about their use in patients with hepatic failure (see Chapter 34) but, besides that, these drugs are rarely contraindicated in most patients. To repeat, however, they will not work well in young healthy dogs and cats when used alone!

Q. What is the clinical difference between midazolam and diazepam?

A. Both drugs work in a similar fashion and produce the same clinical effects. The only important difference is that diazepam is not water soluble and its solvent is propylene glycol. Diazapam is not well absorbed when given IM, but is effective via the IV route. The propylene glycol can sting, especially when diazepam is injected into a catheter that has been in place for a few days. The doses for both drugs are the same (see Table 5.1). Midazolam can be administered both IM and IV. When injected IM, midazolam's chemical structure changes such that it becomes lipid soluble and is readily absorbed into the systemic circulation.

Q. When should ketamine be added to pre-anesthetic medication?

A. Ketamine is a dissociative agent that produces a hypnotic state in animals. Its use for pre-anesthetic medication should be reserved for *chemical restraint* only, and it should not be administered as the sole pre-anesthetic agent. Most commonly, ketamine is included in the premedication "cocktail" for fractious

Table 5.1 Suggested doses for pre-anesthetic sedative drugs.

Dose ranges for pre-anesthetic sedation	IV	IM
acepromazine	0.005–0.02 mg/kg	0.01–0.1 mg/kg
midazolam	0.05–0.1 mg/kg	0.1–0.2 mg/kg
diazapam	0.05–0.1 mg/kg	not useful
ketamine	2–5 mg/kg	5–10 mg/kg
telazol		2–4 mg/kg
medetomidine	2–10 µg/kg	4–20 µg/kg
dexmedetomidine	1–5 µg/kg	2–10 µg/kg
atipamezole (for reversal of alpha-2 agonist sedation)	not recommended	equal volume to administered dose of the alpha-2 agonist (dog); ½ volume of administered dose of alpha-2 agonist (cat)

cats (see Chapter 8). Dogs are reliably sedated with combinations of acepro-mazine, alpha-2 agonists, or benzodiazapines, with opioids, so ketamine is rarely used in dogs for chemical restraint.

Q. What are ketamine's effects? When might it be contraindicated?

A. Ketamine is not a sedative, and its effects on the CNS are actually excita-tory. The animal's pupils will dilate, they will salivate, and they become rigid especially if sedative drugs are not used in combination. Heart rate, contractil-ity, and blood pressure increase. Because heart rate and contractility increase in the face of increased systemic afterload, cardiac oxygen demand goes up as well. The respiratory pattern can be apneustic, which is a slow respira-tory pattern characterized by a long inspiration phase and a relatively short expiratory phase [5]. Ketamine at high doses or when used alone increases intracranial pressure because of increases in cerebral blood flow secondary to an increase in CNS electrical activity and oxygen demand.

Ketamine's use as a pre-anesthetic medication should be reserved for frac-tious cats. Suggested doses are listed in Table 5.1. Because ketamine increases cardiac work, its use in cats with hypertrophic cardiomyopathy should be considered carefully. If possible, ketamine should also be avoided in cats with a history of seizure disorders, increased intracranial pressure from any cause, or increased intraocular pressure from any cause.

In cats, ketamine is cleared by the kidney and is not metabolized by the liver. Therefore, cats with chronic or acute renal failure will experience a prolonged duration of effect from ketamine. In cats with normal renal func-tion, ketamine's anesthetic duration is short, but residual CNS effects, char-acterized by head bobbing, hallucinatory behavior, salivation, and elevated temperature due to increased activity, may be evident for several hours after IM ketamine.

Q. What is telazol?

A. Telazol is a proprietary combination of the dissociative tiletamine and the benzodiazepine zolazepam. Together, they can be given IM to provide some muscle relaxation and chemical restraint. The clinical effects of tiletamine are much like ketamine, so the contraindications are the same.

   The main advantage of telazol is that it can be administered in very small volumes IM to extremely fractious patients. This is sometimes useful in large, very aggressive dogs, where sedation with an opioid/alpha-2 agonist combination may still not be enough to safely handle/examine the patient. Telazol can also be given *per os* in a small meatball if the dog is truly dangerous and cannot be touched or injected by hand or pole syringe. See Table 5.1 for suggested doses.

Q. What are alpha-2 agonists?

A. Alpha-2 agonists are a family of drugs (e.g., xylazine, romifidine, medetomidine, dexmedetomidine) that bind to alpha-2 adrenoreceptors found in the central and peripheral nervous system to produce a myriad of effects on body systems including sedation and analgesia [6].

Q. How are alpha-2 agonists used in veterinary anesthesia?

A. Alpha-2 agonists are most commonly used to provide dose-dependent sedation and analgesia as part of premedication protocols. Newer alpha-2 agonists such as medetomidine and dexmedetomidine may also be administered by continuous rate infusion (CRI) to provide continuous sedation and analgesia, either intra-operatively, where they contribute to provision of a balanced anesthetic technique, or post-operatively [7]. The sedation afforded by alpha-2 agonists is more reliable and profound than sedation provided by other classes of sedative drugs such as benzodiazepines (e.g., midazolam, diazepam) or acepromazine. Sedation and analgesia are enhanced by combining alpha-2 agonists with an opioid and this practice is recommended when alpha-2 agonists are used for premedication (see Chapters 6 and 8).

Q. Are there differences between the alpha-2 agonist drugs?

A. Yes! These drugs differ in their specificity for the alpha-2 receptor and their duration of action. Xylazine is relatively nonspecific for the alpha-2 receptor and administration of xylazine to cats and dogs is not recommended because of significant side effects (cardiovascular collapse, vomiting). Medetomidine is a racemic mixture of dexmedetomidine and levomedetomidine; dexmedetomidine is the active component whereas levomedetomidine is considered to be largely biologically inactive. Dexmedetomidine alone is also available as a licensed preparation for administration to cats and dogs. Romifidine is the longest acting alpha-2 agonist, but is not commonly administered to dogs and cats at the current time [8].

Q. Why would I choose and alpha-2 agonist for pre-anesthetic medication?

A. The reasons for choosing an alpha-2 agonist for premedication are as follows:
   ✓ Reliable sedation that is dose dependent.

✓ Concurrent analgesia, although be aware that the duration of analgesia (approximately 1 h following a 10 mcg/kg dose of dexmedetomidine) is significantly shorter than the total duration of sedation (approximately 3–4 h following a 10 mcg/kg dose of dexmedetomidine). This is another reason why combining alpha-2 agonists with opioids is advantageous.

✓ When used for premedication, there is a profound drug sparing effect on the required dose of induction agent and inhalant, thereby contributing to a balanced anaesthesia technique.

✓ These drugs are reversible through administration of the alpha-2 receptor antagonist atipamezole, shortening the recovery period from anesthesia or sedation.

Q. If alpha-2 agonists have so many advantages, why not premedicate or sedate all cats and dogs with them?

A. Despite their advantages, alpha-2 agonists have profound effects on the function of many other organ systems, particularly the cardiovascular system. This must be considered when deciding which patients are suitable for sedation with an alpha-2 agonist. It is generally not recommended to administer alpha-2 agonists to patients with cardiovascular disease. For a full review of the cardiovascular effects of alpha-2 agonists, see Murrell and Hellebrekers [1].

Q. What are the clinical consequences of these changes in cardiovascular function?

A. Administering an alpha-2 agonist, even at a relatively low dose (e.g., 5 mcg/kg dexmedetomidine IV), will reduce cardiac output to approximately 33–80% of the pre-administration cardiac output [9,10]. This reduction in cardiac output comes at the expense of peripheral organ perfusion, and in healthy animals the blood supply to central organs (e.g., heart, lungs, and kidney) is well maintained, ensuring adequate oxygenation [9]. However this requires utilization of cardiovascular reserve function, which if unavailable (e.g., due to cardiovascular disease), results in a precipitous drop in cardiac output that will compromise oxygenation of vital organs.

Q. If alpha-2 agonists slow down the heart rate, should I use an anticholinergic in combination?

A. It is not recommended to administer alpha-2 agonists with anticholinergics such as atropine or glycopyrrolate. Anticholinergics will block the vagally mediated reflex reduction in heart rate in response to the increased blood pressure that follows peripheral vasoconstriction (phase I cardiovascular response). If heart rate is elevated from the anticholinergic, while peripheral vasoconstriction is present due to the alpha-2 agonist, hypertension and a risk of cardiac arrhythmias can be severe [11].

Q. How do alpha-2 agonists affect respiratory system function?

A. These drugs have minimal effects on respiratory system function. The respiratory rate is often slowed, but this is compensated by an increased depth of respiration, so that normal blood oxygen and carbon dioxide tensions are maintained [12].

Q. How do alpha-2 agonists affect the function of other body organs?

A. ✓ Increase urine production through an effect on the secretion of renin and anti-diuretic hormone (ADH) [13], however this effect is not clinically important when single doses of alpha-2 agonists are administered.

  ✓ Increase blood glucose by decreasing insulin secretion; however, the magnitude of this effect is not sufficient to cause a glycosuria [14].

  ✓ Vomiting is common in animals administered alpha-2 agonists intramuscularly or subcutaneously, particularly cats [15].

  ✓ Gut motility is reduced following alpha-2 agonist administration.

Q. In what types of patients are alpha-2 agonists contraindicated?

A. Alpha-2 agonists are contraindicated in the following patient groups:

  ✓ Animals with significant liver dysfunction; alpha-2 agonists reduce liver blood flow and therefore may further compromise liver function [9].

  ✓ Animals with significant systemic or cardiovascular disease that do not have normal cardiovascular reserve function and are therefore less able to cope with the reduction in cardiac output that accompanies alpha-2 agonist administration.

  ✓ Animals in which vomiting is contraindicated for example (i) patients with increased intracranial or intraocular pressure (or where an increase in intracranial or intraocular pressure is disadvantageous), (ii) patients with reduced cranial nerve reflexes that might be at risk of aspiration should vomiting occur following alpha-2 agonist administration, (iii) patients with a GI foreign body, (iv) patients with spinal disease where vomiting may cause further spinal instability.

Q. What dose of alpha-2 agonist should I use for premedication and sedation?

A. See Table 5.1. Remember that all negative effects are dose dependent but even very low doses of alpha-2 agonists produce a significant decrease in cardiac output.

Q. What is the speed of onset of sedation after alpha-2 agonist administration?

A. Expect the onset of sedation to be within 5 min following IV administration and typically within 20 min following IM administration. Onset of sedation after subcutaneous administration may be more prolonged (30–40 min).

Q. How drug sparing are alpha-2 agonists?

A. These drugs have a significant drug sparing effect on both the dose of induction agent and the dose of maintenance agent (typically an inhalant). It is crucial to keep this in mind in order to avoid anesthetic overdose. The magnitude of this effect depends on the dose of alpha-2 agonist administered, with a greater effect present when higher doses (concurrent with more profound sedation) are used. Expect a 50% reduction in the dose of alfaxalone or propofol required to induce anesthesia; it is *very important* to administer the induction agent intravenously slowly to effect. This is because alpha-2 agonists slow the blood–brain circulation time and therefore it takes longer to see the peak effect of the induction drug. If induction agents are administered quickly anesthetic overdose is more likely. The required dose of inhalant will be reduced by 30–50% dependent on alpha-2 agonist dose; similarly, careful monitoring of depth of anesthesia to avoid anesthetic overdose is mandatory.

Q. Should I always reverse the alpha-2 agonist with atipamezole at the end of anesthesia?

A. Administration of atipamezole will reverse all effects of the alpha-2 agonist and speed return to full consciousness in the recovery period. So, whether to reverse or not depends on the patient, how quickly you want them to wake up, whether residual sedation is at all desirable, and whether you think the patient is likely to have a rough or excitable recovery. A "wait and see" approach to reversal will allow you to assess how that patient is recovering and whether you want to speed it up or not. Atipamezole should be administered IM (the licensed route of administration) because IV administration is associated with a sudden return to wakefulness and excitation is common (i.e., the recovery is too rapid). IV administration of atipamezole can also be associated with a rapid and significant drop in blood pressure.

References

1 Kleine S, Hofmeister E, Egan K. Multivariable analysis of the anesthetic factors associated with time to extubation in dogs. *Research in Veterinary Science* 2014; **97**:592–596.

2 Brock N. Acepromazine revisited. *Canadian Veterinary Journal* 1994; **35(7)**:458–459.

3 Tobias KM, Marioni-Henry K, Wagner R. A retrospective study on the use of acepromazine maleate in dogs with seizures. *Journal of the American Animal Hospital Association* 2006; **42(4)**:283–289.

4 Schwartz M, Munana KR, Nettifee-Osborne JA, *et al*. The pharmacokinetics of midazolam after intravenous, intramuscular, or rectal administration in healthy dogs. *Journal of Veterinary Pharmacology and Therapeutics* 2012; **36**:471–477.

5 Jaspar N, Mazzarelli M, Tessier C, et al. Effect of ketamine on control of breathing in cats. *Journal of Applied Respiratory (Environmental & Exercise) Physiology* 1983; **55(3)**:851–859.

6 Murrell JC, Hellebrekers LJ. Medetomidine and dexmedetomidine: a review of cardiovascular effects and antinociceptive properties in the dog. *Veterinary Anaesthesia and Analgesia* 2005; **32**:117–127.

7 Uilenreef JJ, Murrell JC, McKusick BC, *et al*. Dexmedetomidine continuous rate infusion during isoflurane anaesthesia in canine surgical patients. *Veterinary Anaesthesia and Analgesia* 2008; **35**:1–12.

8 England GC, Flack TE, Hollingworth E, *et al*. Sedative effects of romifidine in the dog. *Journal of Small Animal Practice* 1996; **37**:19–25.

9 Lawrence CJ, Prinzen FW, de Lange S. The effect of dexmedetomidine on nutrient organ blood flow. *Anesthesia and Analgesia* 1996; **83**:1160–1165.

10 Kellihan HB, Stepien RL, Hassen KM, *et al*. Sedative and echocardiographic effects of dexmedetomidine combined with butorphanol in healthy dogs. *Journal of Veterinary Cardiology, in press*.

11 Alibhai HI, Clarke KW, Lee YH, *et al*. Cardiopulmonary effects of combinations of medetomidine hydrochloride and atropine sulphate in dogs. *Veterinary Record* 1996; **138**:11–13.

12 Lamont LA, Burton SA, Caines D, *et al.* Effects of 2 different infusion rates of medetomidine on sedation score, cardiopulmonary parameters, and serum levels of medetomidine in healthy dogs. *Canadian Journal of Veterinary Research* 2012: **76**:308–316.

13 Villela NR, do Nascimento Júnior P, de Carvalho LR, *et al.* Effects of dexmedetomidine on renal system and on vasopressin plasma levels. Experimental study in dogs. *Revista Brasileira de Anestesiologia* 2005; **55**:429–440.

14 Saleh N, Aoki M, Shimada T, *et al.* Renal effects of medetomidine in isoflurane-anesthetized dogs with special reference to its diuretic action. *Journal Veterinary Medical Science* 2005; **67**:461–465.

15 Slingsby LS, Taylor PM, Monro T. Thermal antinociception after dexmedetomidine administration in cats: a comparison between intramuscular and oral transmucosal administration. *Journal of Feline Medicine and Surgery* 2009; **11**:829–834.

6 Opioids and Nonsteroidal Anti-Inflammatory Drugs

An important part of the plan

Lydia Love

Anesthesia Director, Animal Emergency & Referral Associates, USA

KEY POINTS:

- Opioids are the foundation of acute pain management. Side effects, while not inconsequential, can be managed with attention to detail.
- Opioids inhibit second messenger systems, leading to a decrease in transmission and perception of painful stimuli.
- New versions of opioids include sustained-release and transdermal formulations.
- Nonsteroidal anti-inflammatory drugs inhibit cyclooxygenase (COX)-mediated production of prostaglandins (PG).
- Inhibition of PG production leads to both desirable and adverse effects that, because of the ubiquity of COX enzymes, cannot be separated clinically.
- Careful attention to patient selection and clinical monitoring can maximize NSAID safety.

Opioids

Q. What is the nomenclature for opioid receptors?

A. Four opioid receptors are currently included in the opioid-related receptor group and several different naming schemes have been proposed (see Table 6.1). In general, opioid nomenclature is somewhat controversial and the literature can be confusing. The International Union of Basic and Clinical Pharmacology currently recommends conservation of the traditional Greek symbols with the added identification of an opioid peptide (NOP) receptor. The NOP receptor is considered *opioid-like* because it is structurally very similar to opioid receptors but displays a different pharmacologic profile.

Q. How do opioid receptors function?

A. Located centrally and peripherally in the nervous system, opioid receptors are inhibitory G protein coupled receptors, membrane-spanning signal

---

Questions and Answers in Small Animal Anesthesia, First Edition. Edited by Lesley J. Smith.
© 2016 John Wiley & Sons, Inc. Published 2016 by John Wiley & Sons, Inc.

Table 6.1   Various opioid receptor nomenclature schemes.

Greek Symbols[a]	Opioid Peptide[a]	Previous Recommendation[b]
μ or mu	MOP	OP_3
κ or kappa	KOP	OP_1
δ or delta	DOP	OP_2
–	NOP	OP_4

[a]Nomenclature scheme currently recommended by IUPHAR.
[b]This nomenclature may appear in some literature.

transducers that activate second messenger systems within cells. The overall result is to hyperpolarize the cell, decreasing neuronal excitability and reducing transmission of nerve impulses and neurotransmitter release. Inhibitory G proteins interact with various other intracellular signaling cascades with the overall clinical result of analgesia, sedation, respiratory depression, euphoria, and ileus.

Q. What is meant by full μ agonist, partial agonist, antagonist, and mixed agonist–antagonist?

A. A full μ agonist is an opioid that binds efficiently to the μ receptor, resulting in cellular and clinical effects that are dose-dependent. Increased doses do not exhibit a ceiling effect but are limited by the development of adverse clinical side effects. A partial agonist opioid exhibits relatively low intrinsic activity at its receptor and a ceiling effect is demonstrated where escalating doses do not result in intensifying effects. An opioid antagonist has no intrinsic activity at the receptor and available compounds are competitive antagonists that bind to all opioid receptors. A mixed agonist–antagonist has agonistic effects at one receptor and antagonistic effects at another (see Table 6.2).

Q. What are the advantages of using a full μ agonist opioid?

A. Full μ agonist opioids are effective for moderate to severe pain, can be titrated to effect, generally have minimal cardiovascular effects, and are easily reversed. Partial agonist and mixed agonist/antagonist opioids display an analgesic ceiling effect and may not be effective for moderate to severe pain.

Q. Can a full μ agonist and a partial μ agonist or mixed agonist–antagonist be administered together?

A. Yes, but the clinical effects depend on a myriad of pharmacokinetic and pharmacodynamic parameters, including relative timing, doses administered, bioavailability, clearance, species and individual genetic differences, and possibly the nociceptive stimulus. In the USA, it is not uncommon for practitioners to use butorphanol (a κ agonist/μ antagonist) simultaneously with buprenorphine (an opioid with a particularly complicated pharmacologic profile including partial μ & NOP agonism and κ antagonism). The theory is that butorphanol is a fast-acting mild sedative and mild analgesic

Table 6.2   Examples of various types of opioids and doses for dogs and cats

Receptor activity	Drugs	Dosing ranges[b]
Full μ agonists	Fentanyl	2–10 mcg/kg IM or IV
	Hydromorphone	0.05–0.2 mg/kg IM or IV
	Meperidine	2–5 mg/kg SC or IM
	Methadone	0.05–1.0 mg/kg IM or IV
	Morphine	0.25–1 mg/kg IM or IV
	Oxymorphone	0.025–0.1 mg/kg IM or IV
Partial μ agonist	Buprenorphine[a]	0.02–0.05 mg/kg IM or IV
Mixed agonist–antagonists	Butorphanol	0.2–0.8 mg/kg SC, IM, or IV
	Nalbuphine	0.2–0.8 mg/kg SC, IM, or IV
Antagonist	Naloxone	0.005–0.04 mg/kg

[a]Although commonly classified as a partial μ agonist, buprenorphine is also a partial NOP agonist and κ antagonist.
[b]In general, the lower end of the dose ranges presented are administered to cats.

that will eventually be displaced by buprenorphine, which displays high μ receptor affinity and a more effective and longer lasting analgesic profile. Experimental studies have not demonstrated any benefit to the combination, however [1], and it is important that if combinations of opioids are used, the patient is closely and repeatedly assessed for adequate analgesic effect.

Q. What about cats and "morphine mania"?

A. Cats may have increased motor activity and mydriasis upon opioid administration. However, the term morphine mania dates to experimental feline studies carried out in the mid twentieth century with doses of morphine ranging from 15–30 mg/kg and does not occur at clinically relevant doses [2]. If mild excitement or dysphoria occurs with opioid administration, reversal with an antagonist or mixed agonist/antagonist may be considered. As antagonists reverse all effects, including analgesia, consideration should be given to administration of a sedative such as acepromazine or an alpha-2 agonist in painful patients rather than reversal of the opioid drug.

Q. Aren't the respiratory depressant effects of opioids dangerous?

A. Opioids shift the ventilatory response curve downward and to the right – that is, the set point at which an increase in arterial carbon dioxide tension triggers an increase in ventilation is higher, and apnea is possible. However, this effect is much less prominent in dogs and cats than it is in humans and non-human primates and is rarely problematic within the clinical dose range. Ventilation should be monitored when administering μ opioid agonists in combination with sedatives and general anesthetics as respiratory depression will be additive.

Q. What cardiovascular effects might be expected with opioid administration?

A. In general, opioids are hemodynamically very safe, with mild to moderate effects on cardiac output and blood pressure. Bradycardia can result from increases in vagal tone, central inhibition of sympathetic outflow, and minor direct effects of opioids on cardiac conduction. Due to its structural similarity to atropine, meperidine may actually cause tachycardia. Mild vasodilation may occur with opioid administration and can contribute to hypotension, especially in volume-depleted patients. Morphine and meperidine administered intravenously can cause profound vasodilation due to histamine release. Morphine can be administered slowly intravenously but it may be best to restrict meperidine to intramuscular use.

Q. Don't opioids cause a dangerous hyperthermia in cats?

A. Opioids directly affect brainstem thermoregulatory systems and often contribute to hypothermia. In the species of animals that exhibit opioid-induced excitement, mydriasis, and increased motor activity (e.g., cats), hyperthermia may occur. Recent attention has been directed towards hyperthermia in cats following administration of hydromorphone. In one study, temperatures as high as 107 °F (41.7 °C) were recorded [3]. However, hyperthermia in cats has also been associated with buprenorphine, butorphanol, fentanyl, and the dissociative class of anesthetics. In addition, it has been suggested that a rebound effect following intra-anesthetic hypothermia might contribute to post-operative hyperthermia.

Interestingly, even cats with extremely elevated temperatures may not exhibit classical signs of hyperthermia. There has been some debate as to whether aggressive treatment is necessary since clinically relevant consequences are uncommon. The hyperthermia does respond rapidly to reversal with opioid antagonists or, often, the administration of a mixed agonist–antagonist opioid.

Q. What other side effects should I be aware of when administering opioids?

A. Systemic or epidural/spinal opioid administration may cause urine retention. Attention to adequacy of micturition, especially in the peri-anesthetic period, is important to avoid complications such as lower urinary tract infection and bladder atony. Gastrointestinal effects can include nausea, vomiting, and, with longer term use, constipation.

Finally, opioids inhibit aspects of humoral and cellular immunity and potentially affect metastatic and infectious outcomes. Definitive conclusions regarding the immune-modulatory effects of opioids are lacking as many factors, including pain and hypothermia, contribute to peri-operative immunosuppression.

Q. Other than typical injectable administration, how else are opioids administered to animals?

A. Oral administration of opioids generally results in poor bioavailability in cats and dogs, though occasionally oral morphine, hydrocodone, or codeine are prescribed for dogs. Increased plasma concentrations may be obtained by administering some drugs such as buprenorphine and methadone via the oral transmucosal (OTM) route, thereby avoiding first-pass metabolism. Oral

transmucosal administration results in 100% bioavailability of buprenorphine in cats. In dogs, standard dosing (0.02 mg/kg) via the OTM route
results in ~40% bioavailability. Pharmacodynamic studies indicate that
analgesic efficacy is detectable with OTM administration of buprenorphine
in dogs and the author does use this route on an outpatient basis for small
dogs. A compounded sustained release formulation of buprenorphine can
be obtained in the USA (www.wildpharm.com) and provides analgesia for
72 h. In addition, FDA approval has recently been extended for a novel
buprenorphine product that can be administered subcutaneously for cats to
provide 24 h of analgesia (Simbadol™). Fentanyl transdermal patches are
available, though plasma concentrations and clinical efficacy can be variable.
Fentanyl is available as a transdermal gel (Recuvyra™) for dogs in Europe
and the United States.

Q. So to summarize the effects of μ agonist opioids, the list would include?

A. ✓ profound analgesia;
   ✓ mild to profound sedation;
   ✓ bradycardia with no significant decrease in cardiac output;
   ✓ mild respiratory depression that may be additive with anesthetic drugs;
   ✓ urinary retention, GI ileus, vomiting;
   ✓ possible hyperthermia in cats.

Q. To summarize the difference between μ agonist opioids and the partial
   agonists or mixed agonist–antagonist opioids, one would conclude?

A. Partial agonists and mixed agonist–antagonist opioids provide mild–moderate
   dose-related analgesia with a ceiling effect at higher doses. In general, the side
   effects of these opioids are somewhat less than those of the μ agonist opioid
   drugs.

Nonsteroidal anti-inflammatory drugs (NSAIDs)

Q. What are the pharmacologic actions of NSAIDs?

A. Nonsteroidal anti-inflammatory drugs are inhibitors of cyclooxygenases
   (COX). Cyclooxygenase-1 and COX-2 (also known as prostaglandin
   endoperoxide synthases) are enzymes that convert the 20 carbon cell
   membrane breakdown product, arachidonic acid, into biologically active
   lipid compounds including prostaglandins (PG), prostacyclin, and throm-
   boxane. These downstream products (collectively known as prostanoids)
   are autocrine and paracrine effectors of a variety of cell functions, including
   maintenance of the gastric mucosal barrier and regulation of renal blood flow
   and sodium excretion. Many prostanoids are also inflammatory mediators,
   producing vasodilation and sensitization of peripheral nociceptors and
   facilitation of pain transmission centrally. Nonsteroidal anti-inflammatory
   drugs bind to COX enzymes and prevent arachidonic acid from accessing

Table 6.3   Examples of clinically available NSAIDs for *dogs*[a]

NSAID	Dose
Aspirin	10–15 mg/kg PO q12 h
Carprofen	2.2 mg/kg PO, SC, IV q12 h; 4.4 mg/kg PO, SC or IV q24 h
Deracoxib	1–2 mg/kg PO q24 h
Etodolac	10–15 mg/kg PO q24 h
Firocoxib	5 mg/kg PO q24 h
Ketoprofen	1–2 mg/kg SC, IM, or IV q24 h
Mavacoxib	2 mg/kg q14 days twice, then once monthly, for 7 doses
Meloxicam	0.2 mg/kg once, 0.1 mg/kg q24 PO, SC, or IV
Robenacoxib	2 mg/kg SC, followed by 1 mg/kg q24 h PO or SC

[a]Labeled dosing varies amongst countries.

Table 6.4   Examples of clinically available NSAIDs for *cats*[a]

NSAID	Dose
Aspirin	10 mg/kg PO q2–3 days
Carprofen	2–4 mg/kg SC once
Ketoprofen	1–2 mg/kg SC or IV q24 h
Meloxicam	0.1 mg/kg SC or IV; 0.01–0.03 mg/kg POq24 h
Robenacoxib	1 mg/kg SC q24 h

[a]Labeled dosing varies amongst countries.

the catalytic site. Tables 6.3 and 6.4 list commonly available NSAIDs and recommended dosages for dogs and cats.

Q. Where are COX enzymes located and what is the difference between COX-1 and COX-2?

A. Cyclooxygenases are ubiquitous membrane-bound enzymes that are present in every nucleated cell. In general, COX-1 is constitutively expressed, producing prostanoids concerned with homeostatic functions, while COX-2 is inducible during states of inflammation. Cyclooxygenase-2 is, however, expressed constitutively in many tissues, including the kidneys and central nervous system. In addition, COX-1 is expressed by inflammatory cells. Traditional NSAIDs are nonselective in their affinity for COX-1 versus COX-2, whereas recently developed compounds are selective or specific for COX-2. Several amino acid substitutions at the COX-2 catalytic site result in a larger binding site, a feature which is exploited by COX-2 specific NSAIDs [4].

Q. Which pharmacokinetic features of NSAIDs are important clinically?

A. Nonsteroidal anti-inflammatory drugs demonstrate high oral bioavailability in monogastric animals, with the exception of firocoxib. Administration of food with NSAIDs may delay, but generally does not decrease, absorption.

Protein binding of NSAIDs may approach 99% and this facilitates accumulation in protein-rich inflammatory exudate. High levels of protein binding limit glomerular filtration of NSAIDs and elimination is primarily via hepatic metabolism.

Q. What are the adverse effects of NSAIDs?

A. Gastrointestinal (GI) pathology and renal toxicity are most commonly reported in dogs and cats. Via inhibited production of PGE_2 and prostacyclin, NSAIDs cause a decrease in GI mucosal blood flow as well as the amount and quality of the protective mucus layer. In addition, gastric acid secretion is enhanced by PG inhibition. Lesions may include erosions, ulceration, GI bleeding, and perforation. Clinical signs include lethargy, inappetance, vomiting, melena, diarrhea, and death. Disturbingly, it is possible to have significant GI pathology without overt clinical signs.

Both isoforms of COX are constitutively expressed in the kidneys and COX-2 expression is increased during volume-depletion, hypotension, hyponatremia, and in some forms of renal disease [5]. Inhibition of COX by NSAIDs can lead to changes in intra- and total renal blood flow, reduction in the glomerular filtration rate, electrolyte imbalances, and acute renal failure. Hepatotoxicity of NSAIDs is generally idiosyncratic in nature. Serious hepatic complications typically develop in the first few weeks of chronic NSAID use, warranting early intensive clinical monitoring. A report indicating increased incidence of carprofen-induced hepatoxicity in Labrador Retrievers has not been confirmed in adverse drug reports collected since then and may reflect the popularity of the breed [6].

Other potentially undesirable effects of NSAIDs include alterations in hemostasis, hyperkalemia, fluid retention, and hypertension.

Q. Do NSAIDs delay healing?

A. Inflammation is an essential part of the healing process and inhibition of COX-2, whether by NSAIDs or genetic manipulation, delays healing of bones and tendons in experimental animals. The clinical relevance is unclear, however, and robust prospective clinical trials are lacking in any species. Effects of NSAIDs on healing may be partially time dependent. Nonsteroidal anti-inflammatory drugs are efficient analgesics and short-term use of NSAIDs during fracture and/or tendon healing is rational. Long-term use of high doses of NSAIDs should be avoided, especially in patients that are at high risk of delayed healing.

Q. Does sole inhibition of COX-2 result in fewer adverse effects?

A. Although the adverse effect profile may be slightly different for nonselective versus COX-2 specific NSAIDs, all NSAIDs harbor the potential for unwanted side effects. Cyclooxygenase-2 specific drugs result in fewer GI side effects in humans, but there is no demonstrable difference in renal or hepatic adverse events in comparison with nonselective NSAIDs.

Q. What gastro-protectant strategies are available?

A. Caution should be exercised with NSAID use in patients with a history of GI ulceration or those recovering from GI surgery. Consideration may be given to use of a more COX-2 selective agent. Administration of H2-receptor antagonists such as famotidine, or proton pump inhibitors, including omeprazole, may decrease the incidence of NSAID-induced GI pathology, though robust data for dogs and cats is lacking. The prostaglandin E2 analog misoprostol may also be considered.

Q. What drugs may interact with NSAIDs?

A. Glucocorticoids and NSAIDs should not be used concurrently due to the potential for disastrous GI consequences, including GI perforation and death. Contemporaneous use of two different NSAIDs should also be avoided and a washout period consistent with a time period equivalent to 3–5 half-lives of the specific NSAID in question are empirically recommended when switching between NSAIDs.

Nonsteroidal anti-inflammatory drugs may blunt the effects of antihypertensives and diuretics by altering sodium and fluid balance as well as by decreasing production of the potent vasodilator PGI_2. The risk of acute kidney injury may be higher in patients receiving angiotensin converting enzyme inhibitors, diuretics, and NSAIDs due to their combined effects on renal blood flow and glomerular filtration rate.

Nonselective NSAIDs may exaggerate the effects of anticoagulants, whereas COX-2 specific drugs can actually create a prothrombotic state – an effect at least partially to blame for the increased risk of cardiovascular events associated with NSAID use in humans.

Q. What special considerations surround the use of NSAIDs in cats?

A. Extended dosing intervals may be appropriate. Careful patient selection is central to the safe use of NSAIDs in cats. The use of NSAIDs should be avoided in patients dependent on PG production for sufficient renal function, including those that are volume-depleted, hypotensive, hyponatremic, or with chronic renal disease.

Q. Can NSAIDs be administered pre-operatively?

A. General anesthetics cause dose-dependent vasodilation and hypotension, a physiologic situation that precludes the use of NSAIDs. In addition, dehydration and hypovolemia may occur as a result of pre-anesthetic fasting or intra-operative hemorrhage, respectively. However, preemptive NSAID use can be an important part of a balanced preventative analgesic plan. Multiple studies in anesthetized dogs have not demonstrated NSAID-induced changes in creatinine, blood urea nitrogen, or glomerular filtration rate. However, barring catastrophic injury, these parameters are rather insensitive markers of the renal effects of NSAIDs. It is likely that when appropriate monitoring and supportive care are provided to animals with normal renal function, pre-anesthetic administration of NSAIDs is acceptable. If blood pressure monitoring and support are not available, peri-anesthetic use of NSAIDs should probably be limited to administration in the recovery period, after the possibility of drug or hemorrhage-induced decreases in renal blood flow has passed.

Q. Is acetaminophen (APAP) an NSAID?

A. The predominant mechanism of action of acetaminophen is unclear. Inhibition of COX enzymes occurs but rather than binding to the COX catalytic site and preventing access of arachidonic acid, APAP scavenges the reactive oxygen intermediate peroxynitrite, an endogenous activator of COX [7]. This mechanism can be overwhelmed by elevated concentrations of reactive oxygen species, explaining the weak activity of APAP at sites of inflammation. Other mechanisms of action have been proposed, including interference with centrally located COX enzymes (specifically a split variant of COX-1 sometimes referred to as COX-3), interaction with multimodal TRPV-1 nociceptors, or via endogenous serotonergic, opioid, and cannabinoid pathways. Although acetaminophen should not be used in cats at any dose due to toxicity issues, short-term use – even in combination with traditional NSAIDs – can be considered in dogs with normal hepatic function.

Q. Important considerations when using NSAIDs include:
- ✓ analgesia is provided by anti-inflammatory properties;
- ✓ use caution with administration to patients with a risk of intra-operative hypotension, any patient with pre-existing renal or hepatic disease, or any patient at risk of GI ulceration;
- ✓ major side effects include GI mucosal damage, impaired renal blood flow, acute renal failure in susceptible patients, and fluid retention in patients with cardiovascular disease;
- ✓ cats have longer half-lives for some NSAIDs, so dosing intervals should be considered carefully
- ✓ NSAIDs should never be administered concurrently with glucocorticoids.

References

1 Johnson JA, Robertson SA, Pypendop BH. Antinociceptive effects of butorphanol, buprenorphine, or both, administered intramuscularly in cats. *American Journal of Veterinary Research* 2007; **68(7)**:699–703.

2 Sturtevant FM, Drill VA. Tranquilizing drugs and morphine-mania in cats. *Nature* 1957; **179(4572)**:1253.

3 Posner LP, Gleed RD, Erb HN, *et al.* Post-anesthetic hyperthermia in cats. *Veterinary Anaesthesia and Analgesia* 2007; **34(1)**:40–47.

4 Garavito RM, Malkowski MG, DeWitt DL. The structures of prostaglandin endoperoxide H synthases-1 and -2. *Prostaglandins Other Lipid Mediators* 2002; **68-69**:129–152.

5 Rios A, Vargas-Robles H, Gámez-Méndez AM, *et al.* Cyclooxygenase-2 and kidney failure. *Prostaglandins Other Lipid Mediators* 2012; **98(3-4)**:86–90.

6 MacPhail CM, Lappin MR, Meyer DJ, *et al.* Hepatocellular toxicosis associated with administration of carprofen in 21 dogs. *Journal of the American Veterinary Medical Association* 1998; **212(12)**:1895–1901.

7 Schildknecht S, Daiber A, Ghisla S, *et al.* Acetominophen inhibits prostanoid synthesis by scavenging the PGHS-activator peroxynitrite. *FASEB Journal* 2008; **22(1)**:215–224.

7 Anticholinergic Drugs

My heart is racing!

Lesley J. Smith

Department of Surgical Sciences, School of Veterinary Medicine, University of Wisconsin, USA

KEY POINTS:

- Atropine and glycopyrrolate are the two most common anticholinergic drugs in clinical use.
- Both drugs are used primarily to increase heart rate in cases of anticipated or actual bradycardia.
- Neither drug works well in hypothermic patients.
- Neither drug will increase heart rate in patients with 3rd degree heart block.
- Neither drug should be used as a first step in treating bradycardia 2° to alpha-2 agonist administration because of adverse increases in cardiac work and O_2 consumption.
- Atropine has a faster onset of effect, with a shorter duration, than glycopyrrolate.
- Both drugs can be given IM or IV.

Q. What are anticholinergics?

A. Anticholinergics are a class of drugs that work specifically to antagonize acetylcholine (Ach) at muscarinic receptors in the parasympathetic nervous system. Other common terms for these drugs are anti-muscarinics, vagolytics, and parasympatholytics. The two most commonly used anticholinergics in veterinary medicine are atropine and glycopyrrolate.

Q. What is the clinical effect of giving an anticholinergic?

A. The primary clinical effect of these drugs is to increase heart rate and to reduce salivation. All of the clinical effects of these drugs are related to their blockade of Ach at parasympathetic post-ganglionic sites in the body, therefore parasympathetic, or vagal tone, is reduced. Because these drugs do not discriminate between muscarinic Ach receptors, they have other effects in the body that may be undesirable. A list of their clinical effects includes:

✓ increased heart rate/tachycardia;
✓ decreased salivation;

Questions and Answers in Small Animal Anesthesia, First Edition. Edited by Lesley J. Smith.
© 2016 John Wiley & Sons, Inc. Published 2016 by John Wiley & Sons, Inc.

✓ decreased mucociliary transport/decrease airway clearance of debris and mucous;

✓ bronchodilation;

✓ pupillary dilation, decreased tear production (atropine only);

✓ GI ileus, relaxation of gastro-esophageal sphincter → increased risk of GI reflux?

Q. In what situations should these drugs be used?

A. Generally, atropine and glycopyrrolate are used to increase heart rate in the face of actual or anticipated bradycardia, in cases of sinus arrest, or to treat certain bradyarrhythmias. Some clinicians also use them specifically to dry up oral salivary secretions to improve conditions for oro-tracheal intubation. Bradycardia in an animal under anesthesia may be a cause for hypotension, and in these cases atropine or glycopyrrolate can be quite effective at increasing the heart rate, resulting in an increase in cardiac output and blood pressure. Sinus arrest will often respond to a dose of atropine. Bradyarrhythmias that typically respond to these drugs include sinus bradycardia, first and second degree AV block (both Mobitz Type I and II), but not third degree block.

Q. Should I use atropine or glycopyrrolate prior to anesthesia if I am concerned about bradycardia occurring while the animal is anesthetized?

A. This is a controversial area amongst clinical anesthetists. One school of thought is to pre-treat all canine and feline patients with one of these two drugs in the premedication cocktail, as a pre-emptive way to avoid or minimize anesthesia-induced bradycardia. The other school of thought is to take a "wait and see" approach, monitor heart rate and rhythm and blood pressure, and give either drug if the heart rate is low enough to be a cause for hypotension or if significant bradycardia or bradyarrhythmias occur. Either approach is acceptable.

Q. What is the difference between atropine and glycopyrrolate?

A. Atropine has a fast onset of effect, is more likely to increase heart rate quickly, and is more likely to result in tachycardia and potentially tachyarrhythmias. Atropine crosses the blood–brain barrier and the placenta, which is not usually of any clinical consequence unless one is performing a C-section (in which case the newborns will experience the effects of the drug). Because glycopyrrolate does not cross the blood–brain barrier, it is devoid of ocular effects (atropine will cause pupillary dilation and decreased tear production). Atropine has a short duration of action (∼ 30 min after IV administration) on heart rate changes, although ocular changes can persist for days [1].

By contrast, glycopyrrolate's onset of action appears, clinically, to be slower (minutes vs. seconds), heart rate usually increases more slowly, and paradoxical second degree AV block sometimes occurs transiently. Second degree AV block can also be seen after atropine administration, particularly if it is given IM. Controlled studies comparing the onset and duration of glycopyrrolate to atropine are lacking. Generally, glycopyrrolate is a better choice if one wants to increase the patient's heart rate, but not dramatically. Atropine is a better choice if it is an emergency situation where the bradycardia is profound.

Q. By what route should I give these drugs?

A. Both drugs can be given IV or IM. Uptake by the subcutaneous route can be unpredictable particularly if the patient is cold, dehydrated, or hypotensive. Generally the IV route is preferable if a more immediate increase in heart rate is the goal. Low doses IM will increase heart rate gradually, within 10–15 min, but the overall increase can often be less than one would see after IV administration. If using these drugs to pre-emptively prevent bradycardia as part of a premedication cocktail IM, the full dose should be chosen. See Table 7.1 for suggested doses.

Q. Are there situations when these drugs don't have any effect?

A. Clinical experience suggests that these drugs don't work very effectively in patients who are very cold ($< 92\ °F$). Patient rewarming in these instances is more effective at increasing heart rate. Occasionally some patients with very high vagal tone may need a second dose of glycopyrrolate before any effect is appreciated. When glycopyrrolate is given IV, and especially when it is given IM, it can take many minutes before an appreciable increase in heart rate is observed, even in a patient with normal body temperature. Third degree heart block will not respond to these drugs.

Q. Are there situations when these drugs should be avoided?

A. These drugs should be avoided in an anesthetized patient with high blood pressure and a low-ish heart rate, because the result will be a normal–high heart rate and extremely high blood pressure! These drugs should also be avoided, at least initially, to treat bradycardia due to the alpha-2 agonist drugs (medetomidine, dexmedetomidine). This is because the bradycardia seen after alpha-2 agonist administration is reflex bradycardia from the systemic hypertension that is caused by these drugs. The reflex bradycardia is a physiologic response. Increasing the heart rate with atropine or glycopyrrolate increases myocardial work and oxygen consumption. A better approach is to reverse the alpha-2 agonist with atipamezole if an increase in heart rate is desired under these conditions. After reversal, if the heart rate is still too low, then treatment with an anticholinergic may be the next step.

Table 7.1 Suggested doses for atropine and glycopyrrolate in dogs and cats.

Drug	Atropine	Glycopyrrolate
Dose (mg/kg)	0.02–0.04	0.005–0.01
Route	IV/IM	IV/IM

Reference

1 Hendrix PK, Robinson EP. Effects of a selective and nonselective muscarinic cholinergic antagonist on heart rate and intestinal motility in dogs. *Journal of Veterinary Pharmacology and Therapeutics* 1997;**20**:387–395.

8 Time to Premedicate

How do I decide from all these choices?

Lesley J. Smith

Department of Surgical Sciences, School of Veterinary Medicine, University of Wisconsin, USA

KEY POINTS:

- Premedication combinations are used to calm the patient and to provide analgesia in many instances.
- Sedation with acepromazine or an alpha-2 agonist will be more profound than sedation with a benzodiazepine, which may provide little to no sedation but does reduce anxiety.
- Opioids used alone may provide mild to moderate sedation in dogs.
- The addition of an opioid to any of the sedative drugs will result in synergistic sedation.
- Fractious cats may also need to be given ketamine or telazol IM for good chemical restraint.
- NSAIDs will provide analgesia but no sedation and should be used cautiously, when given prior to anesthesia, in patients at risk for reduced renal blood flow or hypotension from any cause.

Q. What am I trying to achieve by my choice of premedication?

A. The main purposes of premedication are to produce a calm and tractable patient, to smooth the induction process, to reduce the required doses of injectable and inhalant anesthetics for better cardiovascular and respiratory stability, and to provide analgesia when needed. The available premedication drugs can produce sedation, anxiolysis, analgesia, and chemical restraint. Which drug or combination of drugs you choose, and the doses of each, will influence where your patient is on the spectrum of premedication results. Temperament, species, breed, health status, and underlying disease will also influence how that patient responds to different premedications.

Q. What is the difference between sedation and anxiolysis?

A. Sedation is characterized by CNS depression and a patient that is generally less aware, or less wary, of its surroundings, but that can still be aroused by painful stimuli or loud/sudden disturbances [1]. Anxiolysis, also referred to by some clinicians as tranquilization, refers to a patient that is rendered more calm and relaxed as a result of the drug, but that is still aware of and

Questions and Answers in Small Animal Anesthesia, First Edition. Edited by Lesley J. Smith.
© 2016 John Wiley & Sons, Inc. Published 2016 by John Wiley & Sons, Inc.

responsive to its surroundings. Acepromazine is a classic drug that provides anxiolysis and, at higher doses, sedation. Benzodiazepines provide anxiolysis but little sedation in most patients. Alpha-2 agonists are generally reliable sedatives.

Q. What is chemical restraint?

A. Chemical restraint refers most specifically to the dissociative drugs ketamine and tiletamine that produce a cataleptic state in which the patient is unaware of its surroundings, unresponsive to stimuli, but with dilated pupils and some reflexes intact. Animals treated with dissociatives often retain a swallow, will salivate profusely, and will have rigid muscle tone if no other drug is given concurrently. Higher doses of alpha-2 agonists can also produce a state of relative chemical restraint.

Q. What is analgesia?

A. Analgesia is reduced or absent pain perception [1]. None of the available pre-medication drugs when administered at clinically relevant doses can reduce pain to non-existent, but some do reduce pain perception. These are most notably the opioids and alpha-2 agonists, with the possible addition of the dissociatives. The NSAIDs also provide analgesia, but do not produce any sedation or anxiolysis.

Q. Should I give my premedications IV or IM? What about subcutaneous routes?

A. The route of administration of your premedications depends on your patient and your technical staff and/or their technical skills. Dogs and cats that are difficult to restrain due to temperament are best premedicated by the IM route, so that IV catheter placement prior to anesthesia is easier to achieve and less stressful for the patient. Less experienced personnel may also benefit from having a sedated patient prior to attempts at IV catheter placement. If IV access is already established, or if it is easy to place a catheter in a tractable, calm patient, then premedications can also be given IV. Generally, doses are reduced when the IV route is chosen. Subcutaneous administration of premedications is also acceptable, but absorption may be slower and less predictable, resulting in lower plasma concentrations of drug and a smaller effect. Subcutaneous administration may be desirable, however, when larger volumes of drug must be given or in animals that are thin with little muscling.

Q. OK, so I have all these choices, where do I start?

A. A good place to start is to evaluate your patient and decide what you want to achieve with your premedication. Do you want heavy sedation? Just a calmer animal? One that is completely immobilized? How much analgesia do you want to add depending on how painful the procedure is anticipated to be? Remember too that all of the premedication drugs have dose-dependent effects – and this means dose-dependent desirable effects (e.g., sedation or analgesia) as well as dose-dependent negative side effects. It might be useful to look at the available sedative and opioid drugs on a spectrum – see Table 8.1.

Table 8.1 Spectrum of premedication effects for a healthy dog or cat.

Minimal sedation but some anxiolysis	Moderate sedation/anxiolysis	Profound sedation
midazolam or diazepam	Low–middle dose acepromazine low dose medetomidine or dexmedetomidine	high dose acepromazine middle-high dose medetomidine or dexmedetomidine
Mild analgesia/sedation	**Moderate analgesia/sedation**	**Profound analgesia/sedation**
butorphanol low dose buprenorphine	high dose buprenorphine low dose morphine, hydromorphone, oxymorphone, methadone, fentanyl	high dose morphine, hydromorphone, oxymorphone, methadone, fentanyl CRI combinations of opioid, lidocaine, ketamine

Note that acepromazine, midazolam, and diazepam provide *no* analgesia! Some analgesia is obtained with medetomidine and dexmedetomidine but the duration of sedation is ~ 3x longer than the duration of analgesia with these drugs [2].

Note also that addition of the opioids will provide synergistic sedation with these sedative drugs. Opioids used alone will provide mild–moderate sedation in healthy dogs, but usually not in healthy cats.

Q. Can you go through some basic case examples to clarify?

A. Yes. Let's start with your everyday healthy, young dog presenting for an ovariohysterectomy and discuss a premedication plan. First choice is whether to give your premedication IM or IV. If it is an energetic dog, it might be easiest on everyone if you go IM. However, if IV access will be easy and not stressful for the dog or personnel, IV administration is fine. Rule of thumb would be to use ~ half the dose of drugs if going IV.

What do you want? A nicely sedated dog, easy to restrain for IV catheter placement, good analgesia that lasts into recovery, and a combination of premedications that reduces your inhalant requirement.

Midazolam? Diazepam? This dog will *not* sedate well with either of these drugs. Benzodiazepines will not provide sedation in young healthy animals and are best reserved for geriatric or sick patients. Remember too that diazepam only works well via the IV route, so IM administration of diazepam is not a good option.

Acepromazine? You'll probably get decent sedation with acepromazine IM or (low dose) IV. The duration of action is long, however, so you need to be prepared for a drowsy dog in recovery that may still be sedate 12 h later. Be prepared for dose-dependent decreases in blood pressure. A low dose of acepromazine (e.g., < 0.05 mg/kg) to a healthy dog will not significantly reduce blood pressure, but will have an additive effect on blood pressure reductions with the inhalant used during surgery. Higher doses of acepromazine will likely result in enough vasodilation to cause low blood pressure during surgery that will be exacerbated by the inhalant.

Medetomidine or dexmedetomidine? Both of these will provide good sedation and some short-lived analgesia. They are reversible. Both cause bradycardia, hypertension, and a decrease in cardiac output and perfusion to peripheral tissues. OK and probably well-tolerated in this healthy dog.

So, appropriate sedation choices for this dog would be acepromazine *or* one of the alpha-2 agonist drugs.

Analgesia? Yes, for this surgery! Which opioid? Butorphanol has a very short duration (45–60 min) so you would need to cover analgesia with other methods for recovery and because butorphanol's analgesic action is mild, the surgeon should be skilled with minimal expected tissue trauma. Buprenorphine might be a good option, again if the surgeon is skilled, because it has a long duration and will last into the recovery period. For any ovariohysterectomy that is expected to produce moderate pain (e.g., unskilled surgeon, deep chested large dog, etc.) a pure μ agonist opioid like morphine, oxymorphone, or hydromorphone is your best bet. Morphine should preferentially be given IM because of histamine release. If morphine is given IV, it should be diluted, given slowly, and at low doses. Fentanyl has an extremely short duration of action (i.e., 20 min) so must be given IV and then continued as a CRI, which may not be practical for the typical ovariohysterectomy. Also, because fentanyl won't last into the recovery period, you will have to add something else into your plan to cover analgesia once the dog wakes up.

To summarize, a good premedication combination for this dog would be:

IM acepromazine (0.02–0.05 mg/kg) + morphine (0.5–1.0 mg/kg) OR hydromorphone (0.1–0.2 mg/kg)

Alternatively, for deeper sedation:

IM dexmedetomidine (5 mcg/kg) + morphine (0.5–1.0 mg/kg) OR hydromorphone (0.1–0.2 mg/kg)

Q. What if the dog in question is fractious or dangerous?

A. Then your best option is probably to use a higher dose of alpha-2 agonist (e.g., dexmedetomidine 10 mcg/kg IM) with a pure μ agonist opioid (e.g., morphine 1 mg/kg) IM.

Even with the higher dose of alpha-2 agonist, exercise caution when handling the patient until it is fully anesthetized. Fractious patients can override the sedative effects of alpha-2 agonists.

Q. How would I change premedications if I have a geriatric dog with elevated renal values that is scheduled for a dental cleaning?

A. Here you have to be more careful. Higher doses of acepromazine or alpha-2 agonists are *not* a good idea because of the hypotension caused by acepromazine and the reduced cardiac output caused by the alpha-2 agonists. If you *must* use one of these drugs because the dog is difficult to handle, then try to stay at the lower end of the suggested dose range.

If the dog is relatively easy to handle, IM midazolam combined with a pure μ agonist opioid is a good choice. The opioid will reduce your inhalant requirement, which is important in this patient because you want to preserve good blood pressure to help keep renal blood flow normal. Even though it is not a painful procedure, the pure μ agonist opioid will be better at sparing the inhalant requirement than butorphanol or buprenorphine in this case.

Q. How are cats different when it comes to premedication choices?

A. Cats really are not that different. The primary difference between cats and dogs when it comes to premedication is that cats do not become classically sedate with opioids. Rather, they will display euphoric behavior, with rolling, paw kneading, and so on. If a sedative like acepromazine or an alpha-2 agonist is included, they will often become quiet, but with dilated pupils. For good chemical restraint in a cat that is young or more fractious, adding ketamine IM will result in a cat that is easy to handle for IV catheter placement.

Q. So what would be a good combination for a healthy cat undergoing an ovariohysterectomy?

A. Good choices would be acepromazine or one of the alpha-2 agonists IM, with an opioid of your choice, +/- ketamine if you want to guarantee good restraint. Depending on surgical skill, if you anticipate mild–moderate pain, your opioid could be butorphanol (but you will have to re-dose for recovery and potentially intra-operatively as well, keeping in mind that the duration of effect is only 45–60 min) or buprenorphine. If you expect more significant pain (e.g., inexperienced surgeon, declaw procedure also being performed) you would want to use a pure μ agonist opioid such as oxymorphone or hydromorphone.

Q. Keeping with the theme above, what if it is a geriatric cat with azotemia having a dental prophylaxis?

A. Same ideas here. You would want to try to avoid acepromazine or the alpha-2 agonists because of their hemodynamic effects and switch to midazolam IM/IV or diazepam IV as your anxiolytic drug, then add your pure μ agonist opioid of choice +/- ketamine if the cat is really fractious. Ketamine should be used cautiously in cats with compromised renal function because the parent drug is partially excreted by the kidney in cats, so its duration may be longer in cats with renal compromise [3].

Q. How do the NSAIDs factor into premedication?

A. The answer to this really depends on your patient. The NSAIDs may work best if given prior to the onset of surgical tissue trauma because of their role in reducing prostaglandin production. If the patient is not anticipated to have *any* problem maintaining good blood pressure during surgery and if you are able to monitor blood pressure and address any significant decreases (i.e., mean arterial pressure < 60 mmHg), then it may be OK to give the NSAID of your choice prior to surgery. The NSAID could be given with the premedication, sometime in advance of premedication, or after anesthetic induction. Some clinicians prefer to play it safe and wait until the patient has recovered from anesthesia, when blood pressure is expected to have returned to normal, before giving the NSAID. Non-selective COX inhibitors may increase the risk of bleeding.

If the patient has a risk for hypotension during anesthesia or if you are not able to monitor blood pressure, then it is wise to wait until the animal is recovered from anesthesia before you administer the NSAID. This is because the NSAIDs contribute to renal damage in the face of reduced renal blood flow $2°$ to hypotension or if renal perfusion is already compromised due to disease [4].

Q. What about adding anticholinergics with my premedication?

A. This is a personal choice. Some clinicians take a "wait and see" approach and only give the anticholinergics if the heart rate drops below acceptable limits. Others pre-emptively give the anticholinergic to prevent decreases in heart rate due to opioids, vagal tone, and so on. The one situation in which anticholinergics should *not* be given with the premedications is when using an alpha-2 agonist. This is because the bradycardia seen with alpha-2 agonist administration is a physiologic reflex to the increase in afterload caused by these drugs due to their effect on systemic vascular resistance. Increasing heart rate with anticholinergics in the face of alpha-2 mediated increases in afterload is not physiologic and increases cardiac work and oxygen consumption.

Table 8.2 Summary of premedication choices for dogs and cats.

Sedative choices	Opioid choices	Dissociative?	NSAID choices	Anticholinergic?
acepromazine	morphine (IM preferred)	ketamine (IM only) [cats only]	carprofen	atropine
midazolam	hydromorphone	telazol IM [fractious dogs or cats]	meloxicam	glycopyrrolate
diazepam (IV only)	oxymorphone		robenicoxib	
medetomidine	methadone		ketoprofen	
dexmedetomidine	fentanyl (IV only, followed by CRI		deracoxib (dogs only)	
	butorphanol (mild analgesia)		firocoxib (dogs only)	
	buprenorphine (mild–moderate analgesia)			

Q. How can I keep track of my different premedication choices?

A. Table 8.2 summarizes the various drugs and their effects when choosing premedication combinations.

References

1 Thurmon JC, Short CE. History and overview of veterinary anesthesia. In: Tranquilli WJ, Thurmon JC, Grimm KA (eds) *Lumb and Jones' Veterinary Anesthesia and Analgesia*, 4th edn. Blackwell Publishing: Ames, IA, 2007:**5**.

2 Murrell JC, Hellebrekers LJ. Medetomidine and dexmedetomidine: a review of cardiovascular effects and antinociceptive properties in the dog. *Veterinary Anaesthesia and Analgesia* 2005: **32**:117–127.

3 Hanna RM, Borchard RE, Schmidt SL. Effects of diuretics on ketamine and sulfanilate elimination in cats. *Journal of Veterinary Pharmacology and Therapeutics* 1988; **11(2)**:121–129.

4 Rios A, Vargas-Robles H, Gámez-Méndez AM, *et al*. Cyclooxygenase-2 and kidney failure. *Prostaglandins Other Lipid Mediators* 2012; **98(3–4)**:86–90.

9 Intravenous Access and Fluid Administration

Water is life

Erin Wendt-Hornickle

Department of Veterinary Clinical Sciences, College of Veterinary Medicine, University of Minnesota, USA

KEY POINTS:

- Most patients benefit from IV fluid administration during anesthesia.
- An IV catheter is important for fluid and drug administration and is critical for emergency situations.
- The majority of patients should receive IV balanced isotonic crystalloids.
- Hypertonic saline should only be used in cases where rapid volume expansion is critical to maintaining life.
- Synthetic colloids can help maintain normal blood pressure in hypotensive patients and also in patients with low total protein or albumin.

Q. What are the indications for intravenous catheter placement?

A. The most common reasons for placing an intravenous (IV) catheter are fluid and drug administration, blood sampling, and emergency preparedness.

Intravascular catheter placement is necessary for IV fluid administration during anesthesia. The American Animal Hospital Association has outlined general guidelines for fluid administration, including recommendations for patients undergoing anesthesia [1]. Fluids given IV help maintain blood pressure, organ perfusion, and normal blood volume.

Intravenous anesthetic induction should be performed via a patent and secure IV catheter. Many induction agents cause adverse effects (tissue damage, pain) when given extravascular; it is important to ensure maintenance of IV access when administering these drugs. Also, having an IV catheter makes giving peri-operative analgesia and antibiotics easier for staff and patients.

Occasionally, blood sampling may be necessary. Though central (jugular) catheters are better suited for this purpose, larger gauge peripheral catheters

Questions and Answers in Small Animal Anesthesia, First Edition. Edited by Lesley J. Smith.
© 2016 John Wiley & Sons, Inc. Published 2016 by John Wiley & Sons, Inc.

can be used for obtaining blood samples without repeatedly performing venipuncture on a patient.

Lastly, IV access is an important aspect of emergency preparedness. In the event of a cardiopulmonary arrest, treatment may be administered quickly and seamlessly if an IV catheter is already in place.

Q. Where can I place a peripheral IV catheter in dogs and cats?

A. There are many options for IV catheter location in small animal patients. The location is dependent upon many factors, including anesthetist experience, patient demeanor, patient health status or pathology, accessibility of the site, overall goals, and the risk of complications.

The cephalic and accessory cephalic veins on the thoracic limbs are options suitable in most small animal patients. There are several advantages to this location. Thoracic limbs are often easier to keep clean. They are also more accessible for surgical procedures that do not involve the cranial third of the patient. The patency of cephalic and accessory cephalic vein catheters may be easier to maintain due to the straight anatomy and limited motion of that area when compared to other locations. In general, a larger gauge catheter can be placed in a patient's cephalic vein than in other peripheral sites. There are a few disadvantages to this location. If the patient is aggressive or fractious, maintaining venous access and also ensuring safety of personnel may be difficult. In these instances, restraint for a saphenous catheter may be safer. Also, if the procedure requires access to the patient's cranial third (e.g., dental prophylaxis, ophthalmic procedures, thoracic limb amputation), this location may not be readily accessible during anesthesia.

Other common choices for intravenous catheter placement include the lateral and medial saphenous veins on the pelvic limbs. Lateral saphenous veins are suitable in most dogs, though they may be more difficult to maintain due to the tortuous nature of the vessel in this area. Medial saphenous veins are suitable in most cats, and are fairly easy to maintain for short periods such as an anesthetic episode. Advantages of catheterization of veins located on the pelvic limb include accessibility if the procedure being performed is on the cranial portion of the patient, and safety of staff if a patient is aggressive or fractious. For fractious patients, an IV extension set filled with saline or heparinized saline can be securely attached to the catheter and then accessed from outside the cage for administration of drugs and so on in the recovery period.

Q. How do I choose which catheter I should use?

A. There are several catheter types available for intravenous use. They include winged needle, over-the-needle, through-the-needle, and guide-wire type catheters. The most common type used in peripheral vessels for anesthesia is an over-the-needle type. They are well suited for maintaining peripheral venous access, inexpensive, and very easy to use. Over-the-needle catheters are useful for administering anesthetic drugs and fluids in the perioperative period, but can be maintained and used for fluid administration for 72 h [2]. The gauge of catheter used depends upon the size of the patient. Hansen suggests the following for maintenance therapies in peripheral vessels: for patients less than 5 kg, a 24-20 gauge catheter is appropriate, for patients 5–15 kg, a 22-18 gauge catheter is appropriate and for patients over 15 kg, a 20-18 gauge catheter is appropriate [2].

The main advantage for choosing a larger gauge catheter is less resistance to flow and the ability to deliver large volumes of fluids or drugs over short amounts of time. This may be necessary in patients during anesthesia. Larger catheters will, however, cause more trauma to the vessel. In general, one should choose the smallest gauge catheter that will effectively achieve the goals of intravenous catheterization.

Q. What reasons are there for intravenous fluid administration during anesthesia?

A. Most patients are fasted for 6–12 h prior to anesthesia. Some may have also inadvertently been held off water or hospitalized overnight, potentially leading to decreased fluid intake. In addition, most anesthetic drugs, and most notably the inhalants, cause cardiovascular depression and/or vasodilation leading to reduced cardiac output, hypotension, and possible decreases in renal blood flow. Fluid losses will continue under anesthesia, for example, via urine and saliva production, evaporation from the respiratory tract and open body cavities. For these reasons, most anesthetized patients should receive IV fluids.

Q. What fluids should I choose for my anesthetized patient?

A. In most cases, a crystalloid solution is the most appropriate choice. Crystalloids are water-based solutions containing electrolytes and other solutes capable of redistributing to all body compartments. There are four types of crystalloid solutions: replacement solutions, maintenance solutions, hypertonic solutions, and dextrose in water. Replacement solutions are the type most commonly chosen for anesthesia because the composition most closely resembles that of plasma. Some examples of replacement-type crystalloids are lactated Ringer's solution, Normosol-R (Abbott Laboratories, Abbott Park, IL), and Plasma-Lyte-148 (Baxter Healthcare, Deerfield, IL).

Q. What kind of crystalloid is hypertonic saline?

A. Hypertonic saline (7.2–23% NaCl) is a crystalloid that is used for increasing intravascular volume quickly in patients that are acutely, severely hypovolemic, such as those with traumatic hypovolemic shock [3,4]. Rapid volume expansion is achieved because of the high sodium concentration and subsequent rapid fluid shifts from the interstitial space to the intravascular space. The recommended volume is 4–7 ml/kg in dogs and 2–4 ml/kg in cats given at a rate of approximately 1 ml/kg/min for maximal effect [5]. The effect on intravascular volume lasts only 30 min [6] so other measures (e.g., isotonic crystalloid or colloid administration) must be taken to replace volume during that time. Contraindications to hypertonic saline administration include dehydration, hypernatremia, hypokalemia, hyperosmolar patients, actively hemorrhaging patients, and patients that may easily develop hypervolemia [7]. Patients with dehydration or electrolyte abnormalities may worsen and patients with active hemorrhage may lose more blood if arterial pressure or intravascular volume increases dramatically prior to successful coagulation.

Q. What are synthetic colloids and when should they be used?

A. Patients with low total protein or albumin, low oncotic pressure, or refractory hypotension during anesthesia may benefit from synthetic colloid administration in addition to crystalloids. Examples of synthetic colloids used in veterinary medicine include hydroxyethyl starch, dextrans, and gelatins. Colloids are larger molecular-weight substances that are restricted to the plasma compartment in normal patients. Colloids increase oncotic pressure and are effective at holding fluids in the vascular space. They increase intravascular volume without dramatically increasing plasma osmolarity or sodium concentrations. The effects can last up to 18 hours or more [8]. Disadvantages of synthetic colloid use include allergic reactions, renal impairment, coagulopathies, and expense [8]. For example, von Willebrand factor and factor VIII can be decreased to 40% of normal after a hydroxyethyl starch administration [8,9] and activated clotting time, activated partial thromboplastin time and platelet plug formation may be prolonged [10,11]. It is important to note that hydroxyethyl starches with a lower molecular weight and molar substitution, such as HES 130/0.4, are less detrimental to coagulation function [12].

Q. What rate of fluid administration is appropriate for anesthetized patients?

A. Current recommendations of initial fluid rates for crystalloids are 3 ml/kg/h in cats and 5 ml/kg/h in dogs [1]. This recommendation is largely anecdotal. Historically, fluid rates up to 10–20 ml/kg/h have been administered in veterinary patients without obvious adverse effects, though a review of the veterinary literature suggests that this rate is probably excessive under most circumstances, especially in cats [13,14]. Patients that may easily become hypervolemic, such as those with heart disease and those with oliguric or anuric renal failure, may need even lower rates [13].

Recommendations for rates of colloid administration vary greatly on the colloid being administered. Most veterinary references cite a maximum dosage of 20–30 ml/kg/day for synthetic colloids (hydroxyethyl starches, dextrans). This recommendation is based on extrapolations from the human literature and from concerns that dosages higher than 20–30 ml/kg/day may have negative effects on coagulation [8,15,16]. Though there have not been any *in vivo* controlled trials in veterinary medicine, formulations of hydroxyethyl starch with lower molecular weight and molar substitution, such as HES 130/0.4, have been given in volumes up to 50 ml/kg/day in humans without adverse effects on coagulation [17]. As such, the recommended maximum daily volume for these products (Vetstarch™, Abbott Animal Health, Abbott Park, IL, USA; and Voluven®, Fresenius Kabi, Australia) is 50 ml/kg/day. Recommendations for synthetic colloid administration in the treatment of anesthesia-related hypotension are a slow administration of 5–10 ml/kg in dogs and 1–5 ml/kg for cats, titrating to effect to minimize vascular overload [1].

Q. How can I practically monitor my patient's volume status?

A. Any time intravascular fluids are being administered, it is important to vigilantly monitor patients' volume status and the need to change the course of treatment. The easiest method for practical assessment is completing serial physical examinations. Changes in pulse rate, pulse quality, capillary refill time, mucous membrane characteristics, and respiratory rate, effort, and lung sounds, should be monitored. Body weight, blood pressure, venous or arterial blood gases, and oxygen saturation are also helpful in guiding treatment.

Laboratory data can also be beneficial. The hematocrit or packed cell volume, total plasma protein concentration, urine specific gravity, blood urea nitrogen, or serum creatinine concentrations evaluated in conjunction with one another are variables that help in determining a patient's volume status.

Measuring urine output and central venous pressure (CVP) allows for more objective assessments in patients' volume status, but may not be practical in most situations. Urine output can be measured by aseptically placing a sterile urinary catheter with a collection bag and keeping track of urine volume over time. Normal urine output is 1–2 ml/kg/hr. Central venous pressure, an estimate of mean right atrial pressure, is also used for clinically monitoring responses to fluid therapy. It is measured by a transducer connected to a port in a jugular catheter in which the distal end has been advanced to the level of the right atrium. Normal CVP is 0–5 cm H_2O. Progressive increases in CVP may be an indication to decrease the rate of fluid administration. There are many variables that may impact CVP values (i.e., surgical procedure being performed, mechanical ventilation, positive end-expiratory pressure), however, and one must be familiar with the limitations and confounding factors when interpreting results. For more detailed information about CVP, the reader is directed to Hansen, 2006 [18].

Q. What are signs of fluid overload during anesthesia?

A. Symptoms of over-hydration may include serous nasal discharge, tachycardia, tachypnea, audible respiratory crackles and pulmonary edema, decreased oxygen saturation, ascites, polyuria, exophthalmos, diarrhea, decreased packed cell volume, and total plasma protein [18,19].

Q. Should I ever *not* administer fluids during anesthesia?

A. Some patients may need greatly reduced rates of fluid administration and there are a few cases when fluid administration should be avoided altogether. The most common scenario is a patient with congestive heart failure. In these cases, the heart is not able to handle the patient's present circulating volume, and adding more intravascular volume is absolutely contraindicated. Patients with anuric or oliguric renal failure also require greatly reduced rates or no administration of IV fluids during anesthesia. These patients are often hypervolemic because of an inability to excrete fluid [13].

References

1 Davis BA, Jensen T, Johnson A, *et al.* 2013 AAHA/AAFP Fluid Therapy guidelines for dogs and cats. *Journal of the American Animal Hospital Association* 2013; **49**:149–159.

2 Hansen B. Technical aspects of fluid therapy. In: DiBartola S (ed.) *Fluid, Electrolyte, and Acid-Base Disorders in Small Animal Practice*, 3rd edn. Elsevier Publishing: Missouri, 2006: 344–376.

3 Razanski E, Rondeau M. Choosing fluids in traumatic hypovolemic shock: the role of crystalloids, colloids and hypertonic saline. *Journal of the American Animal Hospital Association* 2002; **38**:499–501.

4 Schertal LM, Allen DA, Muir WW, *et al.* Evaluation of a hypertonic saline-dextran solution for treatment of traumatic shock in dogs. *Journal of the American Veterinary Medical Association* 1996; **208**:366–370.

5 Muir WW, Sally J. Small-volume resuscitation with hypertonic saline solution in hypovolemic cats. *American Journal of Veterinary Research* 1989; **50**:1883–1888.

6 Mathews KA. The various types of parenteral fluids and their indications. *Veterinary Clinics of North America: Small Animal Practice* 1998; **28**:483–513.

7 Krausz MM. Controversies in shock research: hypertonic resuscitation – pros and cons. *Shock* 1995; **1**:69–72.

8 Hughes D, Boag A. Fluid therapy with macromolecular plasma volume expanders. In: DiBartola S (ed.) *Fluid, Electrolyte, and Acid-Base Disorders in Small Animal Practice*, 3rd edn. Elsevier Publishing: Missouri, 2006:621–634.

9 Thyes C, Madjdpour C, Frascarolo P, *et al.* Effect of high- and low- molecular-weight low-substituted hydroxyethyl starch on blood coagulation during acute normovolemic hemodilution in pigs. *Anesthesiology* 2006; **105**:1228–1237.

10 Madjdpour C, Thyes C, Buclin T, *et al.* Novel starches: single-dose pharmacokinetics and effects on blood coagulation. *Anesthesiology* 2007; **106**:132–143.

11 Wierenga JR, Jandrey KE, Haskins SC *et al.* In vitro comparison of the effects of two forms of hydroxyethyl starch solutions on platelet functions in dogs. *American Journal of Veterinary Research* 2007; **68**:605–609.

12 Epstein KL, Bergren A, Giguere S, Brainard BM. Cardiovascular, colloid osmotic pressure, and hemostatic effects of 2 formulations of hydroxyethyl starch in healthy horses. *Journal of Veterinary Internal Medicine* 2014; **28**:223–233.

13 DiBartola SP. Perioperative management of fluid therapy. In: DiBartola S (ed.) *Fluid, Electrolyte, and Acid-Base Disorders in Small Animal Practice*, 3rd edn. Elsevier Publishing: Missouri, 2006:391–419.

14 Brodbelt DC, Pfeiffer DU, Young LE, *et al.* Risk factors for anaesthetic-related death in cats: results from the confidential enquiry into perioperative small animal fatalities (CEPSAF). *British Journal of Anaesthesia* 2007; **99**:617–623.

15 Concannon KT, Haskins SC, Feldman BF. Hemostatic defects associated with two infusion rates of dextran-70 in dogs. *American Journal of Veterinary Research* 1992; **53**: 1369–1375.

16 Kudnig ST, Mama K. Perioperative fluid therapy. *Journal of the American Veterinary Medical Association* 2002; **221**:1112–1121.

17 Neff TA, Doelberg M, Jungheinrich C, *et al.* Repetitive large-dose infusion of the novel hydroxyethyl starch 130/0.4 in patients with severe head injury. *Anesthesia and Analgesia* 2003;**96**:1453–1459.

18 Cornelius LM, Finco DR, Culver DH. Physiologic effects of rapid infusion of Ringer's lactate solution into dogs. *American Journal of Veterinary Research* 1978; **39**:1185–1190.

19 DiBartola SP, Bateman S. Introduction to fluid therapy. In: DiBartola (ed.) *Fluid, Electrolyte, and Acid-Base Disorders in Small Animal Practice*, 3rd edn. Elsevier Publishing: Missouri, 2006:325–344.

10 Intravenous Anesthetic Induction Drugs

Time for takeoff!

Tanya Duke-Novakovski

Department of Small Animal Clinical Sciences, Western College of Veterinary Medicine, University of Saskatchewan, Canada

---

KEY POINTS:

- There is no single "ideal" induction drug.

- All induction drugs have a rapid onset of action and are redistributed quickly away from the vessel rich organs (brain, heart, lungs, liver, kidney), generally leading to rapid recoveries after a single dose if no other anesthetic drug (e.g., inhalant) is used.

- All induction drugs have some clinically important side effects, which are generally minimized by using the lowest possible dose when inducing anesthesia.

- Anesthetic premedications will allow a much lower dose of induction agent to be used.

Q. What are ideal characteristics of an injectable induction anesthetic drug?

A. ✓ inexpensive;
  ✓ easy to obtain;
  ✓ no record-keeping required;
  ✓ can be obtained in multidose vials;
  ✓ not toxic to tissues;
  ✓ easily titratable;
  ✓ rapid metabolism and recovery;
  ✓ produces good quality of induction and recovery with no apnea;
  ✓ provides cardiovascular stability;
  ✓ has good shelf-life and does not become contaminated once the seal is broken.

Q. Which drugs closely meet these expectations (apart from cost and record-keeping)?

A. No drug meets all the requirements, but propofol, alfaxalone, and ketamine/benzodiazepine combinations are popular because they can meet most of the requirements.

Questions and Answers in Small Animal Anesthesia, First Edition. Edited by Lesley J. Smith.
© 2016 John Wiley & Sons, Inc. Published 2016 by John Wiley & Sons, Inc.

Table 10.1   Suggested doses for IV induction drugs in *healthy* dogs and cats.

Induction drug	IV dose (no premedication)	IV dose (with premedication)	Comment
Thiopental	Cat and Dog: 20–25 mg/kg	Cat and Dog: 5–12 mg/kg	[drug] 2.5% concentration. Do not use in Sighthounds
Propofol	Cat: 6–8 mg/kg Dog: 6–8 mg/kg	Cat: 2–6 mg/kg Dog: 2–4 mg/kg	Heinz body formation in cats with repetitive daily use (>3 days)
Alfaxalone	Cat: 3–5 mg/kg Dog: 2–3 mg/kg	Cat: 1–3 mg/kg Dog: 0.5–2 mg/kg	Pre-anesthetic medication advisable
Ketamine with Diazepam or Midazolam Combination	Cat and Dog: 10 mg/kg of ketamine and 0.5 mg/kg of ben-zodiazepine	Cat and Dog: 2–5 mg/kg ketamine with 0.25 mg/kg of benzodiazepine	Pre-anesthetic medication advisable
Tiletamine/ zolazepam combination	Cat: 4–5 mg/kg Dog: 2–5 mg/kg	Cat: 1–4 mg/kg Dog: 1–2 mg/kg	Lengthy recovery possible with high doses
Etomidate	Cat and Dog: 1–3 mg/kg	Cat and Dog: 0.5–2 mg/kg	Propylene glycol formulation can cause tissue injury and phlebitis Myoclonus without pre-anesthetic medication

Note: It should be noted that these drugs should be given "to effect" and tailored for individual physical health status. Heavy sedation with premedications that include an alpha-2 agonist + opioid will usually lead to induction dose requirements at the lowest end of the suggested dose range.

Q. Which drugs are considered suitable anesthetic induction agents for IV use in veterinary patients?

A. Thiopental, propofol, alfaxalone, etomidate, and ketamine (generally with a benzodiazepine).

Q. What are the suggested doses for the currently available induction drugs?

A. See Table 10.1 for drugs and dosages.

Q. How do injectable anesthetic drugs work?

A. All injectable anesthetic drugs (except ketamine) act mainly upon inhibitory gamma amino-butyric acid (GABA) receptors within the brain to hyperpo-larize the neuron. These receptors normally respond to the indigenous ligand GABA and the anesthetic drug can attach to the receptor in other places and enhance the action of the naturally occurring GABA molecules. Other actions might affect cell-signaling mechanisms, such as those involving calcium and neurotransmitter release, to also cause a state of anesthesia. Ketamine and tiletamine have a different action and mainly produce a "dissociated" state by blocking NMDA receptors. Ketamine "dissociates" the part of the brain responsible for consciousness from the other areas of the brain so the animal is not aware of its surroundings. It is not considered to be true "anesthesia" but rather a cataleptic state. Anesthetic drugs may also have an effect on inhibitory receptors within the spinal cord to produce muscle relaxation or to reduce spinal reflexes.

Q. Why should I use injectable anesthetic drugs for induction and not inhalant anesthetics?

A. Injectable anesthetics require slightly more skill using the intravenous (IV) route because of the need for accurate IV administration, but when administered IV they have a more rapid action compared to inhalant anesthetics. A suitable depth of anesthesia to allow endotracheal intubation can be rapidly achieved and this will reduce the risk of pulmonary aspiration. The excitatory stages of anesthesia are not observed with appropriate dosing and relatively rapid administration, and therefore a suitable depth of anesthesia is achieved efficiently without any potential struggling from the animal. Induction of anesthesia using inhalational techniques in unsedated animals can cause struggling, release of catecholamines, and is potentially riskier to the animal. See Chapter 11 for more information on inhalant inductions.

Q. What are the main anesthetic effects of thiopental?

A. While thiopental is not currently available in the USA, it is available in other countries and may return to the USA at some time in the future. Thiopental is a barbiturate with a reliable onset within 20–30 s following IV administration and is available as a powder for reconstitution with sterile water. Its alkaline nature (pH 11–14) prevents bacterial contamination and it cannot be mixed with other drugs or fluids. Exposure of the solution to carbon dioxide may result in some cloudiness, but otherwise the solution is stable for at least six weeks with only a small decrease in potency with time. It is easily titratable and can produce a rapid recovery if it is only used for induction of anesthesia. If anesthesia is maintained using several injections of thiopental, accumulation can occur and a prolonged recovery will follow. Sighthounds (Afghans, Greyhounds) and other animals with a high muscle mass to fat ratio have clinically relevant prolongation of recovery even with one induction dose just to allow endotracheal intubation [1]. Greyhounds also lack some hepatic enzyme systems required for metabolism of barbiturates. See Chapter 41 for more breed details regarding anesthetic drugs.

Thiopental can cause a decrease in mean arterial blood pressure (MAP) because of vasodilation and the heart rate will increase to compensate (baroreceptor reflex arc). Therefore, good blood pressure is generally preserved in *healthy* animals. Thiopental can also cause induction apnea.

Thiopental can be used without pre-anesthetic medication, but higher doses are required and recovery from these higher doses can result in paddling and an excitable recovery. Thiopental should not be used in concentrations greater than 2.5% in cats and dogs as it can cause tissue irritation, especially if the drug is accidentally administered extravascular. Perivascular administration of thiopental can lead to significant tissue sloughing, especially when more concentrated solutions are used or it is injected into a small peripheral vein.

Q. What are the main anesthetic effects of propofol?

A. Propofol is an alkyl-phenol formulated in a white emulsion (Intralipid®) which can support the growth of bacteria and fungi. Some commercial preparations have preservative, but precautions should be taken to preserve sterility with multidose vials.

Propofol produces a reliable induction within 20–30 s following IV injection and produces a more rapid recovery compared to an equipotent dose of thiopental. The enzyme systems within the liver, gut, kidneys and lungs metabolize propofol. For this reason, it can be used in animals with limited hepatic reserve without impacting recovery time. Several doses of propofol can be administered without prolonging recovery in dogs, including Sighthounds, but some accumulation occurs in cats due to their limited ability to glucuronidize drugs. It can be given without pre-anesthetic medication, but may produce some excitement during recovery when it is used as the sole anesthetic agent; therefore propofol is best used following pre-anesthetic medication. Propofol will reduce blood pressure through vasodilation, but can limit the reflex increase in heart rate that normally allows some compensation. Therefore higher doses of propofol may aggravate hypovolemic conditions. Propofol can also cause induction apnea.

Propofol is not irritating to tissues, but may cause some pain and sudden limb withdrawal reflex if a small or otherwise inflamed vein is used for injection. Dogs and cats may react when propofol is injected via a catheter that has been in place for several days. Some splanchnic blood pooling or unexplained changes within the lung may cause an animal to have a cyanotic appearance following induction, and oxygen should be available.

Q. What are the main anesthetic effects of alfaxalone?

A. Alfaxalone is a neuro-steroid dissolved in a cyclodextrin solution resulting in a clear solution. The 10 ml vial does not contain a preservative, but is not as easily contaminated as propofol [2]. It does not cause tissue irritation and appears to be tolerated when administered into inflamed veins. It is a reliable induction drug with an onset within 20–30 s of IV injection. It can be given without pre-anesthetic medication, but may produce some excitement during recovery and is therefore best used following some sort of pre-anesthetic sedation. Rapid metabolism occurs within the liver, therefore recovery following an induction dose is usually quick in cats and dogs. Accumulation with multiple doses is minimal, even in cats.

Alfaxalone causes vasodilation during induction and an increase in heart rate. It can preserve hemodynamics slightly better compared to propofol, but changes are similar in healthy animals. Induction apnea is possible. Alfax-alone can also be used by the intramuscular (IM) route in cats, but large volumes are required and a poor quality of anesthesia and recovery may be observed.

Q. What are the main anesthetic effects of etomidate?

A. Etomidate is an imidazole and is available in two formulations: one containing high osmolality propylene glycol and the other containing Intralipid (Etomidate-Lipuro®). Etomidate is rapidly hydrolyzed to inactive metabolites by hepatic and plasma esterases. Etomidate should not be used in animals which are immune-compromised, such as those with septicemia or those with adrenal insufficiencies (e.g., Addison's disease) because it is a potent inhibitor of 11-α and 11-β hydroxylases and the activity of the cholesterol side-chain cleavage enzymes responsible for adrenal steroid synthesis (cortisol, aldosterone, corticosterone) is reduced for 2–6 h following an induction dose [3].

Etomidate produces minimal cardiovascular changes in healthy and hypovolemic dogs, therefore it is a good choice for animals with any hemodynamic compromise. The formulation can cause pain on injection and some muscle twitching, and it is recommended that etomidate be used with pre-anesthetic medication. Etomidate can cause induction apnea and dose-dependent respiratory depression. Etomidate also can cause significant nausea, retching, and vomiting at induction, especially in unpremedicated dogs.

The etomidate formulation with propylene glycol can cause tissue irritation if administered perivascularly, due to the propylene glycol. This solvent also stings when given IV and can cause hemolysis and phlebitis when large doses are given because of the high osmolality of solvent.

Q. Can ketamine be used alone?

A. Ketamine was used in cats in the past without any other drugs, but produced a poor quality of anesthesia with limited visceral analgesia. At high doses when used alone, ketamine can produce excitement and seizure-like actions in dogs. Ketamine has poor muscle relaxation properties and for these reasons it should be used alongside other drugs. The best choices of drugs to use with ketamine are benzodiazepines or alpha-2 agonist drugs.

Q. What is the best way to administer ketamine for induction?

A. Ketamine is ideally combined with benzodiazepines, and diazepam and midazolam are popular choices. For IV induction in cats and dogs, ketamine can be mixed with the benzodiazepine of choice or given separately in rapid sequence.

For IM use, especially in cats, ketamine can be combined with alpha-2 agonists (and opioids) to produce profound sedation/anesthesia (see Chapter 8), and higher doses can produce longer periods of anesthesia. Oxygen and ventilatory support may be required with higher doses. Ketamine can be given to extremely fractious or dangerous dogs mixed with alpha-2 agonists and an opioid, but this mainly produces enough sedation for handling, as doses that might produce induction of anesthesia require large volumes and may produce severe cardiopulmonary depression.

Q. What are the main anesthetic effects of ketamine/benzodiazepine combinations?

A. Ketamine mixed with diazepam or midazolam and used for IV anesthetic induction produces good cardiopulmonary stability. Induction apnea may still be possible. There is a minimal reduction in blood pressure and heart rate is generally well preserved. Ketamine increases sympathetic nervous system tone and this is what helps to maintain blood pressure after ketamine inductions. Induction is reliable in well-sedated (aka premedicated) dogs and cats, but ketamine inductions in unpremedicated or poorly sedated animals can cause excitement.

The effects of ketamine may not be noticeable for 60–90 s following IV injection because ketamine crosses the blood–brain barrier more slowly than other induction drugs. This is not ideal if induction is required for emergency intubation and control of the airway. Ketamine-based anesthesia does not cause rotation of the eyeball and, therefore, the cornea is prone to dryness and possible damage. Eye lubrication should be used. Ketamine also increases salivation after induction. Salivary secretions that obscure the larynx for intubation can be cleared with a cotton tipped applicator or gauze sponges on a hemostat in larger animals. Some clinicians advocate the use of anticholinergics to prevent excessive salivation with ketamine, but this may lead to excessive tachycardia.

Ketamine is metabolized in the liver in dogs to its metabolite norketamine, which may have some residual anesthetic action when higher doses of ketamine are used. In cats ketamine is excreted largely as the parent drug. Therefore cats with renal failure may exhibit unexpectedly long recoveries after ketamine administration.

Q. What about the zolazepam/tiletamine combination?

A. A commercial combination of zolazepam (a benzodiazepine) and tiletamine (a dissociative anesthetic similar to ketamine) is available in some countries (Telazol® (USA) or Zoletil® (Continental Europe)) and can be used for induction of anesthesia by using IV injection or larger doses given IM in cats. The formulations contain zolazepam and tiletamine at a ratio of 1 : 1 (250 mg zolazepam, 250 mg tiletamine). For dogs, this drug combination is best used IV as the required volume for IM administration is too high. Recovery may be prolonged and some excitement may be observed. Reconstitution of the powder can be performed using 5 ml of saline, 5% dextrose or sterile water to provide 50 mg/ml of each drug. The combination produces an anesthetic state similar to that of ketamine and a benzodiazepine. After IV injection, induction of anesthesia takes 60–90 s; following IM injection onset of action is 1–7 min. Duration of anesthesia is dose-dependent, but can range from 30 to 60 min. Recovery from anesthesia can be lengthy. This drug is often used for remote/rural or high volume neuter clinics for induction and maintenance of anesthesia in cats.

Q. How does the use of pre-anesthetic medication affect injectable induction techniques?

A. The use of pre-anesthetic medication allows lower doses of induction drugs to be used. Usually, the use of alpha-2 agonists will reduce the required dose of the induction agent more than acepromazine- or benzodiazepine-based drug protocols. The addition of opioids to the premedication reduces induction dose requirements even further, especially in dogs. Inclusion of pre-anesthetic medication reduces the incidence of adverse effects such as excitable induction and recovery and muscle twitching and helps to offset negative hemodynamic effects of the induction drug because a lower dose can be used. High doses of alpha-2 agonists may slow the delivery of the injectable anesthetic drug to the brain and result in a clinically noticeable delay in anesthetic effect. Whenever alpha-2 agonist drugs have been used in the premedication, slow administration of the induction drug will minimize risk of a relative overdose.

Q. How fast should I give IV induction drugs?

A. Most clinicians administer induction drugs IV over 30–60 s. If the drug is given over 60 s in well-sedated animals, it may reduce the incidence of induction apnea, reduce cardiopulmonary depression, and result in a lower total dose of induction drug given. In unsedated or poorly sedated patients, the longer time for injection may result a poor quality of induction with some excitement-like muscle spasms, paddling of legs in dogs and cats, whining in dogs, and explosive behavior in cats.

Q. What is "titration to effect"?

A. One half to a third of the calculated volume of injectable drug is generally given first, depending on the degree of sedation and hemodynamic stability of the patient. The remainder of the drug is given in smaller increments until the desired depth of anesthesia is achieved. Knowing the time to onset of anesthetic effect is desirable in order to correctly give incremental doses of drug.

Q. What are some common problems that I may see with IV induction drugs?

A. ✓ induction apnea
   ✓ paddling or excitement
   ✓ waking up too soon
   ✓ muscle twitching.

Q. What causes induction apnea and how can I prevent it?

A. There may be two distinct reasons for apnea following IV administration of an injectable induction drug. A relative overdose may have been given and respiratory depression may be sufficient to cause apnea. The animal will have concurrent signs of deep anesthesia. Endotracheal intubation and ventilatory support should be provided until the injectable drug leaves the brain during the redistribution phase and the anesthetic depth lightens. In these instances, start with low vaporizer settings of the inhalant.

Alternatively, there may be drug-induced inhibition of the brainstem's response to increased arterial CO_2 tensions. Breathing may be stimulated more by the presence of arterial hypoxemia. When endotracheal intubation occurs and oxygen is administered, hypoxic drive does not trigger breathing, but the central response to CO_2 remains depressed. The animal may have signs which indicate it is lightly anesthetized, (e.g., palpebral reflexes may be vigorous). Therefore increased inspired concentration of inhalant anesthetic may be desirable, otherwise the animal may suddenly waken. Ventilatory support *must* be provided until breathing commences and the animal should be closely monitored during this time. The concurrent use of agonist opioids will have an additive effect to the induction agent on the CNS response to CO_2.

Q. My patient paddles its legs and appears to have seizure-like movements during induction. What is happening?

A. This may occur when the injection is given too slowly, or not enough drug has been administered during the initial bolus. Slightly increase the speed of injection until the bolus is complete. More anesthetic drug may be required to achieve a suitable depth of anesthesia. Be especially aware this might occur if the patient responded poorly to pre-anesthetic sedation drugs or was not premedicated.

Q. My patient wakes up as anesthesia transitions from induction to inhalational anesthesia. What might be happening?

A. This can occur with all the short-acting injectable anesthetic drugs, such as propofol, alfaxalone, etomidate, and ketamine/benzodiazepine combinations, especially with lightly sedated or unpremedicated animals. The transition time from induction drug to inhalant anesthesia is < 3 min due to the rapid redistribution of all the induction agents. If there is a delay in intubation, securing the endotracheal tube, or checking for leaks, the patient might wake up. The inspired concentration of inhalational drug may need to be increased and the lungs ventilated to ensure that gas exchange with the inhalant agent is occurring. It is also prudent to have a small amount of the injectable anesthetic ready to administer IV to prevent the animal from full awakening and coughing out its endotracheal tube. Catecholamine release will be high during this event, and care should be taken to monitor the cardiovascular system for cardiac arrhythmias.

Q. My patient has sporadic, but regular muscle twitching following induction. What might be happening?

A. This phenomenon is quite common after propofol administration in dogs. It may occur because the concentration of injectable anesthetic drug within the spinal cord is becoming low and some excitatory transmission occurs. Usually, the animal is at a suitable depth of anesthesia and is maintained with inhalant anesthetics. This myoclonus usually subsides with time.

Q. What determines how rapidly a patient recovers from one dose of injectable anesthetic drug?

A. Recovery from one dose of injectable anesthetic drug mainly occurs through redistribution of the drug from tissues with a high cardiac output (brain, heart, lungs, kidneys, liver) to those with an intermediate perfusion (muscles) and finally to tissues with low perfusion (fat, skin). Despite low perfusion, adipose tissue will take up a large proportion of the drug from the circulation because all anesthetic drugs are fat soluble. This will effectively remove the drug from the circulation and the brain, and enable recovery from anesthesia. However, if a high amount of the drug is present in fat, the gradual release into the circulation may cause mild sedation and a "hang-over" effect. Metabolism will remove the drug from the circulation and the faster it can be removed, the less likely there will be any sedative effect and the animal returns to full consciousness and is alert (see Figure 10.1). Concurrent use of sedatives and, in some cases, opioids, may delay recovery but are also desirable as they provide a calm, excitement-free, and comfortable recovery for the patient.

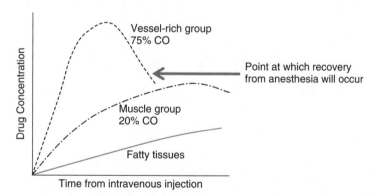

Figure 10.1 Distribution to various tissues of an injectable anesthetic after a single intravenous dose. The dotted line (.......) indicates the drug concentration in the vessel rich groups which receive 75% of cardiac output (CO) and includes the brain, thus producing the anesthetic effect. Recovery from anesthesia occurs as the drug concentration is reduced in the brain, as drug re-enters the circulation to distribute to other tissues with lower CO. The skeletal muscle group drug concentration will rise less rapidly than the vessel rich group (dashed line ..__..__..__), and the drug concentration in fat (as well as connective tissue and bone) will rise even more slowly (solid line _____) due to its low percentage of cardiac output. Release of drug into the circulation from these last 2 groups of tissues can contribute to residual sedation following recovery from anesthesia.

Q. Where can I read more about injectable anesthetics?

A. A thorough review is provided in the *BSAVA Manual of Canine and Feline Anaesthesia* [4].

References

1 Robinson EP, Sams RA, Muir WW. Barbiturate anesthesia in greyhound and mixed-breed dogs: Comparative cardiopulmonary effects, anesthetic effects, and recovery rates. *American Journal of Veterinary Research* 1986; **47**:2105–2112.

2 Strachan FA, Mansel JC, Clutton RE. A comparison of microbial growth in alfaxalone, propofol and thiopental. *Journal of Small animal Practice* 2008; **49**:186–190.

3 Dodam JR, Kruse-Elliot KT, Aucoin DP, *et al.* Duration of etomidate-induced adrenocortical suppression during surgery in dogs. *American Journal of Veterinary Research* 1990; **51**:786–788.

4 Kästner S. Injectable anaesthetics. In: Seymour C, Duke-Novakovski T, de Vries M (eds) *BSAVA Manual of Canine and Feline Anaesthesia and Analgesia*, 3rd edn, British Small Animal Veterinary Association (BSAVA), Gloucester, UK. *In press*.

11 Inhalant Inductions

The last resort?

Lesley J. Smith

Department of Surgical Sciences, School of Veterinary Medicine, University of Wisconsin, USA

KEY POINTS:

- Inductions performed using just inhalants can be extremely stressful to patients.
- Personnel will, by necessity, have to breathe in at least some inhalant.
- There is a delay before the anesthetist can obtain a controlled, patent airway in the patient.
- Monitoring during induction is challenging because the patient is either struggling and moving (mask induction) or hands on monitoring is impossible (chamber induction).
- If inhalant inductions are performed, only the inhalants with the lowest blood-gas solubility (isoflurane, sevoflurane, desflurane) should be used to minimize the induction time.

Q. When would be an appropriate time to consider an inhalant induction?

A. The only time that an inhalant induction should be considered is if the patient is simply too fractious or wild to be handled for an IM injection, or if handling for an IM injection stresses the animal more than a chamber induction might (e.g., unhandled cats). Most domesticated dogs, even if fractious, can be handled at least long enough to hand inject IM drugs that will provide heavy sedation and chemical restraint (e.g., a combination of alpha-2 agonist, opioid, and ketamine or telazol). A combination of this sort will result in a dog that should be amenable to placement of an IV catheter and an injectable induction. Very fractious cats may need to be induced in a chamber/tank if personnel simply cannot get their hands on the cat. The cat may need to be "dumped" into the chamber from a crate or trap. Some exotic pocket pets, (e.g., sugar gliders, hamsters) can be induced using a face mask placed over the animal with delivery of inhalant via the anesthetic circuit. It is also common to mask-induce avian species after they have been sedated, due to the difficulty of IV access in awake birds and the respiratory depressant effects of most injectable anesthetics (see Chapter 44).

Questions and Answers in Small Animal Anesthesia, First Edition. Edited by Lesley J. Smith.
© 2016 John Wiley & Sons, Inc. Published 2016 by John Wiley & Sons, Inc.

Q. Why should inhalant inductions be avoided if possible?

A. Inhalant inductions are a relatively slow method of inducing anesthesia, and in the process the animal will likely go through all of the stages of anesthesia. This includes Stage 1 – which lasts from voluntary movement to loss of consciousness, Stage 2 – which is a state of delirium and involuntary movement, and Stage 3 – which is considered true anesthesia with full unconsciousness, muscle relaxation, and lack of perception [1]. It is during Stages 1 and 2 that the animal will risk hurting themselves as they flail, thrash, vocalize, and struggle. If being induced by mask, personnel will also have to restrain the animal during this time, which can be physically demanding and also puts the person, as well as the animal, at risk for injury. In a chamber or tank, an animal in Stage 2 can obstruct its nares or oral cavity or flex its neck to such a degree that the trachea is obstructed, so airway patency is at risk during this stage. The animal can also physically injure itself during this phase if in a chamber. It is not until the animal reaches Stage 3 that they can be removed from the chamber or mask, and it is only at this point that any hands-on monitoring (e.g., pulse palpation, assessment of membrane color) can be performed. During transition from Stage 1 to Stage 3, because of the stress of this induction method, large amounts of catecholamines are released and the animal may suffer from tachyarrhythmias or even fatal arrhythmias (e.g., ventricular fibrillation), which will go undetected due to the inability to monitor heart rate and rhythm.

Another reason to avoid inhalant inductions is the exposure of personnel and the environment to the inhalant drugs. Scavenging of waste anesthetic can, and should, be performed during a chamber induction, but once the chamber is opened to access the patient, it is almost impossible to properly scavenge the inhalant in the chamber, unless the induction is performed under a fume hood. Similarly, scavenging during a mask induction should be performed via the normal scavenging system of the anesthetic machine, but exposure to the inhalant as it leaks around the mask is virtually unavoidable. Therefore, personnel involved in inhalant inductions will breathe in at least some inhalant gas. While the health risks of exposure to inhalants are somewhat unknown, there is enough evidence to raise concern, especially in personnel with chronic repeated exposure and particularly with more soluble anesthetics (e.g., halothane) and nitrous oxide. Even the headache that some people often suffer after exposure to isoflurane is enough reason to minimize this occurrence.

Q. How do I perform a mask induction in a dog or cat?

A. The mask should be an appropriate size to fit over the muzzle of the animal, and made of clear material that allows the mouth and nostrils to be observed. The diaphragm should fit snugly over the muzzle to minimize leakage of inhalant and oxygen around the mask and to speed the onset of induction. Have enough help so that when the animal starts to struggle it can be safely restrained on a table or gurney. Attach the mask to an anesthetic circuit (either a circle or non-rebreathing) and run your oxygen flow at 3–5 l/min to meet the animal's oxygen demands, to induce anesthesia more quickly, and to meet the peak inspiratory flow demands of the animal while it goes through the excitement phase. A higher fresh gas flow will speed the time constant for delivery of the dialed vaporizer setting of inhalant, but is also more expensive since more inhalant is delivered and then scavenged out of the system. Opinions differ on whether to "sneak" up the inhalant or to start with a high inhalant concentration on the vaporizer dial. If you start with a low vaporizer setting it will take much longer to induce anesthesia, and Stages 1 and 2 will be more prolonged. Some veterinarians feel, however, that starting with a lower setting allows the animal to adjust to the odor of the anesthetic. In this author's opinion, most animals object to the odor of the anesthetic regardless of whether you start high or low on the vaporizer; therefore, in order to speed up the process, a high vaporizer setting (3–5% for isoflurane; 4–6% for sevoflurane) is recommended.

Deliver the anesthetic in oxygen until the animal relaxes, the eyes rotate ventromedial, and breathing becomes regular and slow. At this point, the patient is probably ready to be intubated. Turn off the flowmeter to stop the continued delivery of anesthetic to the circuit, turn off the vaporizer, and quickly intubate. Once intubated, you can return to an oxygen flow rate that meets/exceeds patient metabolic needs (i.e., $\geq$2–10 ml/kg/min if on a circle system) or that provides sufficient wash-out of CO_2 if on a non-rebreathing circuit (i.e., 100–200 ml/kg/min).

Q. How do I perform a chamber induction in a cat or other small mammal?

A. The principles here are similar. It is important that the chamber be made of clear material and that it is big enough to allow the animal to turn around. Typical "chambers" for cats are a 20 gallon fish tank and for small mammals a large canine mask can be used. The chamber should have an intake hole that adapts to the common gas outlet or to the 22 mm internal diameter of the breathing tubes. The intake hole is connected either directly to the common gas outlet via rubber tubing or to the inspiratory limb of the breathing circuit. A second outlet hole on the chamber is connected to the expiratory limb of the breathing circuit or to an absorbent canister such as the F-air for scavenging of waste gas. In a typical chamber used for a cat, high fresh gas flow rates of 3–5 l/min and high vaporizer settings will speed induction time. It is advised to administer oxygen alone for about 5 min before turning on the vaporizer. This allows the animal to adapt somewhat to the chamber and ensures a high inspired oxygen concentration is attained before the animal starts to go into Stages 1 and 2, which increase oxygen demand considerably. Placing a blanket over the chamber during this time will make some cats feel more comfortable as it becomes a "hiding place."

Watch the animal closely in the chamber until it becomes recumbent or relaxed and is breathing regularly and slowly. At this time, it is safe to remove the animal from the chamber, get a quick pulse rate and observe breathing, while transitioning to a mask with a lower concentration of inhalant until the animal is deep enough to intubate. Alternatively, in species where intubation may not be attempted (e.g., small pocket pets) continue maintenance anesthesia on a mask. When getting ready to remove the animal from the chamber, turn off the vaporizer, turn down the O_2 flow rate, quickly remove the patient and have someone remove the tank to a remote area of the working environment so that immediate exposure to a large amount of inhalant in the chamber is somewhat avoided. The patient can then be maintained on oxygen and inhalant as for any other procedure.

Q. How will premedication affect the quality of an inhalant induction?

A. Premedication will definitely smooth an inhalant induction, and also make it go faster. That said, if you were able to administer premedication then, in most circumstances with regard to dogs and cats, an injectable induction technique is preferable!

Q. What are the advantages of an inhalant induction?

A. The only real advantage of an inhalant induction is that it is "hands off." In very fractious or dangerous animals, this may be desirable. See Chapters 43 and 44 for advantages of inhalant inductions in some small mammals and birds.

Reference

1 Muir WW. Considerations for general anesthesia. In: Tranquilli WJ, Thurmon JC, Grimm KA (eds) *Lumb and Jones' Veterinary Anesthesia and Analgesia*, 4th edn. Blackwell Publishing: Ames, IA, 2007:12–15.

12 Induction Techniques for the Really Sick Patient

Do you have any other options?

Berit L. Fischer

Anesthesia Director, Animal Medical Center, New York City, USA

KEY POINTS:

- Stabilize critical patients to the best of your ability prior to inducing anesthesia.
- Try to anticipate complications that may arise and prepare for them ahead of time. Expect the unexpected!
- Pre-oxygenate critical patients prior to induction, when possible.
- Warm hypothermic patients prior to induction.
- IM premedication may not be necessary.
- Benzodiazepine–opioid combinations and low doses of propofol or alfaxalone are good choices in critical patients.

Q. What constitutes a "really sick patient"?

A. A really sick patient is any patient who has an illness or injury that impacts homeostasis to such a degree that there is a constant threat to life. Patients in this category include those suffering from any type of shock (hypovolemic, cardiogenic, obstructive, distributive), severe upper or lower airway diseases (e.g., acute respiratory distress syndrome [ARDS], upper airway obstruction), those that have severe metabolic or electrolyte derangements (e.g., diabetic ketoacidosis or uremia), and patients with severe neurologic disease who may be obtunded or at risk of brainstem herniation.

Q. Does my critical patient require general anesthesia?

A. This depends on the procedure that needs to be performed and why the patient is sick. Consider other options, where practical, such as mild sedation and a block using local anesthetic. This can work well, for example, in blocked cats who are azotemic with electrolyte abnormalities. Systemic butorphanol, hydromorphone, or methadone can be combined with a

---

Questions and Answers in Small Animal Anesthesia, First Edition. Edited by Lesley J. Smith.
© 2016 John Wiley & Sons, Inc. Published 2016 by John Wiley & Sons, Inc.

coccygeal epidural to allow placement of a urinary catheter [1]. On the other hand, some patients may require general anesthesia despite minimally invasive procedures because the effects of sedatives could create more problems. An example is the patient with suspected increased intracranial pressure (ICP), as might occur in a dog hit by car with head trauma. Depending on the level of sedation, patients may hypoventilate, leading to hypercapnia, which can increase ICP. Induction of anesthesia allows the anesthetist to establish an airway and ventilate the patient in order to prevent this from occurring.

Q. If general anesthesia is required, how should I prepare?

A. First things first! Make sure your patient is as stable as possible at the time of anesthesia. This includes ensuring adequate circulating blood volume, administration of blood products to anemic patients (~PCV < 20%) to improve oxygen carrying capacity, correcting acid-base and electrolyte derangements, when possible, and optimizing systemic blood pressure (mean arterial blood pressure (MAP) > 60 mmHg) with fluid support, colloids, and possibly inotropic agents such as dobutamine or dopamine (see Chapter 17).

Unfortunately, some patients may be so ill that stabilization is not possible due to how rapidly their status is declining. A good example is a patient suffering from septic peritonitis that requires an emergency exploratory laparotomy. In these situations, stabilization measures should be ongoing while you are preparing for anesthesia induction.

Q. Do specific diseases require special preparation?

A. Yes! When preparing for each case, you should be thinking about everything that could go wrong at induction and how you can either prevent it or treat it if it occurs. Often, this requires knowing the pathophysiology of the disease and how different anesthetic drugs can affect it.

In general, there are some basics that should be done prior to inducing any critically ill patient:

✓ Perform a thorough physical exam! Pay close attention to the level of consciousness (bright, dull, obtunded, comatose), the cardiovascular system (heart rate, rhythm, pulse quality, mucous membrane color, capillary refill time, hydration, blood pressure), the respiratory system (rate, quality, color, abdominal effort, adventitial sounds), and level of pain. Following your physical exam, evaluate whether any additional stabilization is necessary.

✓ Emergency drugs should be calculated and drawn up. Emergency drugs typically include atropine (0.02–0.04 mg/kg), lidocaine (1–2 mg/kg), and epinephrine (0.01 mg/kg), but may also include naloxone (0.04 mg/kg) or other reversal agents. If your practice has a defibrillator, it should be nearby and plugged in.

✓ Monitoring equipment (blood pressure, ECG) should be attached to the patient and running prior to induction to detect trends early. An assistant can also palpate pulses or auscult the heart as induction is occurring.

✓ A method of keeping the patient warm should be present at the time of induction. Oftentimes, this detail is forgotten and patients enter the operating room hypothermic, thereby increasing morbidity. These drops can be minimized by keeping patients at normal body temperature, to the extent possible, with external warming devices during induction and surgical preparation. These methods are discussed in further detail in Chapter 20.

Q. How should I prepare for critical airway patients?

A. Pre-oxygenation, pre-oxygenation, pre-oxygenation! In situations of upper airway obstruction, be prepared for a difficult airway by having multiple sizes of endotracheal tubes available, two laryngoscopes (in case a light goes out, or for an assistant to hold obstructive tissue/masses out of the way), a guide or "bougie"; a long, flexible, blunt-ended tube that is small enough for the ET tube to fit over (polypropylene urinary catheters work well for this), and equipment for an emergency tracheostomy.

Q. How should I prepare for sick abdominal cases?

A. Pre-oxygenate! These patients have large oxygen demands and compromised tissue oxygen delivery. Dogs with gastric dilatation-volvulus, septic abdomens, and intestinal or gastric foreign bodies are at risk of regurgitation and aspiration at the time of induction. Induction should occur in sternal recumbency with a suction unit ready should passive regurgitation occur. A helper can be instructed to apply pressure to the left side of the larynx during intubation to compress the esophagus and prevent gastric contents from entering the oropharynx. Following intubation, inflate the pilot balloon and ensure there is no leak prior to changing the patient's position.

Methods to support cardiac output in these patients are important since arrhythmias and hypotension are common. Be prepared to administer large amounts of colloids, such as hetastarch, whole blood, or fresh frozen plasma, in combination with crystalloids to address low circulating volume. A second IV catheter or a central line can help accomplish this. Positive inotropes (dopamine or dobutamine), vasopressors (phenylephrine or ephedrine), and anti-arrhythmics should also be considered and prepared ahead of time.

Q. How should I prepare for critical neurologic cases?

A. Patients with suspected increased intracranial pressure should be induced quickly to establish an airway and start ventilation immediately. Induction drugs should be given at doses that make the patient deep enough to prevent coughing or gagging during laryngoscopy, as that will increase ICP. Lidocaine applied topically to the arytenoid cartilages can help to minimize stimulation from intubation.

A capnometer or capnograph are vital pieces of equipment in neurologic cases since hypercapnia (>45 mmHg) can lead to increases in cerebral blood volume and ICP.

Q. What are good anesthetic IM premedications to use in the very sick patient?

A. Many times, patients who are very sick require little, if any, IM premedication. In some patients, excessive premedication can be detrimental, such as those with intracranial disease. On the other hand, patients with respiratory disease may benefit from the anti-anxiety effects of mild sedation (e.g., butorphanol). The need for premedication should be determined on a case-by-case basis and depend on the patients' degree of anxiety and immediate need for analgesia.

If IM premedications are warranted, drugs that minimally affect homeostasis, such as opioids and benzodiazepines, should be used. Benzodiazepines, which often cause excitement in healthy patients, tend to produce good sedation in the sick patient.

Q. What are options for anesthetic induction in really sick patients?

A. The key here is IV premedication with a combination of an opioid and a sedative (often a benzodiazepine) at doses high enough that they "obtund" the sick patient and allow intubation. Fentanyl is an excellent opioid for this type of induction because of its rapid onset and degree of CNS depression. Higher doses (8–10 mcg/kg) combined with midazolam (0.2 mg/kg) IV may produce conditions suitable for intubation on their own; however, a low dose of propofol (1 mg/kg) or alfaxalone (0.5–1 mg/kg) may occasionally be needed to effect full relaxation and reduce the gag reflex.

Etomidate can also be an appropriate induction agent in really sick patients. It is considered "cardiac friendly" because of its minimal effects on cardiac output and blood pressure. It may be less suitable in patients that are anemic, because it can cause hemolysis if the formulation containing propylene glycol is used. Etomidate can also cause retching and may be of concern in patients where regurgitation is likely or increased intracranial pressure is suspected. Its direct suppression of cortisol production should also be considered since really sick patients may be catecholamine-depleted and unable to mount a stress response. Because it can cause pain on injection (again, if the formulation containing propylene glycol is used), combination with a benzodiazepine, lidocaine (dogs), or opioid is recommended.

An induction dose of ketamine in the really sick patient may not always be the best choice despite its ability to support cardiac function. The sympathetic response ketamine induces increased oxygen demand and cardiac work in patients that may already have impaired tissue oxygenation. In catecholamine-depleted patients, it can have the opposite effect and result in direct cardiac depression.

Propofol can be used in this population of patients, but be sure to follow the motto "low and slow." Titrate carefully to effect and use co-induction agents (i.e., fentanyl 5–10 mcg/kg, lidocaine 1–2 mg/kg, midazolam 0.2 mg/kg) to decrease the total dose. This helps to minimize the incidence of apnea, excessive vasodilation, decreased cardiac output, and hypotension.

Alfaxalone is another good choice for induction of the critical patient. At clinically relevant doses, it causes less cardiovascular depression than propofol and has a similar cardiorespiratory profile as a fentanyl-benzodiazepine-propofol combination [2].

Q. Any other pearls of wisdom?

A. ✓ Stay calm and collected when inducing a sick patient. Don't add stress to an already stressful situation, both for you and the patient. Being prepared and having people to assist will help you with this.

   ✓ Don't forget to treat pain! Sick patients deserve analgesia too, but may not be able to demonstrate signs we typically associate with pain. Not only is pain stressful, but it elicits all of the same body responses as shock. Opioids can and should be used liberally in patients who are undergoing painful procedures and can be administered as boluses or as constant rate infusions.

References

1 O'Hearn AK, Wright BD. Coccygeal epidural with local anesthetic for catheterization and pain management in the treatment of feline urethral obstruction. *Journal of Veterinary Emergency and Critical Care* 2011; **21(1)**:50–52.

2 Psatha E, Alibhai H, Jimenez-Lozano A, *et al*. Clinical efficacy and cardiorespiratory effects of alfaxolone, or diazepam/fentanyl for induction of anaesthesia in dogs that are a poor anesthetic risk. *Veterinary Anaesthesia and Analgesia* 2011; **38**:24–36.

13 Inhalant Anesthetics

He's got gas!

Tamara Grubb

Department of Veterinary Clinical Sciences, College of Veterinary Medicine, Washington State University, USA

KEY POINTS:

- Isoflurane is the most commonly used inhalant anesthetic in most countries.

- Sevoflurane and desflurane produce a more rapid onset/offset of anesthetic effects compared to isoflurane because they are less soluble.

- Nitrous oxide is an inhaled gas that is commonly categorized with the inhalant anesthetics but which lacks the potency to produce general anesthesia in animals when used alone.

- Minimal alveolar concentration (MAC) is a measure of inhalant potency that allows determination of "dose" (delivered by the vaporizer) and allows comparison of the physiologic effects of different inhalants at equipotent doses.

- All inhalants cause dose-dependent cardiovascular and respiratory depression.

- Halothane produces more cardiovascular depression, is more likely to produce arrhythmias, and undergoes a greater percentage of hepatic metabolism than isoflurane, sevoflurane, or desflurane.

Q. What inhalant anesthetics are commonly used in veterinary medicine?

A. Isoflurane and sevoflurane are the most commonly used anesthetics in most countries. In the USA, isoflurane is FDA-approved for use in dogs and horses and sevoflurane is FDA-approved for use in dogs only; however, both drugs are routinely used in other species. Halothane is still used in some countries but is not available worldwide. Desflurane is used sporadically but requires a specialized heated vaporizer. Nitrous oxide is an inhaled gas that is commonly categorized with the inhalant anesthetics but which lacks the potency to produce general anesthesia in veterinary patients when used alone.

Q. How are the inhalants supplied and how does this impact delivery?

A. Isoflurane, sevoflurane, desflurane, and halothane are liquids at room temperature and are delivered as a vapor after being volatilized in a precision,

---

Questions and Answers in Small Animal Anesthesia, First Edition. Edited by Lesley J. Smith.
© 2016 John Wiley & Sons, Inc. Published 2016 by John Wiley & Sons, Inc.

agent-specific vaporizer. Nitrous oxide is a gas at room temperature and is delivered from a gas cylinder using a flowmeter during co-administration of oxygen.

Q. Why is it necessary to deliver the inhalants with precision, agent-specific vaporizers?

A. Each inhalant has a specific vapor pressure (see Table 13.1). Vaporizers are calibrated to deliver a specific vapor output (in volume %) that is based on the specific inhalant's vapor pressure. Older inhalants had a very low vapor pressure (e.g., methoxyflurane, 22 mm Hg at 20 °C) and could be delivered in open containers that did not regulate vapor output, but the high saturated vapor pressures of the more modern inhalant anesthetics (e.g., isoflurane, 240 mmHg at 20 °C) would produce a dangerously high inhalant concentration if not regulated by a vaporizer. For instance, if isoflurane was used in an open container at sea level, a concentration of 31.6% would be achieved (240 mmHg/760 mmHg = 31.6%).

Using an inhalant in a vaporizer that is not labeled and calibrated for that specific inhalant can lead to an inadequately low, or lethally high, vapor output, depending on the ratio of the vapor pressure of the inhalant that is meant for the vaporizer to the vapor pressure of the inhalant that is actually in the vaporizer. An inhalant with a lower vapor pressure than the vaporizer is designed for produces a lower concentration than predicted by the vaporizer dial setting, while an inhalant with a higher vapor pressure than the vaporizer is designed for results in a higher than expected vaporizer output.

Precision vaporizers are temperature and flow compensated so that the output remains "precise" within a fairly large range of ambient temperatures and fresh gas flows. The vaporizers should be placed outside the breathing system (vaporizer out of circle or VOC) rather than within the breathing system (vaporizer in the circle or VIC) so that the patient's minute ventilation does not impact the vaporizer's output.

Table 13.1 Vapor pressures and blood-gas solubility of the common inhalants.

Inhalant	Vapor pressure (mmHg) at 20 °C	Solubility (blood : gas partition coefficient)
Isoflurane	240	1.41
Sevoflurane	160	0.69
Desflurane	664	0.42
Halothane	243	2.36
Nitrous oxide	39,500	0.49

Q. How do inhalant anesthetics produce anesthesia?

A. Although inhalant anesthetics have been in use for almost two centuries, the mechanism of action is unknown. There are numerous theories but all are unproven.

Q. What are the beneficial effects of modern inhalants in general?

A. At appropriate doses, inhalants that are in clinical use today produce unconsciousness and muscle relaxation; provide relatively rapid induction to anesthesia; allow rapid control of anesthetic depth; produce fairly rapid recovery because of the need for minimal hepatic metabolism or renal clearance; and have minimal, short-lived residual effects.

Q. What are the adverse effects of inhalants in general?

A. All inhalants cause dose-dependent cardiovascular and respiratory dysfunction, which are primarily manifest as hypotension (which impacts oxygen delivery to tissues) and hypercapnia (which affects acid-base balance and intracranial pressure). Inhalants also contribute to hypothermia because they cause vasodilation, allowing more heat to be lost, and they blunt the shivering reflex or other homeostatic mechanisms that maintain normal body temperature.

Q. What are the pros/cons of using inhalant anesthetics instead of injectable anesthetics for maintenance of anesthesia?

A. Pros:
   ✓ Easy to rapidly and fairly precisely change the anesthetic depth.
   ✓ Minimal to no metabolism so recovery is generally rapid if alveolar ventilation is adequate.
   ✓ By necessity delivered in oxygen, which helps support good oxygenation of the patient under anesthesia.

   Cons:
   ✓ Can take longer to increase anesthetic depth when compared to IV injections of rapidly acting anesthetics.
   ✓ Requires equipment (machine, breathing system, vaporizer) and an oxygen source.
   ✓ Administration of cold, non-humidified gases can contribute to hypothermia and drying of airway secretions.
   ✓ No analgesia is provided.

Q. How is the dose of an inhalant anesthetic determined?

A. The dose is based on the minimal alveolar concentration (MAC) which is a determination of inhalant potency. MAC (see Table 13.2) is defined as the alveolar concentration of an inhalant anesthetic gas at one atmosphere pressure that prevents noxious stimulus-evoked movement in 50% of the patients. This is much like the median effective dose, or ED50, of injectable drugs. Of course anesthesia in only 50% of the patients would be unacceptable and the actual dose of inhalant that produces anesthesia in 95% of patients is generally about 1.5 × MAC in patients having received no other drugs (e.g., premedications) or factors (e.g., certain disease states) that would affect MAC. Clinically, factors that impact MAC (increase it or decrease it) are often present and the clinical dose of the inhalant is generally determined as "MAC multiples," with common dosing occurring at 0.5–2.0 × MAC.

The potency of each inhalant is inversely proportional to the inhalant's MAC value, so isoflurane (MAC 1.3% in the dog) is more potent than desflurane (MAC 7.2% in the dog). Because MAC values are equipotent (i.e., 1 MAC of isoflurane produces the same anesthetic depth as 1 MAC desflurane), the effects of different inhalant anesthetics can be compared at equal dosing.

Q. Is the MAC value different between species?

A. MAC values (Table 13.2) are fairly similar between common mammalian species but do vary slightly.

Q. What factors change MAC [1]? What factors don't change MAC [1]?

A. Factors that decrease MAC:

✓ administration of other CNS depressing drugs (sedative/tranquilizers, opioids, injectable anesthetic drugs, etc.);

✓ geriatric age;

✓ hypothermia;

✓ P_aO_2 < 40 mmHg;

✓ P_aCO_2 > 95 mmHg;

✓ hypotension (MAP <50 mmHg);

✓ pregnancy;

✓ hyponatremia.

Factors that increase MAC:

✓ hyperthermia (up to 42 °C);

✓ hypernatremia;

✓ drugs that cause CNS stimulation (e.g., ephedrine, amphetamines, etc.).

Factors that don't change MAC:

✓ gender;

✓ duration of anesthesia;

Table 13.2 MAC values of the commonly used inhalants for a variety of veterinary species.

Inhalant	MAC value by species		
	Dog	**Cat**	**Horse**
Isoflurane	1.3%	1.6%	1.3%
Sevoflurane	2.3%	2.6%	2.3%
Desflurane	7.2%	9.8%	7.2%
Halothane	0.87%	1.19%	0.88%
Nitrous oxide	188%	255%	205%

✓ variation in P_aO_2 (between 40–500 mmHg);

✓ variation in P_aCO_2 (from 10–90 mmHg);

✓ metabolic alkalosis or acidosis;

✓ moderate anemia;

✓ moderate hypotension (MAP >50 mmHg);

✓ hyperkalemia, hypokalemia.

Q. What determines the uptake of an inhalant anesthetic into the circulation?

A. Uptake is dictated by the alveolar-to-venous partial pressure difference. A variety of factors impact this difference, including:

✓ dose of the inhalant delivered by the vaporizer;

✓ fresh gas flow;

✓ alveolar ventilation;

✓ cardiac output;

✓ solubility of the inhalant.

Q. What role does solubility play?

A. The inhalant anesthetics dissolve into liquids and solids and it is the solubility of the inhalant gas in blood that is a main determinant of the rate of uptake into the blood. This solubility is the blood : gas partition coefficient (PC) listed in Table 13.1. The more soluble the inhalant, the slower its uptake and elimination, thus isoflurane (PC 1.41) uptake and elimination is much slower than that of desflurane (PC 0.42). Changes in cardiac output and alveolar concentration of the inhalant have a greater impact on the uptake of highly soluble inhalants than on the uptake of poorly soluble inhalants.

Q. How are inhalant anesthetics eliminated from the body?

A. Primarily from the lung, thus adequate alveolar ventilation is critical for elimination of the inhaled anesthetics. Delivery to the lung for elimination is also important and this is dependent on solubility, cardiac output, and tissue concentrations of the inhalant. A small percentage of hepatic microsomal metabolism does occur with roughly 0.17% isoflurane, 3% sevoflurane, 0.02% percent of desflurane, 20% halothane, and close to 0% of nitrous oxide metabolized.

Q. Don't some of the inhalants produce by-products?

A. Carbon monoxide can be formed when some inhalants (especially desflurane and to some extent isoflurane) are exposed to desiccated CO_2 absorbent granules containing potassium (KOH) or sodium (NaOH) hydroxide (i.e., Baralyme or soda lime, respectively). The most common clinical scenario is administering these inhalants in a system in which oxygen flow was left on for an extended period of time, dessicating the CO_2 absorbent granules.

Compound A can be formed when sevoflurane is exposed to CO_2 absorbent granules, especially if the granules are hot and the concentration of sevoflurane is high. Compound A is a nephrotoxin but is not produced in toxic amounts with normal clinical use of sevoflurane. Also, newer absorbents are less likely to cause the formation of Compound A.

Q. What are the major cardiovascular effects of the different inhalant anesthetics?

A. Isoflurane, sevoflurane, desflurane, and halothane produce dose-dependent decreases in mean arterial blood pressure, but arterial blood pressure, cardiac output, and systemic vascular resistance are not different in dogs anesthetized with either isoflurane or sevoflurane following premedication with hydromorphone [2]. There is no clinical comparison of desflurane to these inhalants in dogs, but experimentally the cardiovascular effects are similar to those of isoflurane [3]. Halothane causes a greater decrease in cardiac output when compared to isoflurane in horses [4] but the impact of both anesthetics may be similar in dogs [5]. Although not reported in cats, the cardiovascular effects of all four inhalant anesthetics are likely the same as in dogs. Nitrous oxide produces no change or may cause a slight increase in cardiac output through sympathetic stimulation. The first three drugs also commonly cause a slight increase in heart rate (especially desflurane) whereas halothane and nitrous oxide tend to cause no change. The increase in heart rate is due to decreased vagal tone in response to hypotension; halothane inhibits this baroreceptor reflex. Halothane sensitizes the myocardium to epinephrine-induced arrhythmias.

Q. What are the major respiratory effects of the different inhalant anesthetics?

A. Isoflurane, sevoflurane, desflurane, and nitrous oxide all cause a dose-dependent decrease in minute ventilation, increased P_aCO_2, and decreased ventilatory response to increasing P_aCO_2. Although inhalants other than isoflurane may cause increased respiratory rate, the drug-induced depression of tidal volume are the cause of decreased minute ventilation [6]. All of these inhalants also decrease the ventilatory response to hypoxemia. Isoflurane and sevoflurane cause some bronchodilation in patients that are bronchoconstricted. Desflurane, which can cause airway "irritability" and bronchoconstriction, is also pungent, producing increased production of saliva, coughing, breath-holding, and laryngospasm when inhaled directly into the airways (i.e., not delivered via an endotracheal tube). All of the inhalants depress hypoxic pulmonary vasoconstriction (HPV) to some extent, but this is species dependent and, in healthy patients, does not seem to affect oxygenation to an extent that is clinically important.

References

1 Quasha AL, Eger EI 2nd,, Tinker JH. Determination and applications of MAC. *Anesthesiology* 1980; **53(4)**:315–334.

2 Abed JM, Pike FS, Clare MC, *et al.* The cardiovascular effects of sevoflurane and isoflurane after premedication of healthy dogs undergoing elective surgery. *Journal of the American Animal Hospital Association* 2014; **50(1)**:27–35.

3 Warltier DC, Pagel PS. Cardiovascular and respiratory actions of desflurane: is desflurane different from isoflurane? *Anesthesia Analgesia* 1992; **75(4 Suppl)**:S17–29.

4 Grubb TL, Benson GJ, Foreman JH, *et al*. Hemodynamic effects of ionized calcium in horses anesthetized with halothane or isoflurane. *American Journal of Veterinary Research* 1999; **60(11)**:1430–1435.

5 Scheeren TW1, Schwarte LA, Arndt JO. Metabolic regulation of cardiac output during inhalation anaesthesia in dogs. *Acta Anaesthesiologica Scandinavia* 1999; **43(4)**:421–430.

6 Steffey EP, Mama KR. Inhalation anesthetics. In: Tranquilli WJ, Thurmon JC and Grimm KA (eds) *Lumb and Jones' Veterinary Anesthesia and Analgesia*, 4th edn. Blackwell Publishing: Ames, IA, 2007:355–394.

14 Total Intravenous Anesthesia (TIVA)

Who needs gas?

Martin J. Kennedy

Anesthesiologist, MedVet Animal Medical and Cancer Center for Pets, Ohio, USA

KEY POINTS:

- TIVA may be the only anesthetic option for certain procedures.
- TIVA may offer improved hemodynamics compared to inhalation anesthesia, but can still result in significant cardiovascular and respiratory depression.
- Balanced TIVA protocols, that incorporate multiple IV drugs, may offer less cardiovascular depression and a more stable plane of anesthesia compared with inhalant anesthesia.
- The patient should be intubated if possible and the anesthetist should be prepared to assist ventilation and/or provide oxygen.

Q. What is total intravenous anesthesia?

A. Total intravenous anesthesia (TIVA) is the use of one or more injectable anesthetic drugs for the maintenance of general anesthesia instead of using a volatile inhalant (e.g., isoflurane or sevoflurane) for maintenance.

Q. What are the advantages of TIVA compared to inhalant anesthesia?

A. Potential advantages of TIVA include:
- ✓ better hemodynamics;
- ✓ smoother recoveries;
- ✓ better intra-operative analgesia;
- ✓ no potential for personnel or environmental (i.e., ozone depletion) exposure to volatile anesthetics;
- ✓ less specialized equipment is required (i.e., agent specific vaporizer, oxygen source, anesthesia machine, breathing circuit, scavenge, etc.).

Q. What are the potential disadvantages of TIVA?

A. Potential disadvantages of TIVA include:
- ✓ the need for programmable syringe pumps;
- ✓ respiratory depression and hypoxemia without supplemental oxygen;
- ✓ drug accumulation and delayed recoveries with prolonged infusions.

Questions and Answers in Small Animal Anesthesia, First Edition. Edited by Lesley J. Smith.
© 2016 John Wiley & Sons, Inc. Published 2016 by John Wiley & Sons, Inc.

Q. What are some indications for TIVA?

A. TIVA is indicated when the appropriate delivery and/or uptake of inhalant anesthetic may not be possible due to severe respiratory disease or the nature of the procedure being performed (e.g., bronchoscopy, tracheoscopy, laryngeal exam, etc.). TIVA may also be used when the equipment required for inhalant anesthesia is not available, such as field anesthesia during disaster relief efforts or rural veterinary care, or when the equipment may not be compatible with the environment, as in MRI. In critically ill patients, the appropriate TIVA protocol produces less cardiovascular depression than maintenance with inhalant anesthesia [1,2]. TIVA can also serve as an alternative option for procedures of very short duration, such as a bone marrow aspirate or feline neuter. Patients requiring long-term mechanical ventilation in the Critical Care Unit may also require TIVA in order to facilitate controlled ventilation, depending on their disease and the reasons for prolonged ventilation.

Q. What are the goals of TIVA?

A. The general goals of TIVA are the same as for inhalant anesthesia; to provide the appropriate level of unconsciousness, muscle relaxation, analgesia, and immobility in order to allow the completion of a given procedure while minimizing physiologic impairment of the patient. More specific goals for your TIVA plan will depend on the procedure being performed. For example, if you are anesthetizing a patient for bronchoscopy and are unable to intubate that patient, then you will want to provide an adequate plane of anesthesia for the patient to tolerate a fiber-optic scope in the trachea and bronchi. At the same time, however, you will not want to make the patient apneic since assisted or controlled ventilation will not be possible if the patient is not intubated.

Q. What is/are the ideal drug/drugs for TIVA?

A. The ideal drug for TIVA would provide muscle relaxation, analgesia, amnesia, and immobility without cardiovascular or respiratory depression. The ideal TIVA drug would also have a rapid onset and short duration, with no potential for drug accumulation, so as to provide both a rapid induction and recovery regardless of the duration of anesthesia. Unfortunately, there is currently no single drug available that can satisfy all these requirements that would be ideal for TIVA. Thus combinations of drugs are used in order to provide the appropriate muscle relaxation, immobility, and analgesia while minimizing unwanted side effects. This is referred to as balanced TIVA.

Q. How does one formulate an anesthesia plan using TIVA?

A. Designing a TIVA protocol begins with the choice of premedication drugs. In general the premedication drugs will be a sedative and an opioid; the particular drug combination you choose will ultimately depend on the patient, pre-anesthetic evaluation, and the procedure to be performed (see Chapters 5–8). In addition to facilitating IV catheter placement and potentially providing analgesia, premedicating the patient will also significantly reduce the amount of drug required for both induction and maintenance of TIVA, which will help reduce dose-dependent side effects. The induction drug of choice can be any of the commonly used injectable anesthetics; propofol, alfaxalone, or ketamine and midazolam. Anesthesia will then be maintained with continued administration of the injectable anesthetic, in many cases additional drugs will be co-administered to produce more balanced TIVA. Some additional drugs that may be included in the protocol include opioids, alpha2-agonsits, and/or lidocaine. Lidocaine should be avoided in cats, however, when planning TIVA protocols because of the cumulative effect and low tolerance to local anesthetic toxicity in this species.

Q. How does one administer TIVA?

A. The depth of anesthesia produced by injectable anesthetics is directly proportional to the plasma concentration of the given drug. For each anesthetic drug there is a therapeutic range of plasma concentrations; if the plasma concentration falls too low then the patient will not be adequately anesthetized and if the plasma concentration is too high then the patient will be at an excessively deep plane of anesthesia. The goal is to achieve the therapeutic plasma concentration rapidly and then maintain the lowest effective plasma concentration that provides an appropriate plane of anesthesia; clinically this can be accomplished with a loading dose (i.e., induction dose) followed by a constant rate infusion (CRI) of the drug(s). By using a programmable syringe and/or IV fluid pumps to precisely administer drugs we can titrate the patient's depth of anesthesia by either increasing or decreasing the rate of drug administration. When administering multiple drugs it is best to have each drug in a separate syringe or IV pump; this allows for individual drug rates to be increased or decreased accordingly and helps avoid inadvertent over dosage. Note that some syringe pumps need to deliver at least 1 ml/hr for accuracy, thus some drugs may need to be diluted before administration. For example, the commercial formulation of ketamine is 100 mg/ml, and if ketamine is used as part of a TIVA protocol, it may need to be diluted to 10 mg/ml or even 1 mg/ml if the patient is very small.

Q. What are some TIVA protocols?

A. You can design a TIVA protocol using Table 14.1 and Table 14.2. First, select a drug or drug combination from Table 14.1 based on your personal preference and which of these drugs you have on hand at your practice: this gives you your induction and maintenance drug(s) and provides the foundation of a TIVA plan. Next, select one or more drugs from Table 14.2; the purpose of these adjuncts is to produce a more balanced TIVA by providing analgesia and reducing the requirement of the drugs from Table 14.1. The addition of these adjuncts reduces dose-dependent side effects from any single drug used. For example, if you chose propofol and ketamine as your induction/maintenance and fentanyl as the adjunct, your plan would be as follows. Premedicate the patient with 0.005 mg/kg fentanyl IV, a few minutes later give 1–2 mg/kg ketamine IV and then administer propofol to effect

Table 14.1   Drugs for induction and maintenance of TIVA.

Drug(s)	Induction dose (mg/kg)	CRI Range (mg/kg/ min)	Bolus as needed (mg/kg)	Potential side effects
Propofol	2–8	0.1–0.8	0.5–1.0	-respiratory depression -hypotension -no analgesia
Alfaxalone	1–4	0.025–0.2	0.25–0.5	-respiratory depression -hypotension -no analgesia
Propofol Ketamine	2–5 1–2	0.1–0.4 0.05–0.4	0.5–1.0 0.25–0.5	-respiratory depression -improved blood pressure compared to propofol alone -increased heart rate

Table 14.2   Adjuncts for TIVA.

Drug(s)	Loading dose (mg/kg)	CRI range (note units)	Bolus as needed (mg/kg)	Comments
Fentanyl	0.002–0.005	5–20 mcg/ kg/h	0.002–0.004	-minimal cardiovascular effects
Butorphanol	0.2–0.4	0.1–0.4 mg/kg/h	0.1	-only provides mild analgesia of short duration
Lidocaine	1–2	25–50 mcg/kg/min	No bolus!	-not in cats -overdose can be fatal
Ketamine	0.5–1	5–20 mcg/kg/min	0.25–0.5	-somatic analgesia
Midazolam	0.1–0.2	0.1–0.5 mg/kg/h	0.05–0.1	-minimal cardiovascular effects
Dexmedetomidine	0.001–0.003	0.5–3 mcg/kg/h	0.0005–0.001	-significant decrease in cardiac output -do not use in debilitated animals

for induction (~2–4 mg/kg IV). For maintenance you will have the fentanyl CRI at 5–20 mcg/ kg/h and the ketamine and propofol CRIs will both be at 0.1–0.4 mg/kg/min. These dose ranges depend on the desired depth of anesthesia and monitoring depth and physiologic status is important, just as it is during inhalant anesthesia! During the procedure the infusion rates of the various drugs will be adjusted up and down in order to maintain the lightest plane of anesthesia that allows completion of the given procedure. When finished, the infusions are discontinued and the patient will be recovered in the same manner as if inhalation anesthesia had been used.

Q. If I am not going to use an inhalant anesthetic do I still need to intubate the patient? Do I need anything else for respiratory support?

A. If the nature of the procedure allows it, then the patient should be intubated in order to secure the airway and have the ability to provide assisted ventilation in the event of apnea or hypoventilation. An anesthesia breathing circuit is not necessarily required, but at least an AMBU bag should be available to assist with ventilation. Ideally an oxygen source should also be available in case assisted ventilation with room air is not sufficient to maintain adequate oxygen saturation ($SpO_2 \geq 95\%$).

Q. How should I monitor the patient during TIVA?

A. The same patient monitoring guidelines that apply to inhalant anesthesia also apply to TIVA. At a minimum any patient under anesthesia should have temperature, pulse, respiratory rate, blood pressure, and hemoglobin saturation monitored and recorded every 5 min. Ocular reflexes and other physical signs of anesthetic depth should also be frequently assessed. End tidal CO_2 should be monitored in patients that are intubated. High-risk patients should also be monitored with an ECG. See Chapter 15 on anesthetic monitoring for further detail.

References

1 Keegan RD, Greene SA. Cardiovascular effects of a continuous two-hour propofol infusion in dogs: comparison with isoflurane anesthesia. *Veterinary Surgery* 1993; **22(6)**:537–543.
2 Deryck YL, Fonck K, De Baerdemaeker L, *et al.* Differential effects of sevoflurane and propofol anesthesia on left ventricular-arterial coupling in dogs. *Acta Anaesthesiolica Scandinavia* 2010; **54**:979–986.

15 Anesthetic Monitoring Basics

What you don't know can hurt them!

Martin J. Kennedy

Anesthesiologist, MedVet Animal Medical and Cancer Center for Pets, Ohio, USA

KEY POINTS:

- Appropriate frequent monitoring is essential for minimizing anesthetic morbidity and mortality.
- Monitoring should focus on the cardiovascular and respiratory systems.
- Frequent assessment of a patient's physical signs is an important part of monitoring.
- The monitoring plan will vary depending on the procedure and each patient's anesthetic risk.

Q. Who should monitor the patient under anesthesia?

A. The American College of Veterinary Anesthesia and Analgesia (ACVAA) Monitoring Guidelines recommends that a designated veterinarian or technician remain continuously with the patient throughout the anesthetic period and that person be solely dedicated to managing the anesthetized patient [1]. The status of an anesthetized patient can be quite dynamic and changes can occur with little or no warning. Thus, having a person dedicated to continuously monitor the patient can allow early detection of complications or sudden changes in anesthetic depth that could compromise patient care.

Q. Why do I need to monitor?

A. Vigilant monitoring during the peri-operative period (before, during, and after anesthesia) is crucial in order to maximize patient safety and wellbeing. Patient monitoring is needed to assess that there is an adequate depth of anesthesia and minimize any insult to normal homeostasis that can be caused by anesthetic drugs directly, as well as from underlying disease. Monitoring enables early detection of anesthetic complications in order to direct

---

Questions and Answers in Small Animal Anesthesia, First Edition. Edited by Lesley J. Smith.
© 2016 John Wiley & Sons, Inc. Published 2016 by John Wiley & Sons, Inc.

prompt intervention (e.g., fluid bolus, anticholinergic, etc.) to avoid more severe complications. There is no absolute correlation between anesthetic depth and physiologic impairment; a patient can be "too light" but still remain hypotensive or hypoxic, thus appropriate monitoring is always indicated.

Q. What should I monitor?

A. Anesthesia monitoring should primarily focus on the cardiovascular and pulmonary systems – the systems responsible for oxygen delivery to tissues and removal of metabolic by-products from the organism. Patient monitoring involves a combination of repeated assessment of physical signs and objective measurements of cardiovascular and respiratory variables. Unfortunately there is no single variable to monitor, thus it is best to monitor multiple variables and make conclusions based on all available information. At a minimum, any patient under general anesthesia should have pulse, respiratory rate, blood pressure, and hemoglobin saturation monitored and recorded every 5 min, as recommended in the ACVAA guidelines [1]. Ideally, end-tidal CO_2 should also be considered part of basic monitoring. Do not forget to repeatedly assess the patient; your hands, eyes, and ears are your most valuable monitoring tools! A common mistake is for the person monitoring anesthesia to rely too heavily on monitoring equipment. The first thing you should do if you suspect your patient is not doing well is to confirm that there is a pulse and check mucous membrane color!

Q. Do I need to keep an anesthetic record?

A. Yes! The anesthesia monitoring record serves as a legal document that records events during the anesthetic period. The monitoring record documents trends in a patient's physiologic parameters as well as the response to any interventions. It is important to record any drugs administered during the peri-anesthetic period and the patient's response (e.g., premedication drugs and level of sedation). Monitored physiologic parameters should be recorded at least every 5 min, as described above. Any unexpected complications encountered during the anesthetic period should also be recorded (e.g., hemorrhage, inadvertent extubation, etc.). Keeping a detailed anesthetic record is important not only for legal reasons, but it can also serve as a useful reference if the patient requires anesthesia again in the future.

Q. What physical signs should I monitor?

A. Patient heart rate, respiratory rate and character, jaw tone, eye position, muscle tone, and ocular reflexes are important indicators of anesthetic depth. Heart rate can be obtained from pulse palpation or an esophageal or standard stethoscope. Respiratory rate can be determined by watching thoracic movements or movement of the rebreathing bag in medium to large patients. In small patients (e.g., cats) the tidal volume is small enough that movement of the rebreathing bag during inspiration and expiration may be difficult to detect. Keep in mind that jaw tone in some breeds of dogs may be more difficult to assess due to highly developed masseter muscles (e.g., American pit bull). Capillary refill time (CRT) can also offer a subjective assessment of peripheral perfusion; a prolonged CRT (>2 s) can be an indicator of poor peripheral perfusion or excessive vasoconstriction. Anesthetic depth has classically been described as progressing through four stages based on these physical signs [2].

Stage I is the stage of voluntary movement, this stage lasts from the initial administration of anesthetic drug(s) to the loss of consciousness. Patients frequently have high heart rates, increased or irregular breathing, dilated pupils, and can often salivate, urinate, and/or defecate. Muscle tone and reflexes remain normal.

Stage II is defined as the stage of delirium or involuntary movement. This stage begins with the loss of consciousness and continues until a regular pattern of breathing develops. The CNS is depressed but reflexes become exaggerated and patients can react to stimuli with violent struggling and/or vocalization. Respiratory pattern can vary from breath holding to hyperventilation. Heart rate is increased and arrhythmias are possible. The pupils are dilated and the ocular reflexes are prominent. Endotracheal intubation attempts may elicit vomiting, regurgitation, or laryngospasm and thus should be avoided until the patient has obtained Stage III.

Stage III is characterized by unconsciousness with a progressive loss of reflexes and muscle tone. This stage is commonly referred to as "surgical anesthesia" and can further be subdivided into light, medium, and deep planes. Heart rate and respiratory rate are regular and progressively slow as depth increases. In a light plane of Stage III anesthesia the eyes are centrally positioned with medium to normal sized pupils, a sluggish palpebral reflex is present (tactile stimulation of the medial or lateral canthus results in blinking), and there is moderate jaw tone. As anesthetic depth increases from a light to medium plane, the eyes rotate to ventral and medial and the cornea should appear moist and glistening. The palpebral reflex will be absent but the corneal reflex remains (tactile stimulation of the cornea results in blinking) and some jaw tone is present. A medium plane of Stage III is the ideal depth of anesthesia for most surgical procedures. As the plane progresses to deep Stage III, the respiratory pattern will become slow and irregular with a pronounced diaphragmatic component, jaw tone will be absent, the corneal reflex will diminish, and eyes will progressively move back to a central position. The corneal reflex should always be present or the patient is too deep!

Stage IV is characterized by extreme CNS depression. Pulses may be weak or not palpable, respirations may cease, capillary refill time is prolonged, and the eyes will be at a central position with dilated pupils and a dry looking cornea. If the depth of anesthesia is not lightened then cardiovascular and/or respiratory arrest will ensue.

Q. What information do I get from a pulse oximeter?

A. A pulse oximeter provides continuous information regarding the respiratory (oxygen saturation of hemoglobin) and circulatory systems (pulse rate). Pulsatile blood flow in a tissue bed and differing light absorption characteristics of hemoglobin and oxyhemoglobin are used to determine the arterial hemoglobin saturation (S_pO_2). A patient's S_pO_2 should be at least 95%. Patients are most likely to desaturate ($S_pO_2 < 92\%$) on induction and/or recovery from anesthesia, thus these are critical times to monitor S_pO_2!

When S_pO_2 falls below 95% during induction, or shortly after, the endotracheal tube should be checked for proper placement. The combination of low S_pO_2 and an end-tidal CO_2 ($P_E'CO_2$) of zero with spontaneous or assisted ventilation likely indicate esophageal intubation. The combination of a nonzero $P_E'CO_2$ and a low S_pO_2 suggests inadvertent bronchial intubation; the endotracheal tube should be checked for proper placement and backed out as needed.

On recovery from anesthesia patients can desaturate due to hypoventilation; they can have a normal or even increased respiratory rate but their tidal volume is inadequate. Pink mucous membrane color is not enough to ensure an $S_pO_2 > 92\%$, thus S_pO_2 should be monitored until the patient can maintain a normal S_pO_2 while breathing room air. Any patient with a S_pO_2 less than 92% during recovery should receive oxygen supplementation. The human eye can only detect cyanosis when the S_pO_2 falls below 75%, therefore reliance on membrane color alone is not sufficient to ensure adequate oxygenation.

The ability of the pulse oximeter to detect problems with ventilation is limited during maintenance of anesthesia with inhalants delivered in 100% oxygen. This is due to the fact that a patient can have a less than ideal arterial partial pressure of oxygen (P_aO_2) but still have a $S_pO_2 > 95\%$ since the oxygen–hemoglobin dissociation curve is relatively flat when P_aO_2 is greater than 90 mmHg (see Figure 15.1). By illustration, S_pO_2 would not change if the P_aO_2 suddenly dropped from 300 mmHg to 100 mmHg, yet a P_aO_2 of 100 mmHg is less than ideal for a patient breathing 100% oxygen. An arterial blood gas should be used to investigate any suspected problems with ventilation or oxygenation during maintenance with 100% oxygen or when the S_pO_2 accuracy is questionable.

Q. Why do I need to monitor blood pressure?

A. Changes in blood pressure reflect changes in the cardiovascular status of the patient, which ultimately determines oxygen delivery to various tissues. Each contraction of the heart produces a characteristic arterial pressure waveform that yields three distinct pressures: the systolic pressure (SAP) is the peak pressure, the diastolic pressure (DAP) is the minimum pressure, and the mean

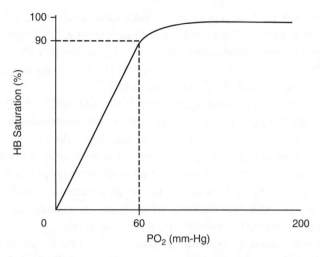

Figure 15.1 Oxygen–hemoglobin dissociation curve. HB: hemoglobin, PO_2: partial pressure of oxygen in the blood. Note that hemoglobin saturation does not significantly change when $PO_2 > 100$ mmHg due to the curve being flat, but hemoglobin saturation drops quickly when $PO_2 < 60$ mmHg.

arterial pressure (MAP) is an integration of the area under the curve that is formed by a pulse pressure waveform between the systolic and diastolic phase; or, in other words, the average pressure that the SAP and DAP oscillate around. The MAP serves as the driving force for organ perfusion and is thus the most important of the pressures [3]. Hypotension is a commonly encountered anesthetic complication and untreated severe or prolonged hypotension (MAP < 60 mmHg) can result in cardiac arrest, blindness or other neurologic dysfunction, and/or ischemic renal injury. Renal blood flow remains constant when MAP is 80–180 mmHg, however, renal blood flow becomes pressure dependent when MAP is <80 mmHg [4]. As a general rule, one should strive to maintain a MAP greater than 60–70 mmHg for healthy normal patients and a MAP greater than 80 mmHg for geriatric patients or patients with renal disease when a baseline MAP cannot be obtained (see "When do I start monitoring?").

Q. What type of blood pressure monitor should I use?

A. Basic noninvasive blood pressure monitoring options include a Doppler or an oscillometric device. Both types of monitors have advantages and disadvantages.

Dopplers are noninvasive, portable and relatively inexpensive, provide a continuous audible pulse rate, and may be the most accurate noninvasive device in patients that are hypotensive or weigh less than 10 kg [5,6]. Changes in pulse quality or pulse rate can be heard by personnel who may not be directly monitoring the patient, alerting them to possible deleterious changes. On the other hand the Doppler requires an operator in order to physically obtain a blood pressure reading, is prone to operator error, and there can be electrical interference from surgical cautery or ultrasonic scaling. The Doppler also only gives one number during a pressure measurement. Doppler gives SAP, which is usually 20–30 mmHg greater than the MAP, thus when using a Doppler the measured pressure should be ≥ 100 mmHg.

Oscillometric devices are automated and report SAP, MAP, and DAP at regular intervals. They are easy to operate and the automated design eliminates many sources of operator error. Nonetheless, the oscillometric monitors are relatively expensive, perform poorly with extremes in heart rate and/or blood pressure, and they provide non-continuous information that will miss rapid changes. For example, if the device fails to detect a pulse, it will continue to cycle several times before alerting "weak signal," so a cardiac arrest may not be detected as quickly as would otherwise be desirable.

Both devices require proper cuff size (cuff width ~40% the circumference of the limb) and proper cuff placement for accurate readings. Cuff placement proximal to the tarsus or carpus provides the most accurate readings [7].

Q. When is invasive blood pressure (IBP) monitoring indicated?

A. IBP is the most accurate method of blood pressure measurement, making it the gold standard. IBP provides continuous real time measurement of SAP and DAP with calculation of MAP. Placement of an arterial catheter (dorsal pedal, coccygeal artery, or less commonly the lingual, femoral, or carpal arteries) can be technically challenging and the additional equipment (i.e., multiparameter monitor) required can be expensive. An indwelling arterial catheter also carries the risk of thrombosis, hemorrhage, inflammation, and/or infection. These additional skills, equipment, and risks limit the indication for the use of IBP to high-risk patients. IBP is indicated for patients that have a significant risk of hypotension due to severe underlying cardiovascular disease, severe dehydration, shock from any cause, anticipated hemorrhage during surgery, or arrhythmias that are ongoing or anticipated due to the procedure.

Q. Why is end-tidal CO_2 ($P_E'CO_2$) important to monitor?

A. $P_E'CO_2$ measurement is a noninvasive means of providing continuous information regarding a patient's ventilation, cardiac output, and tissue metabolism. CO_2 is produced as a by-product of cellular metabolism and then diffuses out of the cells into the blood stream. The heart is a mechanical pump providing the forward flow of blood that delivers the CO_2 to the lungs where it is ultimately expired (see Chapter 19 for further detail). Thus any change in $P_E'CO_2$ can be attributed to a change in ventilation, cardiac output, and/or CO_2 production. The normal range for $P_E'CO_2$ is 35–45 mmHg. An elevated $P_E'CO_2$ can be due to hypoventilation, an increase in cardiac output, an increase in CO_2 production (e.g., malignant hyperthermia, CO_2 insufflation during laparoscopic procedures), or a combination of any of these changes. Likewise a decrease in $P_E'CO_2$ can be caused by hyperventilation, a decrease in cardiac output, a decrease in CO_2 production (i.e., hypothermia), or a combination of changes.

Capnometers measure the $P_E'CO_2$ and then plot $P_E'CO_2$ versus time to produce a waveform called a capnograph. Changes in the capnograph can reflect changes in cardiac output often before these changes will be reflected by alterations in blood pressure, especially when using noninvasive blood pressure monitors. An abrupt decrease in $P_E'CO_2$ is often the first sign of impending cardiovascular collapse. Repeated assessment of the capnograph is also necessary to optimize ventilation and avoid iatrogenic hypoventilation or hyperventilation. Changes in the capnograph can also indicate problems with anesthetic equipment such as breathing circuit leaks, rebreathing of CO_2, faulty one-way valves, or a kinked/occluded endotracheal tube. Capnometry can be used to confirm endotracheal intubation in species with difficult airways, such as rabbits. In human medicine a closed claims analysis revealed that the combination of pulse oximetry and capnometry could prevent over 93% of avoidable anesthetic complications [8].

Q. What does a normal capnograph look like?

A. The normal capnograph is divided into four phases (Figure 15.2) [9]. Phase I occurs during the latter part of inspiration, during which time the CO_2 should be zero (i.e., return to baseline). Phase II is the expiratory upstroke. At the beginning of Phase II most of the gas exhaled is from the conducting airways (trachea, bronchi, etc.) that do not participate in gas exchange and thus do not contain any CO_2, as exhalation continues the alveolar gas from deeper in the respiratory tract starts to mix with the gas from the conducting airways and causes the expired CO_2 concentration to rise. As exhalation continues, the gas from the alveoli makes up a larger portion of the expired gas until all the gas exiting is alveolar gas, marking the end of Phase II. In a normal capnograph, the slope of Phase II should be steep as this change in CO_2 should be rapid. Phase III is the alveolar plateau, the slight slope of Phase III is due to differing rates of emptying between alveoli throughout the lung. The alveolar plateau should be nearly horizontal in a normal capnograph. The CO_2 concentration measured at the end of Phase III is the value reported as the $P_E'CO_2$, representing the final portion of alveolar gas that is exhaled. Phase IV is the first part of inspiration, during which time the CO_2 should fall abruptly to zero as the patient inhales gas devoid of CO_2. The α-angle is between Phase II and III, it is normally 100–110°. The α-angle can become increased with an increase in the resistance to expiratory gas flow (e.g., bronchospasm, occluded endotracheal tube, etc.). Between Phase III and IV is the β-angle, which is normally around 90°. The β-angle will be increased with rebreathing and will be absent with a large leak in the breathing system.

Q. What information do I get from an ECG?

A. An ECG provides information about the electrical activity of the heart; the repeated depolarization of the myocardium produces the heart rate

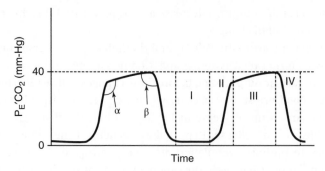

Figure 15.2 Normal capnograph. The various phases are labeled I–IV. See text for details.

and rhythm observed. An ECG can look normal seconds to minutes after a complete cardiac arrest! The ECG does not provide any information regarding mechanical function (i.e., pulse rate) or cardiac output on its own. Thus the ECG is most useful in conjunction with other monitors. For example, how is this abnormal heart rhythm affecting the patient's cardiac output? We need to look at the ECG, MAP, and $P_E'CO_2$ in order to assess the cardiovascular impact of an arrhythmia, decide if treatment is indicated, and then determine if the intervention was successful.

Q. Why do I need to monitor temperature?

A. Mild peri-operative hypothermia can have serious consequences that may extend beyond the peri-operative period. Mild hypothermia has been shown to interfere with immune system function, increase the incidence of surgical infection and prolong wound healing [10], impair platelet function and coagulation [11], decrease drug metabolism, and prolong anesthetic recoveries [12]. The amount of inhalant anesthetic required to maintain a given plane of anesthesia also decreases as temperature decreases [13].

Hypothermia is a common anesthetic complication. Management of normal body temperature in the peri-operative period is covered in Chapter 20. Suffice it to say here that maintaining normal body temperature is important for decreasing anesthetic morbidity and surgical risk. Simple ways to monitor temperature of patients under anesthesia include commercially available esophageal temperature probes and standard rectal thermometers.

Q. When do I start monitoring?

A. The appropriate time to start patient monitoring will depend on the anticipated anesthetic risk for your patient. For healthy animals with relatively low anesthetic risk (i.e., ASA I and II), monitoring begins with pulse palpation immediately after administration of induction agent and intubation, although it is never a bad idea to check pulses and mucous membrane color immediately prior to induction. Once the patient has been connected to the breathing circuit of the anesthesia machine, the oxygen flowmeter turned on, the endotracheal tube secured and leak checked, and the vaporizer set to the desired initial setting, then the pulse oximeter, capnometer, and blood pressure monitor should all be applied and initial measurements obtained.

For higher risk patients (ASA III-IV) monitoring should be implemented prior to induction of anesthesia. When anesthetizing patients with a history of hypertension or renal disease, a few blood pressure measurements should be taken prior to induction in order to establish a baseline. Under anesthesia a hypertensive animal's MAP may be acutely reduced to what would otherwise be considered a normal value; however, for the hypertensive patient this "normal" MAP could result in ischemic renal injury. Therefore it has been recommended that an anesthetized patient's MAP be maintained within 20% of the awake value [14]. For animals that have a suspected arrhythmia or history of an arrhythmia, an ECG should be placed on the patient and assessed prior to and during the administration of any induction drugs. For hemodynamically unstable patients (e.g., dog with a GDV), applying a Doppler blood pressure monitor prior to induction can give immediate audible feedback regarding the patient's heart rate and rhythm during induction. A sudden decrease in the signal strength of a Doppler has been shown to be a reliable indicator of hypotension in anesthetized dogs [15].

Q. When can I stop monitoring?

A. Patients should continue to be monitored until they have adequately recovered from anesthesia. Recovery is a high-risk period with 50–60% of small animal anesthetic related deaths occurring in the first 3 h post anesthesia [16]. Upon recovery, patients may be hypothermic, hypoxic, painful, and/or distressed or dysphoric; it is crucial that patients are continually assessed so that ongoing supportive care can be administered as needed. An animal is usually adequately recovered when they are able to sit sternal or stand, they are showing minimal signs of pain and/or distress, they respond appropriately to interaction, and their temperature, pulse, and respiratory rates are back within the normal physiologic range.

Q. My patient has a high risk of substantial hemorrhage, so how will this affect my monitoring plan?

A. When anesthetizing a patient for a procedure that has a significant risk for hemorrhage (e.g., splenectomy, liver lobectomy, abdominal mass removal, amputation, laminectomy, etc.) begin with your basic monitoring (physical signs, TPR, pulse oximetry, blood pressure, $P_E'CO_2$) and build on it. Ideally you would add IBP for its accuracy and ability to detect rapid changes in MAP. If you are unable to have IBP then a Doppler would be the next choice since it offers continuous information; a sudden fade in the Doppler signal can warn of decreasing MAP even when the anesthetist is not taking a measurement. When significant hypotension is present the Doppler can often obtain a blood pressure reading when oscillometric devices only give error messages.

In addition to the conventional monitoring, the anesthetist also needs to keep track of blood loss. Intra-operative blood loss can be estimated by watching the contents of the suction bucket, given known amounts of saline that might be part of the content, and by counting surgery sponges. A soaked "4 × 4" sponge holds approximately 10 ml of blood, while a soaked laparotomy sponge will hold approximately 50 ml of blood. Counting sponges is especially important in cases where there are small amounts of hemorrhage over a prolonged period of time because the total volume of blood lost may accumulate to a significant portion of the patient's blood volume even though it seems as if the animal never experienced a major bleeding episode. Volumes of blood that seep down surgical drapes can be hard to estimate; in these cases evaluating patient status is even more important. Trends in pre-operative and intra-operative packed cell volume (PCV) and total protein (TP) can also be used to assess blood loss.

References

1 American College of Veterinary Anesthesia and Analgesia. Anesthesia Monitoring Guidelines. http://www.acvaa.org/acvaa-anesthesia-monitoring-guidelines.pml (accessed October 21, 2014).
2 Muir WW. Considerations for general anesthesia. In: Tranquilli WJ, Thurmon JC, Grimm KA (eds) *Lumb and Jones' Veterinary Anesthesia and Analgesia*, 4th edn. Blackwell Publishing: Ames, 2007:7–30.
3 Haskins SC. Monitoring anesthetized patients. In: Tranquilli WJ, Thurmon JC, Grimm KA (eds) *Lumb and Jones' Veterinary Anesthesia and Analgesia*, 4th edn. Blackwell Publishing: Ames, 2007:533–558.
4 Shipley RE, Study RS. Changes in renal blood flow, extraction of inulin, glomerular filtration rate, tissue pressure and urine flow with acute alterations of renal artery pressure. *American Journal of Physiology* 1951; **167**:676–688.
5 Gains MJ, Grodecki KM, Jacobs RM, *et al.* Comparison of direct and indirect pressure measurements in anesthetized dogs. *Canadian Journal of Veterinary Research* 1995; **59**:238–240.
6 Simmons JP, Wohl JS. Hypotension. In: Silverstein DC, Hopper K (eds). *Small Animal Critical Care Medicine*, 1st edn. Saunders Publishing: St. Louis, 2009:27–30.
7 Garofalo NA, Teixeira Neto FJ, Alvaides RK, *et al.* Agreement between direct, oscillometric and Doppler ultrasound blood pressured using three different cuff positions in anesthetized dogs. *Veterinary Anaesthesia and Analgesia* 2012; **39**(4):324–334.
8 Tinker JH, Dull DL, Caplan RE *et al.* Role of monitoring devices in prevention of anesthetic mishaps. A closed claims analysis. *Anesthesiology* 1989; **71**:541–546.
9 Dorsch JA, Dorsch SE. Gas monitoring. In: Dorsch JA & Dorsch SE (eds) *Understanding Anesthesia Equipment*, 5th edn. Lippincott Williams & Williams: Philadelphia, 2008:685–727.
10 Bremmelgaard A, Raahave D, Beir-Holgersen R, *et al.* Computer-aided surveillance of surgical infections and identification of risk factors. *Journal of Hospital Infections* 1989; **13**:1–18.
11 Staab DB, Sorensen VJ, Fath JJ, *et al.* Coagulation defects resulting from ambient temperature-induced hypothermia. *Journal of Trauma* 1994; **36**:634–638.
12 Pottie RG, Dart CM, Perkins NR *et al.* Effect of hypothermia on recovery from general anaesthesia in the dog. *Australian Veterinary Journal* 2007; **85**:158–162.

13 Eger E, Saidman L, Brandstater B. Temperature dependence of halothane and cyclopropane anesthesia in dogs: correlation with some theories of anesthetic action. *Anesthesiology* 1965; **26**(**6**):764–770.

14 Stafford-Smith M, Shaw A, George R, Muir H. the renal system and anesthesia for urologic surgery. In: Barash PG, Cullen BF, Stoelting RK, *et al.* (eds) *Clinical Anesthesia*, 6th edn. Lippincott Williams & Williams: Philadelphia, 2009:1346–1375.

15 Dyson D. Assessment of 3 audible monitors during hypotension in anesthetized dogs. *Canadian Veterinary Journal* 1997; **38**:564–566.

16 Brodbelt DC, Blissitt KJ, Hammond RA *et al.* The risk of death: the confidential enquiry into perioperative small animal fatalities. *Veterinary Anesthesia and Analgesia* 2008; **35**:365–373.

16 Normal Values for Anesthetized Patients

Are there any rules?

Lesley J. Smith

Department of Surgical Sciences, School of Veterinary Medicine, University of Wisconsin, USA

KEY POINTS:

- Many drugs and co-existing diseases will influence what may be considered a normal value in anesthetized dogs and cats.

- The anesthetist should look at the whole picture when assessing whether a particular value is normal or cause for concern.

- Trends in the parameters being monitored may be more important than a single value.

- Signs of excessive anesthetic depth are always cause for concern and steps should be taken to lighten the anesthetic plane.

Q. Why can't I just rely on my vaporizer setting to tell me that my patient is at a good anesthetic plane?

A. While the minimum alveolar concentration (MAC) of inhalant anesthetics provides some guideline as to where the vaporizer should be set to attain a surgical plane of anesthesia, *many* other factors influence how deep or light that patient may be. In general, all premedications will reduce inhalant anesthetic requirement, resulting in a substantial reduction in the required vaporizer setting. Other ancillary drugs that are given as constant rate infusions during anesthesia (see Chapter 22) can decrease required inhalant concentrations significantly. Underlying disease state, co-morbidities, and regional analgesia will influence the required inhalant concentration. For example, a healthy dog undergoing an orthopedic procedure where an effective local block was performed, and premedications included an opioid such as hydromorphone, may require an isoflurane vaporizer setting of <0.8% during the maintenance phase of anesthesia [1]! In addition, the vaporizer setting does not equal the inhaled concentration of anesthetic: during the early phase of anesthesia when the patient has just been connected to the circuit the inhaled concentration of anesthetic will be much less than that delivered

Questions and Answers in Small Animal Anesthesia, First Edition. Edited by Lesley J. Smith.
© 2016 John Wiley & Sons, Inc. Published 2016 by John Wiley & Sons, Inc.

from the vaporizer, while during the recovery phase when the vaporizer has been turned off, the exhaled concentration of inhalant will be much higher than that of the circuit. When using a circle system, increasing the fresh gas flow rate will speed the equilibration time between the vaporizer delivered concentration, the circuit concentration, and the inhaled/exhaled inhalant concentration of the patient. Finally, always remember that vaporizers can deliver inaccurate concentrations of inhalant, especially if they are not calibrated regularly or have been tipped or dropped! Never just trust the number on the dial!

Q. So what should I look for at an ideal anesthetic plane?

A. This would be referred to as Stage 3 of anesthesia. There should not be spontaneous movement or purposeful movement that is avoidance behavior from a stimulus. These would both indicate that the patient is too light. Some drugs, notably propofol and sometimes etomidate, can cause muscle twitching, often of the triceps and neck muscles, and this should not be interpreted as spontaneous movement. This twitching is usually transient and goes away once the animal is transitioned to inhalant. Ketamine will make the animal appear rigid with dilated, central pupils, but this should not be interpreted as either an animal that is too light (increased muscle tone) or too deep (dilated pupils), and these effects also tend to disappear as the patient is transitioned to inhalant.

Jaw tone may be moderate at an ideal plane of anesthesia, and tight jaw tone indicates a light plane. There are exceptions, however: dogs with heavy mandibular muscling always appear to have quite a bit of jaw tone regardless of anesthetic depth and puppies/kittens will have almost absent jaw tone even at light planes [2]. The animal should not be swallowing or gagging.

Sudden increases in heart rate, blood pressure, or respiratory rate can indicate a change in anesthetic depth where the animal has suddenly become too light, often in response to the onset of surgical stimulation or a more painful part of the surgery. Conversely, a trend downwards in blood pressure, heart rate, or a change to an abdominal breathing pattern can sometimes indicate that the animal is becoming too deep. Again, there are caveats to this general rule. For example, blood pressure may trend down due to blood loss regardless of any change in anesthetic depth and heart rate may trend down as the animal gets cold.

The patient should have a slow or absent palpebral reflex, the pupil should rotate ventro-medial so that only the sclera is visible when the eyelids are parted, and the cornea should appear moist with some tear production. If the cornea is lightly touched from under the lower lid, the patient should have a slow blink in response.

Q. What is a "normal" heart rate for a dog or cat under anesthesia?

A. The answer to this question varies a huge amount on the individual patient, what drugs they've received, their body temperature, and their breed/size (in the case of dogs). Generally, in a dog with a physiologically slow heart rate due to fitness, a slower heart rate under anesthesia is tolerated. Dogs or cats that have received alpha-2 agonists should be expected to be bradycardic due to the effects of these drugs. Opioids will also decrease heart rate, while ketamine will increase it. A general rule of thumb is to consider the heart rate in light of the patient's blood pressure under anesthesia and whether the heart rhythm is normal or not. If the heart rate is considered slow and blood pressure is also low, then it might be wise to increase the heart rate with an anticholinergic (see Chapter 17). If bradyarrythmias are present (e.g., 2° AV block or ventricular escape beats), then an anticholinergic is also warranted. Remember that if the patient received an alpha-2 agonist, first consideration should be given to reversal with atipamezole to effect an increase in heart rate. Normal resting physiologic ranges for heart rate in dogs is 60–120 bpm and for cats 120–180 bpm. Under anesthesia, a heart rate <55–60 bpm in most dogs and <80–100 bpm in most cats would be considered too slow.

Q. What is normal capillary refill time (CRT)?

A. The capillary refill time should be < 2 s. If the animal is vasoconstricted due to hypothermia, volume loss, or alpha-2 agonist administration the CRT may be prolonged. If the patient is vasodilated due to hyperthermia or vasogenic/analphylactic shock then the CRT will be shorter.

Q. What is "normal" respiratory rate for a dog or cat under anesthesia?

A. Probably more important than the rate is to watch the breathing pattern to help assess anesthetic depth. Panting can be a sign that the animal is too light, although animal's that are too warm under anesthesia (often iatrogenic with over-zealous warming methods) will pant as well, even at a good plane of anesthesia. A slow, shallow respiratory rate with an abdominal pattern indicates the patient is too deep. Ideally, the breaths should be regular, thoracic in origin, with good movement of the rebreathing bag or the chest wall. Monitoring end-tidal CO_2 ($P_E'CO_2$) with capnometry is the best way to assess the adequacy of ventilation. Normal physiologic ranges for respiratory rate in dogs and cats are approximately 6–12 breaths/min and 12–20 breaths/min, respectively. Apnea is never normal and should be addressed by assisting ventilation and assessing depth.

Q. What is normal temperature for a dog or cat under anesthesia?

A. Temperature under anesthesia should be maintained at or near the normal for an awake animal. Efforts should be made to keep core body temperature above 96 °F (36 °C) and below 104 °F (40 °C). Within those ranges of temperature there are not deleterious effects in anesthetized animals [2]. Animals that are at less than ideal body temperature (99 °F) may shiver at recovery, which increases oxygen consumption.

Q. What is normal blood pressure in an anesthetized dog or cat?

A. Again, there are many caveats here, but there are a few rules. In general, in healthy small animal patients the *mean* arterial pressure (MAP) should be above 60 mmHg to prevent damage to visceral organs such as the liver or kidney due to poor perfusion and poor oxygen delivery. A good goal is to maintain mean arterial pressure $\geq$60–70 mmHg in healthy patients and $\geq$ 80 mmHg in patients with renal disease or with baseline hypertension in order to optimize renal perfusion in these patients. In anesthetized patients, given the cardiovascular depressant effects of so many anesthetic drugs, this is a lofty goal, and hypotension is a common occurrence even at reasonably appropriate, or even light, anesthetic planes (see Chapter 17).

Q. What should my pulse oximeter be reading?

A. The pulse oximeter should read between 95–100%. At values <95%, the probe should be checked for placement and reasons for possibly hypoxemia should be explored. Remember that the pulse oximeter only tells you the % saturation of hemoglobin with oxygen, not the adequacy of oxygen delivery to the tissues! If you're not also measuring blood pressure, then a good pulse oximeter reading for the duration of anesthesia is meaningless with respect to organ perfusion and oxygen delivery!

Q. What should I strive for with $P_E'CO_2$ readings?

A. The end-tidal CO_2 on a capnometer is generally about 5–10 mmHg lower than the true arterial CO_2, depending on whether you are using a mainstream or side-stream device and what type of circuit the animal is on (rebreathing vs. non-rebreathing). A side-stream device attached to a non-rebreathing circuit will provide a very diluted CO_2 reading and the arterial CO_2 is likely much higher. Conversely, with a circle system and a mainstream device, the $P_E'CO_2$ will quite accurately reflect the arterial CO_2. Normal arterial CO_2 in dogs ranges from 35–45 mm of Hg. In cats, normal arterial CO_2 is somewhat lower, i.e., 30–35 mmHg. This means that the $P_E'CO_2$ on your capnometer should read between 30–40 mmHg, as a general rule of thumb. Elevations above that range indicate hypoventilation or excessive CO_2 production due to fever or, rarely, malignant hyperthermia or reduced CO_2 elimination due to exhausted sodasorb, incompetent one-way valves, or a fresh gas flow that is too low on a non-rebreathing circuit to wash away exhaled CO_2 (see Chapter 19).

References

1 Smith LJ. Comparison of epidural analgesia provided by bupivicaine alone, bupivicaine + morphine, or bupivicaine + dexmedetomidine for pelvic orthopedic surgery in dogs. *Veterinary Anesthesia and Analgesia* 2013; **40(5)**:527–536.

2 Haskins SC. Monitoring anesthesia. In: Tranquilli WJ, Thurmon JC, Grimm KA (eds) *Lumb and Jones' Veterinary Anesthesia and Analgesia*, 4th edn. Blackwell Publishing: Ames IA, 2007: 552–553.

17 Troubleshooting Hypotension

A common complication

Lesley J. Smith

Department of Surgical Sciences, School of Veterinary Medicine, University of Wisconsin, USA

KEY POINTS:

- High inhalant concentrations are the most common reason for hypotension.

- Hypotension can lead to organ dysfunction and devastating CNS abnormalities after anesthesia.

- Geriatric patients should be treated more aggressively for hypotension because of their more limited organ "reserve."

- A combination of fluid therapy and decreased inhalant by using ancillary analgesic drugs is often an easy and effective way to increase blood pressure.

- Inotropes (dobutamine, dopamine) increase contractility and thereby blood pressure, but should not be the first line of defense.

- In cases of intractable hypotension, "pressor" agents like vasopressin or norepinephrine may be used, but should be the last resort.

Q. What is considered "low" blood pressure in anesthetized animals?

A. Mean arterial pressure (MAP) is the driving force for blood flow (perfusion) through capillaries that supply oxygen to organs and tissue beds of the body. In healthy dogs, cats, and other small mammals, mean arterial pressures <60 mmHg result in compromised perfusion of visceral organs and peripheral tissues, potentially leading to cellular or whole organ oxygen deprivation. In all species, mean arterial pressures <40 mmHg are associated with inadequate perfusion of vessel-rich organs such as the heart, lungs, and CNS. Prolonged hypotension can have obvious and devastating effects on organ function that are not apparent until the recovery period. Post-anesthetic blindness is an unfortunately common example.

Q. How important is it to treat a mean arterial pressure <60 mmHg?

A. The answer to this depends a bit on your patient. A young healthy animal can probably tolerate a MAP <60 mmHg for quite a bit of time (minutes,

---

Questions and Answers in Small Animal Anesthesia, First Edition. Edited by Lesley J. Smith.
© 2016 John Wiley & Sons, Inc. Published 2016 by John Wiley & Sons, Inc.

not hours) without suffering obvious or sub-clinical organ impairment. Very young animals (<6 months of age) have physiologically lower blood pressure, so a MAP of 60 mmHg in adolescent animals can be considered "normal." In geriatric patients, sub-clinical organ impairment that may not yet reveal itself in abnormal chemistry values should have a high index of suspicion. For this reason, in geriatric patients a MAP <60–70 mmHg should be treated earlier and more aggressively.

Q. What are the major risks posed by hypotension?

A. Significant hypotension that lasts for minutes to hours can lead to renal failure, delayed metabolism and clearance of drugs, ventilation/perfusion mismatch and hypoxemia, delayed recovery from anesthesia, and CNS abnormalities after recovery from anesthesia that may or may not resolve with time and supportive care. Untreated hypotension can lead to cardiac and respiratory arrest.

Q. How can I estimate MAP from systolic blood pressure?

Mean arterial pressure = diastolic pressure + 1/3(systolic pressure - diastolic pressure). Most indirect blood pressure monitors provide data for systolic pressure (e.g., Doppler method) or systolic, diastolic, and mean arterial pressure (e.g., oscillometric devices). Roughly, the mean arterial pressure is 20–30 mmHg less than the measured systolic pressure on a Doppler in most species. Thus, a Doppler reading of 80–90 mmHg correlates with a mean arterial pressure that would be considered hypotensive. The exception to this rule is cats, in which the Doppler reading correlates most closely with mean arterial pressure [1]. For more information on blood pressure monitoring, see Chapter 15.

Q. What determines MAP?

A. Mean arterial pressure = cardiac output (CO) × systemic vascular resistance (SVR). Cardiac output = heart rate (HR) × stroke volume (SV). Thus, a drug that reduces contractility (e.g., isoflurane) will lower stroke volume and can then contribute to a lower cardiac output, which may result in low mean arterial pressure if systemic vascular resistance has not increased. Figure 17.1 summarizes the factors that influence mean arterial pressure.

Q. Which factors decrease systemic vascular resistance and thus might lead to hypotension?

A. ✓ acepromazine;
  ✓ thiobarbiturates;
  ✓ propofol;
  ✓ isoflurane;
  ✓ sevoflurane;
  ✓ desflurane;
  ✓ hemorrhage;
  ✓ any type of shock (cardiogenic, septic, neurogenic, anaphylactic);

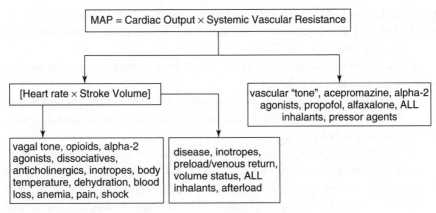

Figure 17.1 Factors that influence Mean Arterial Pressure (MAP)

✓ dehydration;

✓ inadequate volume administration or replacement;

✓ histamine release from any cause (e.g., mast cell degranulation);

✓ severe hypercapnia;

✓ significant hyperthermia.

All of the above listed drugs decrease SVR in a dose-dependent fashion. Thus, higher doses of acepromazine, as might be used for pre-anesthetic sedation in a nervous dog, could lead to hypotension because of a profound decrease in SVR. The injectable anesthetics decrease SVR transiently because of rapid redistribution. High inhalant settings will profoundly decrease SVR and lead to hypotension.

Q. What common factors might decrease heart rate?

A. These include:

✓ physiologic bradycardia (e.g., athletic dog);

✓ increased vagal tone (GI disease, brachycephalic breeds, oculo-cardiac reflex);

✓ hypothermia;

✓ intracranial disease, especially space-occupying lesions that elevate intracranial pressure;

✓ electrolyte imbalances;

✓ opioids;

✓ alpha-2 agonists;

✓ acetylcholinesterase inhibitors (e.g., edrophonium);

✓ anticholinesterases (transient, paradoxical; increase in heart rate usually follows).

As with drugs that decrease SVR, bradycardia caused by anesthetic drugs is usually dose-dependent and will be most profound in animals that have pre-existing bradycardia.

Q. What factors reduce preload, and thus indirectly reduce stroke volume?

A. ✓ Reduced blood volume from blood loss, dehydration, inadequate fluid replacement.

✓ Vasodilation and "relative" hypovolemia from peripheral vascular pooling (e.g., inhalant anesthesia).

✓ Compression of vessels of venous return (e.g. large deep chested dog in dorsal recumbency, positive pressure ventilation, surgical manipulations, abdominal distension).

A common cause of reduced preload in anesthetized animals is positive pressure ventilation, including ventilation by hand. During the inspiratory phase of positive pressure ventilation, peak airway pressure is reflected as peak intra-thoracic pressure which may be high enough to compress the cranial and caudal vena cava during inspiration. Right atrial filling during inspiration is then reduced and a lower stroke volume will occur on the subsequent ventricular contraction.

Q. Afterload and stroke volume are inversely related. What factors might increase afterload and thus reduce stroke volume?

A. ✓ high sympathetic tone;

✓ pheochromocytoma;

✓ hyperthyroidism;

✓ cardiac outflow tract stenosis (e.g., pulmonic/aortic stenosis, heartworm disease);

✓ exogenous epinephrine administration;

✓ phenylephrine;

✓ alpha-2 agonists;

✓ ketamine, tiletamine (telazol).

Q. What factors decrease contractility and thus decrease stroke volume?

A. ✓ inhalants (halothane>isoflurane=sevoflurane>desflurane);

✓ thiobarbiturates;

✓ propofol;

✓ alpha-2 agonists;

✓ intrinsic cardiac disease (e.g., dilated cardiomyopathy);

✓ pericardial disease;

✓ severe sepsis or endotoxemia;

✓ electrolyte imbalances, especially Ca^{2+};

✓ severe acidemia;

✓ beta-blocking drugs (e.g., propranolol, esmolol, atenolol);

✓ profound hypothermia.

Drug-related decreases in contractility are dose dependent. Among the commonly administered anesthetic drugs, inhalants probably have the most profound effect on contractility, with reductions of up to 50% at surgical planes of anesthesia. The induction drugs listed also reduce contractility, but their effect is more transient and less profound than that seen with the inhalants.

Q. What is a logical treatment plan for my hypotensive patient?

A. When faced with a hypotensive patient look for drugs or physio-logic/pathologic factors as listed above that may reduce (i) SVR, (ii) heart rate, (iii) stroke volume (primarily preload and contractility).

Q. What are the treatment steps in addressing hypotension?

A. See Figure 17.2 for a treatment plan.

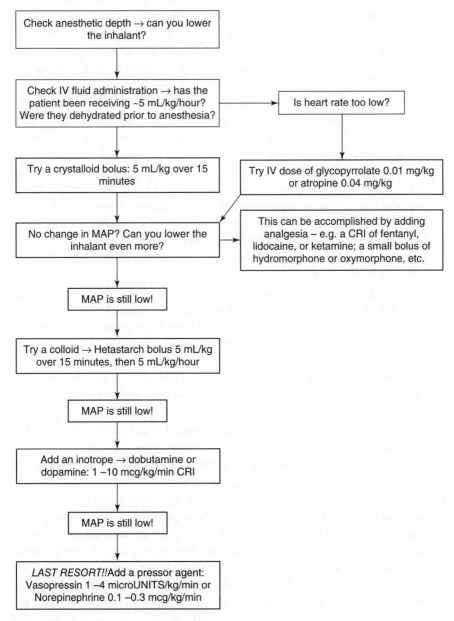

Figure 17.2 Flow Chart for treatment of Hypotension

Q. What are recommended settings for my isoflurane or sevoflurane vaporizer?

A. Premedication drugs will greatly affect how low you can set your vaporizer. Refer to Chapters 5, 6 and 8 for a more thorough discussion of premedication choices and doses. Generally, if an animal has been premedicated with an opioid +/- a sedative, you should be able to keep your isoflurane vaporizer at ~1.5% and your sevoflurane vaporizer at ~2–2.3%. If regional analgesic blocks have been used (e.g., dental block, epidural) your inhalant setting can be even lower. For example, in dogs undergoing TPLO surgery a recent study demonstrated that isoflurane settings could be kept as low as 0.7–0.8% if the patient had received an epidural containing bupivacaine prior to surgery [2].

Q. Isn't my patient going to get light and move on the table if the first thing I do is turn down the gas?

A. You should assess anesthetic depth before you make a major change in your vaporizer setting. Generally, patients who are hypotensive are too deep. *Cats, however, love to ride the roller coaster of Hypotensive ← → Awake!*

If you're turning down your gas, have some propofol or other induction agent handy in case the patient really moves, and plan to give about 25% of an induction dose IV. Usually, if you can't keep the inhalant low and the blood pressure has not improved, adding one of the suggested adjunctive analgesics listed in Figure 17.2 really will help smooth your anesthetic plane, maintaining lower inhalant settings and better blood pressure.

Q. What are risks of crystalloid fluid administration and what are the limits to how much I can give?

A. In a normal patient with a healthy heart, it is safe to give up to 90 ml/kg in a dog and 70 ml/kg in a cat. Rapid fluid administration in a normally hydrated patient is not advisable, so limit your fluid boluses to 5–10 ml/kg over 15-min increments. Fluid administration should be *much* more conservative in patients with cardiac disease (see Chapter 32) and in patients who are anemic or hypo-albuminemic. In these patients, treatment of hypotension often involves the adjunctive analgesics to keep the inhalant low and an earlier move to an inotrope.

Q. What drugs and doses of adjunctive analgesics should I use in order to lower my inhalant?

A. The suggested analgesics should be given IV for the more immediate effect desired. Table 17.1 summarizes suggested doses.

Q. What do I have to consider if I'm adding an adjunctive analgesic?

A. Any of the recommended adjunctive analgesics will decrease inhalant requirement. An opioid such as fentanyl will decrease inhalant requirement approximately 50%, depending on the dose used; and in combination with lidocaine and ketamine, a fentanyl CRI can reduce the isoflurane requirement up to 97% [3]. Some clinicians avoid using lidocaine CRIs in cats because of the fear of toxicity of this drug in this species. Lidocaine CRIs

Table 17.1 Adjunctive drugs: note different units for different drugs.

DRUG	Fentanyl	Lidocaine**	Ketamine	Hydromorphone	Oxymorphone
DOSE	1–10 mcg/kg/h	25–50 mcg/kg/min	2–10 mcg/kg/min	0.05–0.1 mg/kg bolus	0.02–0.05 mg/kg bolus

Note: caution with Lidocaine in cats due to lower toxic dose. Recommend limiting lidocaine to dogs only.

should be carefully calculated and monitored, as a lidocaine overdose in any species can be fatal. These CRIs should be tapered down to the lower recommended doses near the end of the procedure in order to facilitate a relatively rapid recovery. If the patient is expected to be painful, however, maintain the CRIs at a low dose through extubation when the patient can be assessed for pain. A more complete discussion of the many drugs that can be used for constant rate infusions can be found in Chapter 22.

Q. Are there risks to treating bradycardia with anticholinergics?

A. Administration of anticholinergics can result in tachycardia. Severe tachycardia may worsen hypotension, since diastolic filling and stroke volume are compromised. However, if tachycardia develops after anticholinergic administration it usually resolves within 10–20 min. Other side effects of anticholinergic administration include ileus, decreased salivation (which may or may not be desirable in a given patient), pupillary dilation (with atropine), bronchodilation, and reduced mucociliary transport in the trachea.

Q. What are the risks of colloid administration and how much can I give?

A. Colloids increase oncotic pressure and help to act as a "sponge" to hold fluid in the vascular space. They are especially effective in patients that may have low oncotic pressure due to low total protein or from blood loss before or during surgery. Their positive effect on blood volume is more long-lived than that of crystalloids, that is ~12–18 h compared to 25 min with crystalloids. Disadvantages include the rare anaphylactic reaction, coagulopathies after high-volume administration, and renal damage with high volume administration. Current recommendations for hetastarch 130/0.4 (Vetstarch) are to limit volume administration to <50 ml/kg/day.

Q. How do the inotropes work?

A. Inotropes such as dopamine and dobutamine can be given to increase contractility. However, these drugs should not be used without ensuring adequate fluid administration as well. Additionally, before administration of an inotrope, one should seek to minimize inhalant doses as described above. Dopamine and dobutamine stimulate B-1 receptors in the myocardium, thus improving ventricular contractility. These drugs are given as infusions, at a dose range of 1–10 mcg/kg/min. Individual animal sensitivity varies greatly, so always start with the lowest recommended dose. The half-life of these drugs is short (3–5 min) so their effect is short-lived once the infusion is discontinued. Do *not* give these drugs as a bolus, as severe tachycardia and hypertension will result!

Q. Are there risks associated with giving inotropes?

A. Dobutamine is a synthetic catecholamine, while dopamine is a precursor to epinephrine and norepinephrine. As such, these drugs exert effects similar to endogenous catecholamines. The most common side effect noticed in anesthetized animals when these drugs are given are tachycardia (especially with dopamine) and occasionally atrial and ventricular arrhythmias. Because the half-life of these drugs is short, stopping or decreasing the dose of the infusion usually resolves these complications.

Q. When should I consider a pressor agent?

A. The pressor agents, vasopressin and norepinephrine, primarily increase blood pressure by vasoconstriction and arterio-constriction. They should only be given by slow IV infusion and only after all other methods to increase blood pressure have been exhausted. They will increase SVR and potentially improve venous return because of contraction of vascular beds in the periphery, thereby increasing central circulating volume. However, their constrictive effects include possible reductions in visceral organ blood flow, notably of the GI tract, kidney, and liver.

Q. How common is hypertension under anesthesia?

A. Hypertension (definitions vary, but generally most clinicians would consider MAP >120 mmHg hypertension) is pretty rare in anesthetized patients. The usual causes are inadequate anesthetic depth, pain, or iatrogenic over-administration of inotropes. Some patients with hypertensive disease states may continue to be hypertensive under anesthesia.

Q. How can I prevent hypotension when I plan anesthetic management for my patients?

A. ✓ Ensure adequate volume status prior to anesthesia.
   ✓ Correct underlying acid-base and electrolyte abnormalities.
   ✓ Correct underlying pathologic states if possible.
   ✓ Use the lowest possible dose required of acepromazine or alpha-2 agonists, or eliminate them altogether.
   ✓ Premedicate with agonist opioids for reduction of inhalant requirement.
   ✓ Reduce induction drug requirements with IV benzodiazapines and opioids immediately prior to induction.
   ✓ Consider supplemental analgesics during anesthetic maintenance, as needed.
   ✓ Look for alternative methods to provide analgesia for surgery, such as epidurals, local blocks, and so on.
   ✓ Give IV crystalloids to all patients receiving inhalant anesthetics.
   ✓ Monitor blood pressure!

References

1 Caulkett NA, Cantwell SL, Houston DM. A comparison of indirect blood pressure monitoring techniques in the anesthetized cat. *Veterinary Surgery* 1998; **27**:370–377.
2 OO , Smith LJ. Comparison of epidural analgesia provided by bupivicaine alone, bupivicaine + morphine, or bupivicaine + dexmedetomidine for pelvic orthopedic surgery in dogs. *Veterinary Anesthesia and Analgesia* 2013; **40(5)**:527–536.
3 Aguado D, Benito J, Gomez de Jegura IA. Reduction of the minimal alveolar concentration of isoflurane in dogs using a constant rate of infusion of lidocaine and ketamine combined with either morphine or fentanyl. *Veterinary Journal* 2011; **189(1)**:63–66.

18 Troubleshooting Hypoxemia

Blue is bad!

Rebecca A. Johnson

Department of Surgical Sciences, School of Veterinary Medicine, University of Wisconsin, USA

KEY POINTS:

- Oxygenation can be assessed non-invasively (pulse oximetry) or invasively (arterial blood gas), each with their own advantages/disadvantages.
- Mechanisms underlying hypoxemia include:
  - ✓ hypoventilation
  - ✓ ventilation-perfusion inequalities
  - ✓ pulmonary or cardiac shunting of blood
  - ✓ impairments to gas diffusion
  - ✓ decreased inspired oxygen levels.
- Treatment of hypoxemia depends on the underlying cause but frequently includes enriching inspired O_2 levels, improving ventilation, and minimizing ventilation-perfusion abnormalities.

Q. How is adequacy of oxygenation determined and quantified?

A. Oxygenation can be determined in three ways, depending on the specific information required: (i) the partial pressure of oxygen dissolved in arterial plasma (P_aO_2; mmHg), (ii) the percent of arterial hemoglobin (Hb) saturated (bound) with oxygen (S_aO_2; %), and (iii) the arterial blood oxygen content (C_aO_2), calculated by:

$$C_aO_2 = (1.34 \times Hb \times S_aO_2) + (0.003 \times P_aO_2)$$

Although C_aO_2 depends on both Hb and P_aO_2, Hb concentration is quantitatively the most important contributor to oxygen content. It follows that overall tissue oxygen delivery is therefore the product of oxygen content and cardiac output [1].

Q. How do anemia and hypoxemia affect O_2 content?

A. Table 18.1 can be used as an example to determine the relative effects of Hb, PO_2, and SO_2.

Questions and Answers in Small Animal Anesthesia, First Edition. Edited by Lesley J. Smith.
© 2016 John Wiley & Sons, Inc. Published 2016 by John Wiley & Sons, Inc.

Table 18.1   Examples of the effects of anemia and hypoxemia on total oxygen content.

	F_IO_2	P_aO_2 (mm Hg)	S_aO_2 (%)	Hb (g/dl)	C_aO_2 (ml/dl)
Normal	0.21	100	98	15	19.9
Anemia	0.21	100	98	5	6.9
Hypoxemia	0.21	50	85	15	17.3
Hyperoxemia	1.0	500	99	15	21.6
Anemia + Hyperoxemia	1.0	500	99	5	8.2
Anemia + Hypoxemia	0.21	50	85	5	5.8

Anemia (i.e., low Hb levels) has a significantly greater effect on C_aO_2 and O_2 delivery than does hypoxemia, manifest as low PO_2 levels. O_2 therapy (inspired fraction of O_2 [FIO_2 = 1.0]) does little to improve C_aO_2 in the anemic patient. The combination of anemia and hypoxemia results in the lowest levels of C_aO_2 and should be treated aggressively in the clinical patient [2,3].

Q. How is hypoxemia detected in anesthetized animals?

A. Hypoxemia, defined as an abnormally low level of O_2 in the blood, is typically detected by a combination of the patient's clinical signs as well as the use of specific monitoring equipment. Physiologic abnormalities of mild hypoxemia include tachycardia and hypertension due to reflex sympathetic stimulation; however, these reflexes may be blunted in patients under general anesthesia. Patients with severe hypoxemia (<5 g/dl deoxygenated Hb) will be cyanotic and may have bradycardia (or continued tachycardia), cardiac depression, and circulatory collapse. However, to definitively diagnose hypoxemia, arterial blood gas analysis should be performed. Although pulse oximetry easily and non-invasively measures the percent saturation of hemoglobin with oxygen (S_pO_2), oximetry only provides an *estimate* of P_aO_2, it assumes the oxyhemoglobin curve is not shifted, and it assumes abnormal forms of hemoglobin (i.e., carboxyhemoglobin) are not present. Thus, although clinical signs and S_pO_2 may aid in the detection of hypoxemia, PaO_2 values are essential in determining the presence and degree of clinical hypoxemia [4].

Q. What are the major mechanisms underlying hypoxemia?

A. There are five main contributors to patient hypoxemia: (i) hypoventilation, (ii) ventilation-perfusion inequalities, (iii) right-to-left pulmonary or cardiac shunting of blood, (iv) impairments to gas diffusion, and (v) decreased inspired oxygen levels [5].

Hypoventilation is defined as an elevation of arterial carbon dioxide levels (P_aCO_2; see Chapter 19) relative to CO_2 production. When alveolar CO_2 levels rise (P_ACO_2), the alveolar (and arterial) PO_2 must be reduced based on the *alveolar gas equation*, especially when breathing room air [6]:

$$P_AO_2 = P_IO_2 - (1.25 \times P_ACO_2)$$

When lung regions exhibit low ventilation with normal or near-normal perfusion (e.g., bronchospasm, alveolar fluid accumulation, atelectasis, etc.) or have areas ventilated normally with little perfusion (e.g., dead space ventilation, low cardiac output states), the overall ventilation-perfusion relationships are altered, which frequently contributes to hypoxemia. Increasing inspired O_2 levels may improve oxygenation in these patients. However, if small airway and alveolar collapse are *severe*, a state of pulmonary shunting exists where alveoli are perfused with blood circulating from the right side of the heart, but there is no oxygen uptake due to the lack of ventilation in that area of the lung. This is a similar situation to patients with anatomic disorders of cardiac right-to-left shunting where blood travels from the right heart to left heart without exchanging O_2 in the lungs. In these situations, O_2 supplementation will not improve hypoxemia.

Diffusion impairment due to dramatic thickening of the alveolar/pulmonary capillary interface is uncommon in veterinary medicine. Similarly, low inspired O_2 levels are infrequently encountered in anesthesia since high levels of O_2 are routinely used (approaching 100%) as a carrier gas during inhalant anesthesia. However, if nitrous oxide is concurrently delivered, inadvertent administration of hypoxic mixtures may occur. Likewise, TIVA without supplemental oxygen delivery can result in inhalation of a hypoxic mixture. Other causes of a low inspired O_2 level would include a disconnection of the fresh gas inlet from the anesthesia machine, a disconnection between the endotracheal tube and anesthetic breathing circuit or from the anesthetic circuit to the anesthesia machine, an esophageal intubation, an exhausted O_2 source (e.g., empty E cylinder), and inadvertent lowering of the fresh gas flow knob down to an O_2 flow that is less than that which meets the patient's minimum O_2 requirements for metabolism. Correction of the underlying cause will correct the hypoxemia in these cases.

Q. If I have an anesthetized patient with a pulse oximeter reading of < 95% (S_pO_2), what are the steps I should take to treat it?

A. First, double check your patient's mucous membrane color. Remember that cyanosis is only apparent to the human eye when S_pO_2 is < 75%. Next, check that the pulse oximeter probe is securely located on a tissue bed where it can pick up pulsatile flow (i.e., non-pigmented skin such as the tongue, a toe web, or a vulvar fold). Then, check that your O_2 source is adequate, that everything is connected correctly from the anesthesia machine to the patient, and that the patient is breathing 100% O_2. Check that the patient is appropriately intubated (in the trachea), and that the endotracheal tube is not inserted so far that the distal end may be in a bronchus. Cats, especially, are very intolerant of endo-bronchial intubation and will desaturate quickly despite delivery of 100% O_2. This can be assessed by pre-measuring the length of your endotracheal tube so that you can estimate how far to insert it such that the distal end is located at the thoracic inlet. This can be checked by taking another endotracheal tube and, using the numbers along the side of the tube that indicate length, hold it next to the proximal end of the inserted endotracheal tube with the numbers aligned to estimate where the distal end is located. Deflating the cuff and pulling the tube out a few centimeters often corrects the hypoxemia. Then leak check and re-inflate the cuff again an appropriate amount. Finally, if you have done all these things, treatment may consist of: increasing inspired O_2 levels, increasing minute ventilation (respiratory frequency and/or tidal volume), optimizing ventilation-perfusion inequalities using techniques such as positive end-expiratory pressure (PEEP), or by increasing cardiac output [7] (see Chapter 17 for details).

Q. If my patient is in recovery and extubated, but hypoxemic, how can I deliver O_2 to address this?

A. Enriched O_2 levels can be supplied via a tight-fitting mask, O_2 cage, or via nasal insufflation through unilateral or bilateral cannulas advanced to the medial canthus of the eye. A humidified O_2 flow rate of 50 to 100 ml/kg is usually used.

Q. What are normal blood gas values in dogs and cats? How do these numbers change if the animal is breathing 100% O_2?

A. Normal mean arterial blood gas values (range) reported in dogs and cats breathing room air are shown in Table 18.2.

Q. How should I interpret pulse oximetry readings in peri-operative patients on varying levels of inspired O_2?

A. SpO_2 may not discriminate between a patient with adequate oxygenation and one experiencing relative hypoxia (or less than ideal oxygenation) when inspiring an enriched O_2 mixture. For example, the predicted P_aO_2 of a healthy animal is ~500–600 mmHg when inspiring ~100% O_2. With respiratory compromise, such as hypoventilation or ventilation-perfusion inequalities, the P_aO_2 may drop significantly, for example from 500 mmHg to 100 mmHg. Although the difference between a P_aO_2 of 500 and 100 mmHg is extremely important to the patient physiologically, the corresponding

Table 18.2 Normal blood gas values in the dog and cat breathing room air (F_iO_2 ~ 21%). However, when breathing ~100% O_2 (as during anesthesia), PO_2 values in both dogs and cats are expected to approach 500–600 mmHg with ideal gas exchange [8].

	Dog	Cat
pH	7.41 (7.35–7.46)	7.39 (7.31–7.46)
P_aCO_2 (mmHg)	36.8 (30.8–42.8)	31.0 (25.2–36.8)
HCO_3^- (mEq/l)	22.2 (18.8–25.6)	18.0 (14.4–21.6)
P_aO_2 (mmHg)	92.1 (80.9–103.3)	106.8 (95.4–118.2)

Brunson DB, Johnson RA. Respiratory disease. In: Culp-Snyder LB, Johnson RA (eds) *Canine and Feline Anesthesia and Co-Existing Disease*, 1st edn. Wiley: Hoboken NJ, 2014:55–70.

decrease in S_pO_2 from 99 to 98% would hardly be noticed since the S_pO_2 measurements are still positioned on the upper plateau of the oxy-Hb dissociation curve.

Therefore, to truly assess oxygenation, an arterial blood gas is necessary to detect abnormalities in P_aO_2. If the pulse oximeter is reading > 95%, the only thing you can conclude is that the patient has a P_aO_2 of ~ 100 mmHg or higher. An oxygen saturation > 95% is adequate for normal delivery of oxygen to tissues (assuming the patient has normal hemoglobin levels and good blood pressure), but without a blood gas you cannot detect trends in oxygenation between the "ideal" of 500–600 mmHg on 100% O_2 and that which is minimally required to maintain normal hemoglobin saturation (90–100 mmHg).

Q. How do dyshemoglobinemias affect hemoglobin saturation?

A. Carboxyhemoglobin will absorb light similar to oxyhemoglobin at 660 nm but minimally at 940 nm (just as the patient with carboxyhemoglobin toxicity from smoke inhalation shows the classic "cherry red" appearance). This will increase the apparent hemoglobin saturation as read by the pulse oximeter. Methhemoglobin absorbs light at both the 660 and 940 nm wavelengths and tends to push the pulse oximeter reading toward 85% (underestimating measurements when S_aO_2 is above 85% and overestimating it when below 85%) [9].

References

1 West JB. Gas Transport by the Blood. In: West JB (ed.) *Respiratory Physiology – The Essentials*, 9th edn. Lippincott Williams & Wilkins: Baltimore, 2012:78–82.

2 Haskins S. CanWest Veterinary Conference. Proceedings. http//canadawestvets.com/symposium2011/ (accessed May 6, 2014).

3 West JB. Gas Transport by the Blood. In: West JB (ed.) *Respiratory Physiology – The Essentials*, 9th edn. Lippincott Williams & Wilkins: Baltimore, 2012:92.

4 West JB. Respiratory Failure. In: West JB (ed.) *Pulmonary Pathophysiology – The Essentials*, 8th edn. Lippincott Williams & Wilkins: Baltimore. 2013:130–131.

5 West JB. Ventilation-Perfusion Relationships. In: West JB (ed.) *Respiratory Physiology – The Essentials*, 9th edn. Lippincott Williams & Wilkins: Baltimore, 2012:56–62.

6 Hedenstierna G. Respiratory Physiology. In: Miller RD (ed.) *Miller's Anesthesia*, 7th edn. Churchill Livingstone: Philadelphia, 2010:373.

7 Kerr CL, McDonell WN. Oxygen Supplementation and Ventilatory Support. In: Muir WW, Hubbell JAE (eds) *Equine Anesthesia*, 2nd edn. Saunders: St. Louis, 2009:341–346.

8 Brunson DB, Johnson RA. Respiratory Disease. In: Culp-Snyder LB, Johnson RA (eds) *Canine and Feline Anesthesia and Co-Existing Disease*, 1st edn. Wiley: Hoboken NJ, 2014:55–70.

9 Kirson LE, Koltes-Edwards R. Pulse oximetry. In: Duke J (ed.) *Anesthesia Secrets*. 4th edn. Mosby: Philadelphia, 2011:168–174.

19 Troubleshooting Hypercapnia and Hypocapnia

Just breathe!

Rebecca A. Johnson

Department of Surgical Sciences, School of Veterinary Medicine, University of Wisconsin, USA

KEY POINTS:

- Alterations in patient CO_2 can be assessed non-invasively (capnometry) or invasively (blood gas), each with their own advantages/disadvantages.

- Hypercapnia is associated with CO_2 production in excess of alveolar ventilation; hypocapnia is associated with alveolar ventilation in excess of CO_2 production.

- In normal patients, end-tidal (capnometry) values for CO_2 only differ by 1–5 mmHg from arterial CO_2 levels; abnormal pulmonary physiology results in a much larger gradient (~5–10 mmHg).

- Hypercapnia associated with respiratory depressant drugs is extremely common in anesthetized patients.

- Treatment of hypercapnia/hypocapnia depends on the underlying cause; however, hypercapnia is frequently treated by increasing alveolar ventilation either via assisted or controlled ventilation.

Q. How is carbon dioxide (CO_2) carried in the blood?

A. CO_2 is produced in the tissues and diffuses down a concentration gradient until it enters the blood where it is carried in three ways: (i) dissolved in solution (~5% in arterial blood), (ii) as bicarbonate (~75–80% in arterial blood), and (iii) combined with proteins such as carbamino compounds (~15–20% in arterial blood) [1,2].

Bicarbonate is the main type of CO_2 found in the blood and is formed by the *carbonic anhydrase equation*:

$$CO_2 + H_2O \leftrightarrow H_2CO_3 \leftrightarrow H^+ + HCO_3^-$$

The first reaction is slow in plasma but fast in the red blood cell due to the presence of carbonic anhydrase. The second reaction occurs quickly. The HCO_3^- diffuses out of the red blood cell but the H^+ ions become trapped since the cell membrane is relatively impermeable to cations. Chloride ions

---

Questions and Answers in Small Animal Anesthesia, First Edition. Edited by Lesley J. Smith.
© 2016 John Wiley & Sons, Inc. Published 2016 by John Wiley & Sons, Inc.

move into the cell from the plasma (the *chloride shift*) to maintain electrical neutrality. Carbamino compounds are formed by the chemical combination of CO_2 with terminal amine groups of proteins such as hemoglobin, resulting in carbaminohemoglobin [1,2].

Q. How are O_2 and CO_2 transport in the blood related to each other?

A. O_2 and CO_2 transport in the blood have mutual interactions via the Bohr and Haldane effects. For example, some of the H^+ ions produced from the carbonic anhydrase equation above bind to reduced hemoglobin (Hb) and displace O_2:

$$H^+ + HbO_2 \leftrightarrow H^+Hb + O_2$$

Thus, in the O_2-enriched lungs, Hb is a poor buffer, which aids in the unloading of CO_2, termed the *Haldane effect*. In the tissues, the high level of CO_2 reduces the affinity of Hb for O_2 and consequently aids in the unloading of O_2, termed the *Bohr effect* [1,2].

Q. How is CO_2 related to ventilation?

A. Hypo- and hyperventilation are defined by alterations in the partial pressure of arterial CO_2 (P_aCO_2). Whereas hypoventilation is associated with hypercapnia, i.e., increased P_aCO_2 values (and respiratory acidosis), hyperventilation results in hypocapnia, i.e., decreased P_aCO_2 levels (and respiratory alkalosis). Normal P_aCO_2 is somewhat species dependent but is approximately 31–37 mmHg in small animals (see: normal blood gas values in Chapter 18) [3]. The determinants of PCO_2 are based on the *alveolar ventilation equation* (simplified below), which describes the relationship between ventilation and CO_2 production ($\dot{V}CO_2$):

$$P_aCO_2 = (\dot{V}CO_2/\dot{V}A) \times K$$

Where $\dot{V}A$ = alveolar ventilation and K = constant to equate dissimilar units for $\dot{V}CO_2$ and $\dot{V}A$.

In general, alveolar ventilation and P_aCO_2 are inversely related when CO_2 production is held constant [4,5]. In the normal awake animal, P_aCO_2 is held relatively constant by respiratory center-driven changes in alveolar ventilation, despite situations of vastly increased CO_2 production, as during exercise. This CO_2 response curve is generally linear over physiologic P_aCO_2 levels. However, many respiratory depressant drugs used in anesthesia, such as inhalants and opioids, shift the response curve to the right, resulting in a higher P_aCO_2 being required for a given response in ventilation. In addition, the slope is reduced, indicating that ventilation is less responsive to changes in P_aCO_2 (Figure 19.1) [6].

Q. What are the relationships between CO_2 production ($\dot{V}CO_2$), partial pressure of CO_2 (PCO_2), and alveolar ventilation ($\dot{V}A$)?

A. At a constant $\dot{V}A$ (alveolar ventilation), increased CO_2 production ($\dot{V}CO_2$) would predictably result in an increase in P_aCO_2. In a normal patient,

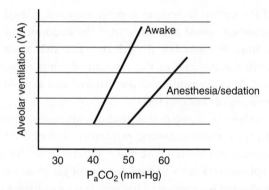

Figure 19.1 Relationship between arterial CO_2 and ventilation in the awake state and after opioid sedation in mammals.

increased $\dot{V}CO_2$ leads to an increase in ventilation and the patient maintains their P_aCO_2 close to normal. However, patients with moderate/severe lung disease may not be able to increase their ventilation appropriately to compensate for the increase in $\dot{V}CO_2$ and the P_aCO_2 may rise [7].

Q. How are alterations in CO_2 levels detected in anesthetized animals?

A. Clinical signs of hypocapnia are usually caused by the underlying disease process and not necessarily the hypocapnia itself [5]. However, hyperventilation, hypotension, and cardiac arrhythmias may be present in patients experiencing hypocapnia [5]. In contrast, acute, severe hypercapnia can result in concomitant hypoxemia, especially if the patient is not breathing 100% O_2, and these two together can be an immediate threat to life [5]. A more gradual onset of hypercapnia, as would be common in a deeply anesthetized patient experiencing depressed ventilation, results in sympathetic nervous system stimulation, thereby increasing circulating catecholamine levels which can lead to sympathetically-mediated arrhythmias [8]. In addition, increased heart rate and cardiac output, altered ventilatory patterns, and "flushed" or "brick red" mucous membranes are common [5]. Despite these findings, however, clinical evaluation of the patient alone is not reliable in making a diagnosis of hypo- or hypercapnia. Monitoring devices such as capnometers, or arterial blood gas analysis, are required to make the definitive diagnosis of hypo- or hypercapnia. Due to its relatively low expense and its non-invasive technology, capnometry is more frequently used in veterinary patients at this time.

Q. What is the difference between capnography and capnometry?

A. Capnometry refers to the measurement of CO_2 in respiratory gases and display of the values in numerical form only. Capnography refers to the continuous measurement and display of CO_2 in respiratory gases; frequently it is associated with a real-time waveform. Because of the waveform display, capnography allows more information to be gathered from this type of CO_2 monitor.

The infrared absorption technique is most commonly used for monitoring CO_2 with the sensor placed near the end of the endotracheal tube (end-tidal CO_2). The technique is based on the principle that CO_2 absorbs infrared light energy of specific wavelengths; the amount of energy absorbed is directly related to the CO_2 concentration in the inspired and expired gases.

Q. What are the types of capnometers?

A. There are two types of capnometers: mainstream and side-stream [9]. However, both measure the inspiratory, expiratory, and end-tidal (which is the closest to arterial) gas values. The main difference is the sensor location. *Side-stream* capnometers draw a fixed volume of gas from the respiratory circuit. The sampled gas is transported through tubing into the measuring sensor then is released to the atmosphere or returned to the breathing system. To improve accuracy, sampling should be performed as close to the patient's endotracheal tube as possible; if the sampling rate exceeds the expiratory flow rate of the patient, inspired gas will also be sampled and erroneously low end-tidal CO_2 values will be reported (e.g., small patients such as cats). *Mainstream* capnometers have the infrared sensor located within the respiratory circuit, at the end of the endotracheal tube. Gas is not removed from the system and they are frequently used in very small patients to provide more accurate information than side-stream monitors. To avoid condensation on the sensor, it must be warmed and may add additional weight to the breathing apparatus; care should be taken not to inadvertently cause traction on the endotracheal tube.

Q. How do CO_2 levels determined from an arterial blood gas differ from end-tidal CO_2 values measured by capnometry?

A. In normal patients, the $P_E'CO_2$ generally underestimates the P_aCO_2 by 1–5 mmHg due to a small amount of alveolar dead space which functions to slightly dilute the CO_2 being expired from the alveoli [9,10]. However, in patients with increased alveolar dead space (e.g., chronic obstructive pulmonary disease, acute respiratory distress syndrome, etc.) this difference widens and the $P_E'CO_2$–$PaCO_2$ gradient is usually 5–10 mmHg [9,10].

Q. What are the major causes of hypercapnia in anesthetized patients?

A. The most common cause of hypercapnia in anesthetized patients is inadequate ventilation relative to CO_2 production, because of the respiratory depressant nature of many drugs used in anesthesia, most specifically the inhalants. Induction drugs are also potent respiratory depressants. Opioids shift the CO_2 response curve to the right, so higher CO_2 levels are needed to stimulate an increase in ventilation. Other possible causes for hypercapnia in anesthetized patients include:

✓ Airway obstruction (tracheal collapse, asthma, laryngeal paralysis).

✓ Intrinsic pulmonary or small airway disease (pulmonary thromboembolism, edema or pneumonia, acute respiratory distress syndrome, chronic obstructive pulmonary disease, fibrosis).

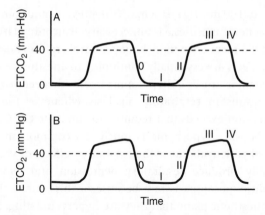

Figure 19.2 (a) (top graph). Capnograph waveform appearance during hypercapnia. Note that Phase 3 is elevated above the normal value of 40 mmHg. (b) (bottom graph). Capnograph waveform when hypercapnia is secondary to inspired CO_2, as, for example, with exhausted CO_2 absorbent or malfunctioning one-way valves.

✓ CNS depression (pharmacologically-induced, neurologic disease).

✓ Increased production with impaired ventilation (iatrogenic over-heating, malignant hyperthermia).

✓ Restrictive extrapulmonary disorders (diaphragmatic hernia, pneumothorax, pleural effusion).

✓ Marked obesity (Pickwickian Syndrome).

✓ Surgical positioning in a "head down" or Trendelenburg position.

✓ Iatrogenic increased extrathoracic pressure (bandaging, a surgeon's arm).

✓ Increased inspired CO_2 with ineffective ventilation (exhausted CO_2 absorbent, ineffective one-way valves, excess mechanical dead space).

✓ Fever, shivering (increased CO_2 production).

Q. How does the capnography waveform appear during the causes of hypercapnia?

A. $P_E'CO_2$ will be elevated above normal values with any of the aforementioned causes (Figure 19.2a) if the alveolar ventilation falls behind the CO_2 production. If the baseline is elevated above zero, inspired CO_2 is also present, as would be the case with exhausted CO_2 absorbent (Figure 19.2b) [10].

Q. What are the physiological effects of hypercapnia?

A. Hypercapnia results in respiratory acidosis due to accumulation of CO_2 in the body. These acid-base derangements shift the oxyhemoglobin dissociation curve to the right. Due to activation of the sympathetic nervous system, catecholamines are released, the renin–angiotensin system is activated, cardiac output is increased and tachyarrhythmias can also be seen [5]. Any associated neurologic signs depend on the degree and rapidity of the development of hypercapnia; acute increases can cause cerebral vasodilation, consequently increasing cerebral blood flow and intracranial pressure. P_aCO_2 levels approaching 70–100 mmHg result in CNS depression and coma; at P_aCO_2 levels this high, general anesthesia is unnecessary! If an animal hypoventilates to this degree in the recovery period, it may not waken from anesthesia because the high CO_2 levels are essentially continuing to anesthetize the patient [5]!

Q. What are the major causes of hypocapnia in anesthetized patients?

A. Hypocapnia results in respiratory alkalosis whenever the magnitude of alveolar ventilation exceeds that required to eliminate the CO_2 produced by cellular metabolism. Hypocapnia is much less common than hypercapnia in anesthetized patients because the respiratory effects of various anesthetic drugs generally produce respiratory depression and elevated P_aCO_2 is expected. True hypocapnia is rare because of this, unless the patient is at such a light anesthetic plane that they are hyperventilating. Some causes of low measured $P_E'CO_2$ include:

✓ Overzealous mechanical or assisted ventilation.

✓ Panting, where mostly dead space ventilation is being measured.

✓ Extreme hypothermia.

✓ Decreased cardiac output.

✓ Capnometer errors (e.g., side-stream capnometer on a very small patient, capnometer attached to a non-rebreathing circuit where fresh gas flow dilutes the expired sample).

✓ Esophageal intubation, inadvertent tracheal extubation, endotracheal tube obstruction, and anesthetic circuit leak or disconnection will also cause low capnometer readings (arterial levels may be unaffected).

Q. Why do low cardiac output states result in hypocapnia?

A. In these situations, the arterial CO_2 tension may also be normal or high, but because cardiac output is so low, arterial CO_2 is not delivered back to the lung for gas exchange. $P_E'CO_2$ readings of <10 mmHg are associated with impending cardiac arrest.

Q. How does the capnography waveform appear with causes of hypocapnia?

A. The $P_E'CO_2$ will be reduced below baseline in any of the aforementioned causes. However, the appearance of the waveform over time will vary, depending on the underlying cause. For example, $P_E'CO_2$ abruptly decreases to near zero from an acute event such as tracheal extubation, esophageal intubation, complete breathing system disconnection, ventilator malfunction or a completely obstructed tracheal tube. If the decrease is gradual, but also approaches zero, sudden, severe hypotension or circulatory arrest with continued ventilation or pulmonary thromboembolism may be considered. However, if the CO_2 decreases gradually but does not reach near-zero levels, a leak or partial disconnection of the breathing system or a partial tracheal tube obstruction may be causative [10].

Q. How do I treat clinical hypocapnia and hypercapnia?

A. Treatment of either hypo- or hypercapnia is directed at the suspected underlying cause. Respiratory stimulants, such as doxapram, should never be used as a substitute for appropriate assisted or controlled ventilation. Controlled or assisted mechanical ventilation techniques may be used to correct hypercapnia during anesthesia or in patients with significant pulmonary disease (see Chapter 31).

References

1 West JB. Gas transport by the blood. In: West JB (ed.) *Respiratory Physiology – The Essentials*, 9th edn. Lippincott Williams & Wilkins: Baltimore, 2012:82–86.

2 Robinson NE. The respiratory system. In: Muir WW, Hubbell JAE (eds) *Equine Anesthesia*, 2nd edn. Saunders: St. Louis, 2009:29–30.

3 Brunson DB, Johnson RA. Respiratory disease. In: Culp-Snyder LB, Johnson RA (eds) *Canine and Feline Anesthesia and Co-Existing Disease*. Wiley: Hoboken, *In press.*

4 Hedenstierna G. Respiratory physiology. In: Miller RD (ed.) *Miller's Anesthesia*, 7th edn. Churchill Livingstone: Philadelphia, 2010:361–391.

5 Johnson RA, de Morais HA. Respiratory acid-base disorders. In: DiBartola SP (ed.) *Fluid, Electrolyte, and Acid-Base Disorders*, 4th edn. Elsevier: St. Louis, 2012:293–298.

6 Ciarallo CL. Opioids. In: Duke J (ed.) *Anesthesia Secrets*. 4th edn. Mosby: Philadelphia, 2011: 82–89.

7 MD Nexus. http//mdnxs.com/topics-2/pulmonary-and-critical-care/hypercapnia/ (accessed May 6, 2014).

8 Brofman JD, Leff AR, Munoz NM, *et al.* Sympathetic secretory response to hypercapnic acidosis in swine. *Journal of Applied Physiology* 1990; **69**:710–717.

9 Eskaros SM, Papadakos PJ, Lachman B. Respiratory monitoring. In: Miller RD (ed.) *Miller's Anesthesia*, 7th edn. Churchill Livingstone: Philadelphia, 2010:1425–1428.

10 Dorsch JA, Dorsch SE. Gas monitoring. In: Dorsch JA, Dorsch SE (eds) *Understanding Anesthesia Equipment*, 5th edn. Lippincott Williams & Wilkins: Philadelphia, 2008:712–719.

20 Troubleshooting Hypothermia and Hyperthermia

Brrrr is bad too!

Lysa Pam Posner

North Carolina State University, USA

KEY POINTS:

- Hypothermia occurs in most anesthetized animals.
- Hypothermia causes many physiologic disturbances, so should be prevented and/or treated.
- Preventing heat loss is easier than treating hypothermia.

Q. What is normal body temperature in dogs and cats?

A. Normal rectal temperature in dogs is $39 \pm 0.5\,°C$ ($102 \pm 1\,°F$) and in cats is $38.5 \pm 0.5\,°C$ ($101.5 \pm 1\,°F$) [1]. Unlike, humans, body temperature can vary ($\sim 0.5\,°C$ ($1\,°F$)) and is known as the inter-threshold range. Body temperatures within this range do not trigger any thermoregulatory responses.

Q. What is the difference between core temperature and peripheral body temperature?

A. Core body temperature is the temperature at which vital organs (e.g., brain, heart) are maintained. Peripheral body temperature is measured from structures located in the periphery (e.g., skin, mouth, rectum). Core and peripheral body temperatures can vary by up to $4\,°C$ [2]. Core body temperature can be accurately measured at the tympanic membrane, nasopharynx, esophagus, and the pulmonary artery. Although rectal temperature can more easily be measured, it can lag behind changes in core body temperature. Skin is not a reliable indicator of core temperature as it is often $2–4\,°C$ lower than core temperature [2].

Normally, there is a heat gradient between the periphery and the core. In general, core temperature is more constant and peripheral body temperature varies (because it buffers core temperature changes). This gradient from core to periphery allows the skin to act as a gate for heat dissipation and conservation. Arteriovenous anastomoses present in the skin are major contributors to

---

Questions and Answers in Small Animal Anesthesia, First Edition. Edited by Lesley J. Smith.
© 2016 John Wiley & Sons, Inc. Published 2016 by John Wiley & Sons, Inc.

thermoregulation. Dilation of these shunts allows for large amounts of heat to be lost to the environment from the core and conversely, vasoconstriction of these shunts prevents heat loss from the core.

Q. How is body temperature regulated?

A. Thermoregulation is a complex interaction between thermal sensing, central processing in the hypothalamus, and behavioral and physiologic responses. The hypothalamus regulates temperature by "comparing" current body temperature with the threshold temperatures that trigger thermoregulatory responses (i.e., those temperatures that are outside the inter-threshold range).

If the body temperature has exceeded the threshold temperatures (either above or below) a series of behavioral and physiologic responses will be triggered. For example, behavioral responses to decreasing body temperature can include a more compact posture or heat seeking behavior (e.g., sun seeking). Autonomic responses to declining body temperature include vasoconstriction in arteriovenous anastomoses and activation of the sympathetic nervous system (SNS) which increases thermogenesis. The ability to tightly control thermoregulation declines with age.

Q. How is body heat generated?

A. The production of heat (thermogenesis) is primarily accomplished by increases in metabolism (e.g., muscle movement or by non-shivering thermogenesis). Shivering is a major source of heat production and occurs when muscle groups involuntarily contract in small movements, creating warmth by expending energy. Shivering can increase metabolic rate 2–3-fold from normal. Similarly, vigorous exercise can increase heat production 30–40-fold compared with resting muscle [3].

Non-shivering thermogenesis includes increased metabolic rate via increased sympathetic tone or increased thyroid hormone or chemical thermogenesis. Chemical thermogenesis occurs by increased metabolism of brown fat and enhances heat production. Chemical thermogenesis has been shown to occur in infants, but the contribution in adults is less clear [3].

Regardless of pathway, thermogenesis is metabolically expensive as it increases consumption of oxygen, ATP, and glucose.

Q. What are the types of heat loss?

A. Heat loss is generally divided into five types; radiation, convection, evaporation, respiration, and conduction. Radiation and convection are the most important causes of heat loss and can account for 80% of the total heat losses in a patient [4].

✓ Radiation: Heat loss from radiation occurs when a hot object emits radiation waves. These waves carry energy (heat) away from the body and cause it to cool. Fifty percent of body heat loss can be from radiation [4]. Keeping the air temperature around your patient warmer will decrease radiative losses.

✓ Convection: Losses from convection occur when the warmed air surrounding the body (from radiation) rise and is carried away from the body (how fans cool patients). Keeping your patient covered (with a towel or blanket) prevents convection losses.

✓ Evaporation: Evaporative heat loss occurs due to the loss of the latent heat of vaporization (the heat created by changing from liquid to vapor), and can increase with large surgical exposures, as in an abdominal exploratory or thoracotomy. Evaporative losses are difficult to prevent.

✓ Respiration: Respiratory heat loss occurs when gases are warmed and humidified by the body. Normally respiratory heat loss is less than 10% of total heat loss; however, during anesthesia the inspiration of dry cooled gases can increase heat loss through respiration. Respiratory losses are also hard to prevent, but there are some advanced techniques that can decrease heat loss via respiration, such as the use of a heat and moisture exchange device (HME).

✓ Conduction: Conduction losses occur by way of heat energy being transferred through a substance and normally accounts for minimal losses. However, metal surgical tables can increase heat loss through conduction. Limiting contact with conductive surfaces, such as placing a towel or blanket over a metal surgical table, will help limit conductive losses.

It should be noted that most types of heat loss are dependent on the amount of exposed skin. Thus if skin exposure is minimized, heat loss can be minimized too.

Q. Why do anesthetized animals frequently become hypothermic?

A. Anesthesia inhibits thermoregulation in a dose-dependent manner and routinely results in hypothermia. The effects of anesthesia on thermoregulation are multifactorial and include: the loss of normal behavioral responses, the enlargement of the inter-threshold range which alters the trigger at which normal thermoregulatory responses occur, and the effects of anesthetic drugs.

✓ Loss of normal behaviors: Anesthetized animals are unable to perform heat sparing behaviors such as curling in a circle, avoiding cold conduction areas (metal surgical tables) or moving towards warmth.

✓ Body temperatures outside of the inter-threshold range normally trigger a response from the hypothalamus: Anesthetic drugs (e.g., opioids, propofol) can blunt the hypothalamic sensing of temperatures outside normal range, which effectively increases the inter-threshold range, lowering or abolishing the threshold for shivering.

✓ Inhalant anesthetics (e.g., isoflurane) cause vasodilation which contributes to heat loss. Regional anesthetics also can lead to loss of thermoregulatory control due to vasodilation at sites blocked (potentially large surface areas), loss of ability to shiver, and altered thermal sensors at the blocked sites. Furthermore, many patients are sedated, in addition to the regional blocks, which can contribute to loss of thermoregulation.

In humans, the inter-threshold range can increase 3–4-fold from normal with regional anesthesia [5].

Q. When are anesthetized animals most likely to become hypothermic?

A. Loss of core body temperature occurs in three phases. The first phase occurs during the first hour of anesthesia. Due to redistribution of heat from the core to the periphery, there is a large drop in body temperature which is then easily lost. Dogs without supplemental heat can lose almost 2 °C in the first hour of anesthesia [6]. The second phase occurs over the next 2–5 h. There is a slow linear drop in temperature due to the increase in heat loss compared to heat production. The final phase occurs late in the anesthetic period, ~3–5 h after the beginning of anesthesia. During this time there is a thermal plateau, or steady state, where core temperature remains fairly unchanged.

Q. What are the physiologic consequences of hypothermia?

A. Subnormal body temperature decreases basal metabolic rate and oxygen consumption and can be used clinically for those advantages (e.g., preventing myocardial or CNS ischemia) [7]. However, unintentional hypothermia is associated with a host of unwanted and potentially-life threatening complications. Effects of hypothermia include the following.

✓ *Immune system/healing*: Hypothermia impairs the immune systems by decreasing oxidative killing by neutrophils, reduction of phagocytosis, suppression of leukocyte migration, protein wasting, and decreased synthesis of collagen. Furthermore, vasoconstriction and increased viscosity decreases oxygen delivery to tissues which can contribute to poor wound healing. In humans, hypothermia triples wound infection rates compared with normothermic patients [8].

✓ *Hematology and coagulation*: Hypothermia causes an increased viscosity of blood and slows enzymatic reactions of intrinsic and extrinsic coagulation pathways. There is reduced platelet function and a reversible prolongation of coagulation times [9]. In humans, hypothermic patients lose more blood and require more transfusions than equally matched normothermic patients [10].

✓ *Cardiovascular*: Hypothermia decreases cardiac output, increases norepinephrine release, and causes vasoconstriction. With rewarming, increased capacitance (vasodilation) can unmask hypovolemia or relative hypovolemia and precipitate shock-like episodes. In dogs, arrhythmias are likely at a core body temperature of ~31 °C (87.8 °F) and ventricular fibrillation is likely with temperatures below 30 °C (86 °F) [11].

✓ *Metabolism*: Hypothermia is associated with decreased liver and renal blood flow. This results in decreased liver metabolism and renal excretion. The slowed metabolism of anesthetic drugs can lead to prolonged recovery times and the potential for relative overdosing.

✓ *Consequences of shivering*: Shivering increases metabolism (2–3-fold) and can increase heat production by 500%. Although it is effective in raising body temperature, shivering increases myocardial oxygen demands, glucose needs, and raises intra-cranial and intra-ocular pressure. Aside from the metabolic demands of shivering, humans often describe it as the most unpleasant memory of their perioperative experience.

✓ *Increased morbidity*: Human studies have repeatedly shown that even mild intra-operative hypothermia is associated with increased time in ICU and total increased hospitalization times [8]. Although no veterinary studies have looked at the morbidity associated with hypothermia, it is reasonable to believe that similar increases in morbidity might occur.

✓ *Shift in the oxygen dissociation curve*: Hypothermia is associated with a left shift to the oxygen dissociation curve. This shift results in greater binding of oxygen to hemoglobin and less offloading of oxygen at the tissue level. It is possible that the poor offloading in conjunction with vasoconstriction will decrease tissue oxygenation. As the patient rewarms, the oxygen dissociation curve will return to normal and more offloading can cause a decrease in peripheral hemoglobin saturation.

✓ *Decrease in MAC*: Decreased body temperature is associated with a decrease in minimum alveolar concentration (MAC) of volatile inhalant anesthetics. The decreased requirement for inhalants coupled with slowed metabolism can increase the risk of anesthetic overdose.

✓ *Acidemia*: Poor tissue perfusion, from vasoconstriction, decreased cardiac output, and shifting of the oxygen dissociation curve can result in anaerobic metabolism and the production of lactic acid. With rewarming, lactic acid from poorly perfused areas mixes with core blood and results in a systemic metabolic acidosis. Derangements in acid/base status can be detrimental if not monitored and addressed.

Q. Is it easier to prevent hypothermia or to treat it?

A. Prevention of peri-operative hypothermia is easier than treatment. Pre-induction skin warming is the only way to prevent redistribution of core heat to the skin (redistribution hypothermia) [12]. Since the skin is the major source of heat loss during anesthesia, cutaneous heat loss can be decreased by 30% by simply covering the skin. A warm ambient temperature can help maintain normothermia but can cause discomfort for hospital staff. It also is important to know which anesthetic drugs can inhibit thermoregulatory responses. For example, meperidine can abolish the shivering response.

Q. What are best ways to warm a hypothermic patient during or after anesthesia?

A. Treatment of hypothermia should be directed at preventing further heat loss as well as providing active warming. Prevention of heat loss could include covering of non-essential exposed skin, the administration of warmed fluids, and exposure to a warm environment when possible. Skin covering can be accomplished with blankets, plastic, metallic/reflective sheets, or a combination. Heat and humidity exchangers can be used in the anesthetic circuit to prevent the body from having to warm and humidify cold dry anesthetic gases.

Active warming increases the total heat content by the net transfer of heat to the body via external heating source. Such heating sources can include forced warm air blankets, electrical heating blankets, circulating warm water blankets, and heat lamps. Circulating warm water blankets are more effective when placed over the patient as they provide external warmth as well as prevent radiative heat loss. Cotton or reflective blankets can be placed over circulating water or forced air blankets to increase insulation. Caution should be used with any heating source to assure that the patient cannot be burned or become dehydrated.

The transfer of body heat to cold intravenous fluids can contribute to loss of core body temperature. The amount of heat loss is dependent on the temperature and the amount of fluid infused. Thus warming intravenous fluids can minimize heat loss.

In cases of extreme hypothermia, peritoneal and pleural irrigation with warm saline can effectively change core body temperature. Cardiopulmonary bypass has been used successfully in humans as a means to actively rewarm a patient with excellent long-term outcomes.

Q. Can anesthetized animals become hyperthermic?

A. Although hypothermia is common in animals under anesthesia, occasionally hyperthermia is observed. Hyperthermia can result from anatomical or breed differences in patients, (e.g., long-haired breeds, fat animals), excessive external heat supply, drug reactions, or hypermetabolic disease states (e.g., fever, malignant hyperthermia). Careful temperature monitoring of all anesthetized patients will identify animals that need more or less thermal support. Panting may be misinterpreted as a sign that the animal is light; in these instances body temperature should be checked to ensure that the patient is not, in fact, too hot!

Q. Why do some cats become hyperthermic following anesthesia?

A. All opioids can result in an elevated body temperature in cats. The degree of hyperthermia appears to be more associated with full mu opioid agonists (e.g., hydromorphone) and in cats that have been anesthetized. Although not proven, it is likely that opioid drugs alter the thermoregulatory set point in cats and that cats that become cold during anesthesia have an exaggerated response and "overshoot" their temperature set point. Affected cats have been documented to have body temperatures in excess of 41.7 °C (107 °F). Interestingly there has not been any documented morbidity and mortality in these cats. The hyperthermia is transient and normally resolves within 3–4 h (about the duration of the opioid drugs).

Interestingly, treatment of hyperthermia in cats with NSAIDs does not lower body temperature; however, reversal of the opioid drugs does (supporting the opioid causation) [13,14]. Treatment of hyperthermia is primarily supportive. Hyperthermic cats should have external heating sources removed and should be monitored for signs of distress and dehydration. Reversal with naloxone or butorphanol can be considered if the hyperthermia is severe. For cats that have had an opioid reversal, other methods of analgesia need to be provided.

References

1 Kahn CM, Line S (ed.). Reference guides. In: *The Merck Veterinary Manual*, 9th edn. Whitehouse Station, NJ: Merck & Company, 2010: 2582.

2 Matsukawa T, Sessler DI, Sessler AM, *et al.* Heat flow and distribution during induction of general anesthesia. *Anesthesiology* 1995; **82(3)**:662–673.

3 Marieb EN, Hoehn K. Nutrition, metabolism, and body temperature regulation. In: *Anatomy & Physiology*. 3rd edn. San Francisco CA: Pearson Education, 2007:871–872.

4 Davis P, Parbrook G, Kenny G. Temperature. In *Basic Physics and Measurements in Anesthesia*. 4th edn. Boston MA: Butterworth Heinemann, 2002:115–124.

5 Sessler DI. Mild perioperative hypothermia. *New England Journal of Medicine* 1997; **336(24)**:1730–1737.

6 Tan C, Govendir M, Zaki S, *et al.* Evaluation of four warming procedures to minimise heat loss induced by anaesthesia and surgery in dogs. *Australian Veterinary Journal* 2004; **82(1–2)**:65–68.

7 Wass CT, Lanier WL, Hofer RE, *et al.* Temperature changes of > or = 1 degree C alter functional neurologic outcome and histopathology in a canine model of complete cerebral ischemia. *Anesthesiology* 1995; **83(2)**:325–335.

8 Kurz A, Sessler DI, Lenhardt R. Perioperative normothermia to reduce the incidence of surgical-wound infection and shorten hospitalization. Study of Wound Infection and Temperature Group. *New England Journal of Medicine* 1996; **334(19)**:1209–1215.

9 Ao H, Moon JK, Tashiro M, *et al.* Delayed platelet dysfunction in prolonged induced canine hypothermia. *Resuscitation* 2001; **51(1)**:83–90.

10 Schmied H, Kurz A, Sessler DI, *et al.* Mild hypothermia increases blood loss and transfusion requirements during total hip arthroplasty. *Lancet* 1996; **347(8997)**:289–292.

11 Mortensen E, Berntsen R, Tveita T, *et al.* Changes in ventricular fibrillation threshold during acute hypothermia. A model for future studies. *Journal of Basic and Clinical Physiology and Pharmacology* 1993; **4(4)**:313–319.

12 Camus Y, Delva E, Sessler DI, *et al.* Pre-induction skin-surface warming minimizes intraoperative core hypothermia. *Journal of Clinical Anesthesia* 1995; **7(5)**:384–388.

13 Posner LP, Pavuk AA, Rokshar JL, *et al.* Effects of opioids and anesthetic drugs on body temperature in cats. *Veterinary Anaesthesia and Analgesia* 2010; **37(1)**:35–43.

14 Niedfeldt RL, Robertson SA. Postanesthetic hyperthermia in cats: a retrospective comparison between hydromorphone and buprenorphine. *Veterinary Anaesthesia and Analgesia* 2006; **33(6)**:381–389.

21 Common Arrhythmias in Anesthetized Patients

Is that ECG normal?

Benjamin M. Brainard and Gregg S. Rapoport

College of Veterinary Medicine, University of Georgia, USA

KEY POINTS:

- A normal ECG tracing consists of a P wave followed by a QRS and T wave for every beat.
- Ventricular tachycardia can compromise cardiac output and should be treated.
- AV block is common with high vagal tone, opioid administration, and alpha-2 agonist administration.
- Sinus tachycardia may occur in patients that are too light, need more analgesia, or are volume depleted.
- Pulseless electrical activity (PEA) is a cardiopulmonary arrest rhythm and CPR should be initiated immediately.

Q. What is the appropriate placement for ECG leads in a small animal?

A. For purposes of anesthesia, the main utility of ECG monitoring is to display a rhythm strip so the anesthetist can evaluate the rate, regularity, and pattern of cardiac conduction. Classically, this is accomplished in small animal patients by following a lead II trace, with the right arm (white) lead placed in the right axilla, or on the right leg, of the patient. The left arm (black) lead may be placed on the left leg in a similar manner. The hind limb (red) lead is placed on the left hind limb or in the inguinal area. Because the ECG is a galvanometer, it will display the electrical activity of whatever is placed between the two electrodes. In the context of surgery where a limb might not be easily available (e.g., amputation), the leads can be positioned so that the heart lies between the white and red electrode (e.g., by placing a lead on the lateral thorax), or other ECG options (e.g., lead I or III) may be evaluated to find the tracing that best displays the waves of the ECG pattern and allows for diagnosis of arrhythmias during anesthesia.

Questions and Answers in Small Animal Anesthesia, First Edition. Edited by Lesley J. Smith.
© 2016 John Wiley & Sons, Inc. Published 2016 by John Wiley & Sons, Inc.

Q. What are the parts of an ECG tracing?

A. Each ECG tracing should have a P wave (corresponding with atrial electrical activity), a QRS complex (corresponding to ventricular electrical activity), and a T wave (representing ventricular repolarization). The general appearance of these waves, in a lead II tracing, are illustrated and labeled in Figure 21.1a.

Q. How can you calculate the heart rate from an ECG tracing?

A. When the ECG is run at 25 mm/s (the usual paper speed for small animal patients), each large box on the paper is equal to 1/5 of a second, and each set of 5 large boxes (usually indicated by a black mark at the base of the grid) is equivalent to 1 second of ECG. To calculate the rate, a 3 s interval (3 sets of large boxes, or three black marks) is chosen and the number of QRS complexes in that interval is counted. This number is multiplied by 20 to calculate the beats per minute. At 50 mm/s, 3 sets of large boxes is equivalent to 1.5 s and the number of QRS complexes should be multiplied by 40 to calculate beats/min. Commercially available ECG monitors with variable speeds and

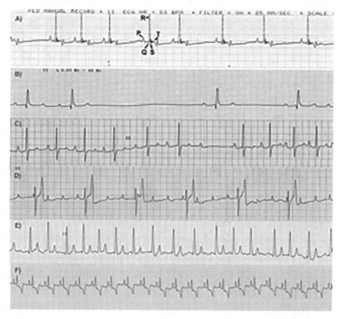

Figure 21.1 Sinus Rhythms. **A.** Normal Sinus Rhythm. **B.** 1st degree AV Block. Note the prolonged interval between the P and QRS complex, but every P wave is followed by a QRS. **C.** 2nd degree AV Block. Note that some P waves are not followed by a QRS and the overall rate is slow **D.** 3rd degree AV block. Note that the P waves occur independently and the QRS complexes have a wide and bizarre appearance with a slow rate **E.** Atrial Fibrillation. Note the undulating baseline, absence of discernable P waves, and the irregularly irregular pattern to the rhythm. **F.** ST segment depression. Note the abnormal "slurred" appearance of the ST interval.

printer functions are available and these allow traces to be printed out and the heart rate calculated more easily in patients with extreme tachycardia or rapidly changing rhythms.

Q. What is a step-wise method for analyzing the ECG tracing?

A. ✓ Calculate the rate. In awake animals, tachycardia may be considered as a rate greater than 160 beats/min in a dog and greater than 200 beats/min in a cat, while bradycardia is considered a rate less than 45 beats/min in a dog, and less than 160 beats/min in cats. Due to the influence of anesthetic drugs, animals may display relative bradycardia during anesthetic events that may be considered normal or appropriate.

✓ Note the regularity of the QRS complexes and characterize the rhythm as regular or irregular. Patients that have respiratory sinus arrhythmia (rhythmic variation as a consequence of changes in intrathoracic pressure that occur with breathing) have a regularly irregular rhythm, in that it is irregular in a predictable way. Dogs with atrial fibrillation have an irregularly irregular rhythm, without any discernible pattern to the irregularity.

✓ Evaluate the tracing for P waves. Verify that a P wave precedes every QRS complex. Also, evaluate the distance between the P wave and each QRS and verify that it is equal for all complexes. In patients with AV block, the P–R interval may vary or some P waves may not correspond reliably with a QRS complex. In patients with ventricular or junctional arrhythmias, a QRS complex will occur without an associated P wave.

✓ Verify that there is a QRS complex for every identified P wave. QRS complexes without P waves may be ventricular in origin or they may arise from the AV junction (the portion of the conduction systemic including the AV node plus the bundle of His).

Q. How do I distinguish artifacts on an ECG from real cardiac activity?

A. True premature complexes generally disrupt the underlying sinus rhythm. Artifacts which "masquerade" as premature complexes do not disturb the underlying rhythm. Artifacts that are generated by the ECG machine may also occur at random points throughout the ECG trace, while ECG tracings representing true cardiac electrical activity will generally happen at the same point in each cardiac cycle. Additionally, ECG artifacts will not cause a pulse deficit if pulses are being palpated, nor will they cause a pulse deficit in a displayed pulse oximeter waveform or direct arterial blood pressure trace. True ECG activity will be associated with a pulse wave for every observed QRS complex. A common source of ECG artifact is 60 cycle "noise" from other electrical devices in the operating room. This will look like a finely jagged baseline on the ECG.

Q. What is the appropriate diagnostic and therapeutic approach for a patient demonstrating sinus tachycardia under anesthesia?

A. Sinus tachycardia (ST), usually defined as a sinus rhythm greater than 160 beats/min in a dog and greater than 200 beats/min in a cat, occurs frequently in animals under anesthesia. The conformation of the ECG is normal, but the rate is too rapid. Observation of ST should prompt an immediate assessment of the patient, including blood pressure, capillary refill time (CRT), and depth of anesthesia. ST may result from inadequate anesthetic depth or inappropriate analgesia, and these aspects should be evaluated as well. Additionally, equipment malfunction that causes elevations in arterial CO_2 (e.g., malfunctioning valves or expired CO_2 absorbent) or a kinked endotracheal tube can result in ST because of the associated catecholamine release. Intra-operative occurrences, such as hemorrhage or a pneumothorax, can also cause ST. Iatrogenic ST can also occur with inadvertent boluses of inotropes (e.g., dopamine or dobutamine) or after treatment of bradycardia with atropine or glycopyrrolate. Once appropriate depth of anesthesia and analgesia have been confirmed, the volume status of the animal should be assessed; hypovolemia will result in ST as the heart compensates for decreased stroke volume with an increased heart rate. In this case, the CRT is prolonged as well. Chapter 17 outlines treatment strategies for hypovolemia and hypotension.

Q. What is the difference between first-, second-, and third-degree AV block?

A. First-degree AV block (Figure 21.1b) describes a prolonged interval between the P wave and start of the QRS complex (i.e., greater than 130 ms in the dog and 90 ms in the cat). In anesthetized patients, first-degree AV block is not considered pathologic. Second-degree AV block (Figure 21.1c) describes a situation where some P waves are not followed by QRS complexes, due to intermittent lack of conduction through the AV node. There are two types of second-degree AV block. Mobitz type I second-degree AV block (also known as Wenckebach rhythm) includes a progressive prolongation of the P–R interval, eventually leading to a "dropped beat" with no QRS complex. In cases of Mobitz type II second-degree AV block, P–R intervals are of fixed duration. Second-degree AV block is commonly seen secondary to high vagal tone, and may be caused by alpha-2 agonist or opioid drugs. Third-degree AV block (Figure 21.1d) is one form of AV dissociation, wherein there is no relationship between atrial depolarization (P waves) and ventricular depolarization (QRS complexes). Specifically, the QRS (ventricular) rate is comprised of a slower escape rhythm, while the P wave (atrial) rate is faster and generated from the SA node. In most dogs, the escape rhythm usually originates in the ventricles, generating wide QRS complexes at a slow rate. In fewer dogs and in most cats with third-degree AV block, the escape rhythm arises from the AV junction (which includes the AV node and bundle of His), generating QRS complexes that are narrow and normal in appearance. The majority of dogs with this bradyarrhythmia are symptomatic and require artificial pacemaker implantation. Some cats have a high enough escape rate (e.g., 100–120 beats/min) that they remain asymptomatic and do not require therapy.

Q. When should the anesthetist treat AV block?

A. First-degree AV block does not require therapy. Second-degree AV block that results in hypotension or unacceptable bradycardia may require treatment. If the AV block is due to elevated vagal tone (e.g., during ophthalmologic surgery, from an oculocardiac reflex, or secondary to the use of potent opioid analgesics), an anticholinergic medication is indicated. Both atropine and glycopyrrolate are appropriate treatments. Anticholinergics may initially worsen the bradyarrhythmia before heart rate increases. Occasionally, a second dose of anticholinergic may be required. Second-degree AV block caused by alpha-2 agonists should *not* be treated, as a first step, with anticholinergics (see Chapters 7 and 17).

Q. What are the ECG characteristics of atrial fibrillation? What medications can be used to slow the rate? What underlying diseases are usually associated with atrial fibrillation in dogs?

A. Atrial fibrillation is a supraventricular tachyarrhythmia in which electrical impulses are rapidly and chaotically generated by non-nodal atrial tissue, rather than the SA node (Figure 21.1e). Because of the supraventricular site of origin, QRS complexes are generally narrow and appear normal. Conduction of impulses through the AV node is also haphazard, which results in an irregularly irregular rhythm. Heart rate is generally high although exceptions do occur. Due to a lack of coordinated atrial depolarization, P waves will be absent, replaced with fibrillation waves, or an undulating baseline between the QRS complexes. Atrial fibrillation in dogs most often results from diseases that induce significant atrial enlargement, notably dilated cardiomyopathy and advanced mitral valve insufficiency. Atrial fibrillation *can* occur in the absence of significant structural heart disease and is typically seen in larger dog breeds such as Irish wolfhounds and Newfoundlands. This "normal" atrial fibrillation may occur without tachycardia ("slow a-fib"). Atrial fibrillation is less frequently seen in cats but can occur with severe heart disease. Treatment of atrial fibrillation in small animals is generally focused on slowing the ventricular response rate. Diltiazem is the most common drug utilized for this purpose, with digoxin and beta-adrenergic blocking drugs (e.g., atenelol) being other options. The latter may result in negative inotropy and should only be used if the patient can tolerate a decrease in cardiac output. Beta-blocking drugs are also contraindicated in cases with congestive heart failure.

Q. Following a lead-II ECG rhythm, you note that the P waves are either no longer visible or have disappeared. What can you do to verify the lack or presence of P waves?

A. Most ECG machines have the ability to display leads I through III of a standard ECG; if the patient has moved or the P wave amplitude is not visible in one lead, checking the other two leads may provide an adequate tracing for rhythm analysis. Alternatively, it may be necessary to replace one or more of the leads to improve the orientation with respect to the cardiac electrical

activity. If P wave flattening or absence is suspected or confirmed, then hyperkalemia should be quickly ruled out as a potential cause. ECG changes associated with hyperkalemia, and treatment of this electrolyte abnormality, are
covered in Chapter 36.

Q. What is the significance of ST segment depression on the ECG?

A. ST segment depression (Figure 21.1f) may be associated with myocardial
hypoxia, such as might result from shock or myocardial infarction. At any
point where myocardial oxygen demand exceeds delivery, ST segment
depression may be seen. If an ECG shows a new ST segment depression, the
anesthetist should evaluate the patient's oxygen delivery parameters (blood
pressure, S_pO_2, PCV).

Q. What is the ECG appearance of bundle branch block? What is the diagnostic
significance?

A. Bundle branch block refers to a rhythm in which the initiating impulse originates in the SA node as usual (thus there is a P wave for each QRS complex)
but is "blocked" as it travels through one of the bundle branches. Since the
ventricle on the blocked side is not activated through the normal, fast conduction system, and instead must be depolarized via slow cell-to-cell conduction, the QRS complex is markedly widened (Figure 21.2a). Conditions that
can cause a bundle branch block may include myocardial ischemia or scar-
ring, inflammatory changes in the myocardium, neoplasia, or infection. Right
bundle branch block may also occur as an idiopathic and incidental finding.
Treatment should be directed at the underlying condition.

Q. What is the difference between an idioventricular rhythm and ventricular
tachycardia?

A. Both of these are wide-complex arrhythmias, due to the fact that the impulses
generating them arise from within the ventricles and are transmitted outside
of the normal cardiac conduction system. This generates the classic wide and
bizarre appearance of a ventricular premature complex on ECG. Ventricular tachycardia (VT) is generally regarded as a series of at least four complexes of ventricular origin, occurring at a rate greater than 160 beats/min
(Figure 21.2b). An accelerated idioventricular rhythm has a similar morpho-
logic appearance but occurs at rates less than 160 beats/min (but greater
than a ventricular escape rate, which is generally ~ 40 beats/min in the dog)
(Figure 21.2e).

Q. When should ventricular rhythms be treated?

A. Ventricular tachyarrhythmias may warrant anti-arrhythmic therapy. While
the decision to treat (or not treat) requires case-by-case evaluation, criteria
favoring treatment include the presence of one or more of the following: ventricular tachycardia, multiform VPCs (which describe ventricular
complexes suspected to originate from different areas of the ventricle
based on differing morphology; see Figure 21.1c), R-on-T phenomenon
(which describes the initiation of ventricular depolarization prior to full

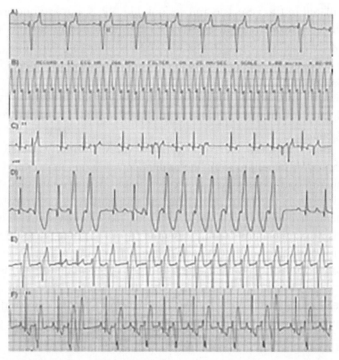

Figure 21.2 Ventricular Abnormalities or Arrhythmias. **A.** Bundle Branch Block. Note the widened base of the QRS complex, sometimes with a step-like appearance at the upstroke of the Q or downstroke of the S components. **B.** Ventricular Tachycardia. Note the fast rate, absence of P waves, and rapid bizarre looking QRS complexes. **C.** Multi-form Ventricular Premature Complexes (VPC). Note that the wide and bizarre appearance of the VPCs changes along the sample strip. **D.** R-on-T phenomenon. Note that the T wave occurs very early and during completion of the QRS complex, rather than after it. **E.** Accelerated idioventricular rhythm. Note the presence of some P waves, and the relatively normal rate of the VPCs (i.e. > 45 beats/min and < 160 beats/min). **F.** Ventricular Bigeminy classic for thiobarbiturate drugs. Note that a normal beat (P-QRS-T) alternates with a VPC. This rhythm is usually transient and resolves a few minutes after thiobarbiturate administration.

repolarization of the previous complex; see Figure 21.2d), and ventricular rhythms that result in adverse hemodynamic consequences such as systemic hypotension. Generally, therapy for ventricular tachyarrhythmias can begin with a class I anti-arrhythmic such as lidocaine or procainamide, both of which can be administered IV. Oral drugs like sotalol (a mixed class II/III agent) may be used if the arrhythmia persists once the animal is awake. Accelerated idioventricular rhythms (Figure 21.2f) generally do not require anti-arrhythmic therapy due to their typically benign features and hemodynamic stability. Animals with third-degree AV block will have a very slow idioventricular rhythm, or a ventricular escape rhythm, and P waves that are not followed by normal QRS complexes. These beats also are initiated in the ventricle and so look like VPCs, but are not premature. Ventricular anti-arrhythmic agents are contraindicated in patients with this bradyarrhythmia, and pacemaker therapy should be considered.

Q. What arrhythmias are associated with the use of thiobarbiturates for anesthetic induction?

A. Ventricular premature complexes, classically manifesting as ventricular bigeminy (alternating sinus-origin and ventricular-origin complexes (Figure 21.2f).

Q. What does pulseless electrical activity (PEA, formerly called electromechanical dissociation) look like on ECG?

A. During cardiopulmonary arrest, electrical impulses may continue to be transmitted through the heart, even though this activity is not translated into ventricular contraction. The ECG will look like normal sinus rhythm, but there is no cardiac output and, consequently, no palpable pulses. If monitoring with capnometry, the CO_2 will decrease to $\leq$ 10 mm Hg. This condition should be treated as a cardiac arrest, and the appropriate therapy is to institute cardiopulmonary resuscitation. As cardiac arrest persists, the relatively normal looking initial PEA tracing will develop a wider QRS and eventually appear as a slow QRS rate with no identifiable P waves, which generally progresses to either ventricular fibrillation or asystole.

22 Constant Rate Infusions

Just drip it in!

Carolyn Kerr

Department of Clinical Studies, Ontario Veterinary College, University of Guelph, Canada

---

KEY POINTS:

- A CRI of a drug or drugs provides more steady-state plasma concentrations than intermittent bolus administration.
- CRIs are commonly used to provide supplemental analgesia and to reduce inhalant requirements.
- Common opioids that are administered as a CRI include fentanyl, morphine, and hydromorphone.
- A loading dose of drug ensures that effective plasma concentrations are reached quickly.
- Ketamine CRIs can also be used, alone or in combination, to provide analgesia.
- Lidocaine CRIs also provide analgesia and reduce inhalant requirement, but should be reserved for use in dogs only.

Q. What is a constant rate infusion?

A. A constant, or continuous, rate infusion (CRI) refers to the continuous administration of a dose of drug per unit of time. In veterinary medicine, CRIs are mostly commonly administered via the intravenous route with infusion doses and rates expressed as (mcg or mg)/kg/min or (mcg or mg)/kg/h. The goal of administering a drug as a CRI is to achieve and maintain a constant target concentration of drug in the blood for a desired period of time. As drugs have different patterns of distribution, metabolism, and excretion from the body (pharmacokinetic properties), they are administered at either a fixed rate or a variable rate to achieve constant plasma concentrations.

Q. Why administer drugs as a CRI?

A. Although the drugs we administer as a CRI in the peri-anesthetic period do not exert their effect in the vascular space, but rather at an effect (or receptor) site, the plasma concentrations generally correlate with clinical effects. Above a certain plasma level, the effect is excessive and below a certain level, the effects are inadequate. The traditional method of administering intermittent

---

Questions and Answers in Small Animal Anesthesia, First Edition. Edited by Lesley J. Smith.
© 2016 John Wiley & Sons, Inc. Published 2016 by John Wiley & Sons, Inc.

boluses of a drug intravenously results in peaks and valleys in that drug's plasma concentrations, with corresponding waxing and waning of clinical effect. By administering a drug as a CRI, a near-constant plasma concentration of drug within the therapeutic range can be achieved, thereby producing a more consistent clinical effect and minimizing the risk of drug under- or overdosing. Moreover, it may be easier to titrate the administration of a drug to achieve the desired clinical effect compared with an intermittent bolus technique. When a drug is given as a CRI versus intermittent boluses, less quantity of drug is administered overall and the time from discontinuation of drug administration to termination of drug effect is generally more rapid and predictable.

Q. What are common reasons to administer anesthetic/analgesic drugs by CRI?

A. In veterinary medicine, some of the more common reasons for administering injectable drugs as infusions in the peri-anesthetic period include:

✓ providing and/or improving analgesia;

✓ reducing inhalant anesthetic requirements;

✓ producing a more stable anesthetic plane;

✓ providing hemodynamic support.

Q. What is a loading dose and how do I know if I need to administer one if I plan on performing a CRI?

A. When a clinician starts a CRI, the goal is generally to achieve target drug levels in a short period of time. The half-life of a drug is the sole factor that influences the rise in plasma concentrations to achieve the desired plasma concentrations at steady state when a drug is administered as an infusion [1]. When a drug is administered as a CRI, after five half-lives 97% of the desired plateau concentration will have been achieved. Clearly, the shorter a drug's half-life, the faster the desired steady-state plasma concentration is reached. For many drugs it would take a considerable amount of time to achieve the desired blood concentrations if the initial method of administration was only a CRI without a loading dose. For example, the half-life of morphine is approximately 60 min in the dog; therefore, it would take 5 h to achieve the desired plateau concentration if the mode of administration was via a CRI alone. Recommended hourly rates of CRI drug administration generally assume the infusion is being administered following a loading dose of the drug that is being administered as an infusion. There are exceptions; for example, dopamine, dobutamine, and norepinephrine are drugs that do not need a loading dose to rapidly achieve desired concentrations due to their extremely short half-lives (see Chapter 17).

Loading doses can be administered as either a bolus or short-duration infusion to minimize the acute side effects associated with rapid increases in plasma concentrations of a drug. The loading dose is calculated as the desired plasma drug concentration multiplied by the volume of distribution at peak effect

[2]. In veterinary medicine, the desired plasma concentrations or the volume of distribution at peak effect for individual drugs are rarely known, but clinical experience and extrapolation from research data has resulted in recommended doses that can be used as the loading dose.

Q. How is an infusion rate determined?

A. The recommended infusion rate for a drug is calculated by multiplying the desired plasma drug concentration by the clearance [1]. Pharmacokinetic data may have resulted in published recommended infusion rates for some drugs that are administered in veterinary patients. When published infusion rates are not available, an alternative approach for the clinician is to divide the effective dose by the typical duration of effect. For example, hydromorphone can be administered as a CRI. The typical dose recommended in the canine is 0.1–0.2 mg/kg and its duration of effect is approximately 4 h. The hourly infusion rate would therefore be 0.1–0.2 mg/kg divided by 4 h resulting in an infusion rate of 0.025–0.05 mg/kg/h [3].

While pharmacokinetic data or clinical experience can be used to determine an approximate infusion rate, they should be used only as a guide and each patient receiving a CRI should be assessed individually for their response to treatment, both desirable and undesirable. One of the major advantages of using a CRI is the ability to "fine tune" the dose of drug administration without inducing major changes in the degree of the desired effects, as might occur with a bolus administration.

Q. When a drug CRI is terminated, how long will the effects of the drug last?

A. Ideally, when a drug CRI is stopped, the plasma concentration declines and effects diminish in a predictable manner. The decrease in plasma drug concentration at the end of the CRI is dependent on the elimination of drug from the plasma [1]. Elimination includes distribution out of the plasma as well as removal by metabolism and excretion. The context sensitive half-time is the time for the plasma concentration to decrease by 50% after an infusion of specified duration is terminated. This variable is a good predictor of the duration of effect following the termination of an infusion.

Q. Are there different methods by which a CRI can be delivered?

A. The short answer is that most CRIs are delivered by syringe pump or by adding the drug(s) to a bag of IV fluids. In general, when contemplating using a CRI, start by considering the anticipated duration of administration, the patient's ideal body weight, and the dose. Infusions should be administered through a secure intravenous catheter. While some systems of delivery may have alarms to indicate a delivery failure, it is highly recommended that the site of the catheter be routinely inspected, as extravascular administration will result in treatment failure.

Advantages of syringe pumps include safety, convenience, ease of adjusting the infusion rate, and minimization of drug wastage, as the quantity of drug prepared can be closely matched to the quantity required. Syringe pumps are available with many different options including syringe size compatibility, alarm settings, and programmability. With some pumps there is the ability to enter the patient weight, dose, and drug concentration, which reduces the probability of mathematical errors by the operator. Quick verification of the accuracy of a pump can be determined prior to use by setting the pump to deliver a volume and rate similar to that anticipated for your patient and observing the delivered volume over 15–30 min. Individuals responsible for monitoring patients receiving infusions should be directed to verify that the desired administration volume has been delivered on a regular basis.

In many instances, the commercially available preparation of the drug is used. In some instances, however, the drug may need to be diluted with saline to accommodate suitable syringe sizes for the pump and limitations of the pump in the minimal volume that can be delivered in a given time. For example, ketamine at 100 mg/ml is often diluted to 10 mg/ml for dogs and to 1 mg/ml for cats or very small dogs in order for the syringe pump to accurately deliver the dose in mcg/kg/min.

The second option of adding CRI drugs to IV fluids allows the patient to receive both their IV fluid therapy and the adjunctive CRI drugs via the same IV line and without the expense of a syringe pump. The concentration of drug to allow delivery of the hourly fluid rate and the appropriate drug dose will need to be calculated. Risks of combining drugs into intravenous fluids include the potential of creating fluctuations in drug delivery due to inadequate mixing of drug with the intravenous fluid or (rarely) incompatibility of the drug with the fluid used as the diluent. Once drugs are added to intravenous fluids, ideally they are administered as a CRI using a fluid pump to accurately control drug delivery. Even with a fluid pump, accuracy of drug delivery is not 100% ensured. A recent case report detailed an overdose of lidocaine delivered by fluid pump to a dog [4]. If a fluid pump is not available, the drug concentration and drip set should be selected to permit a reasonable estimate of drops per second for delivery of the desired dose of the drug and fluid. If a prolonged duration of administration is not anticipated, a buretrol can be used to permit adjustments in drug delivery in short time periods. In this instance, the fluid administration volume for a set time period such as an hour (depending on patient size and buretrol size) can be placed in the buretrol with the appropriate quantity of drug.

Q. What drugs are commonly administered as a CRI with the goal of providing analgesia?

A. Drugs most commonly administered as a CRI to provide analgesia, in either the conscious patient or the patient under anesthesia, include opioids, ketamine, and lidocaine. The latter is only recommended for use in dogs. An opioid analgesic is generally selected first with other agents added as

Table 22.1 Recommended intravenous loading and infusion rates of drugs administered as analgesics in dogs and cats.

Drug	Loading dose	Infusion dose
Fentanyl	3–10 mcg/kg	5–10 mcg/kg/h
Hydromorphone	0.05–0.2 mg/kg	0.0125 – 0.05 mg/kg/h
Ketamine	0.5–2 mg/kg	2–10 mcg/kg/min (0.012–0.6 mg/kg/h)
Lidocaine(Canine only)	1 mg/kg	25–100 mcg/kg/min (1.5–6 mg/kg/h)
Morphine	0.1–0.2 mg/kg	0.1–0.25 mg/kg/h

needed to achieve the desired level of analgesia. Specific drugs administered as a CRI to provide analgesia and their recommended loading doses and infusion rates are outlined in Table 22.1. Further details on dose selection are provided below.

Q. Can more than one agent be administered as a CRI at a time to a patient to increase analgesia?

A. Many times, clinicians elect to use more than one agent to provide optimal analgesia with minimal side effects. Two basic approaches are used when more than one type of agent is being administered as an infusion to a patient. Drugs can be added sequentially to a treatment regime as needed to achieve a desired level of analgesia or agents can be combined and administered concurrently. For example, in the former approach, the clinician typically starts by administering an opioid analgesic and if the level of analgesia were inadequate despite dose adjustments, ketamine would be added to the patient's treatment regime. If inadequate analgesia were achieved with the combination of an opioid and ketamine, lidocaine would also be added to the analgesic regime. An example of the latter approach would be the administration of a mixture of fixed doses of morphine, lidocaine, and ketamine.

Q. What are some advantages and disadvantages of opioid analgesics typically administered as a CRI to dogs and cats?

A. Overall, drugs within the opioid group are highly effective analgesics that are suited to administration as a CRI pre-operatively, intra-operatively and post-operatively. When administered in the anesthetic period, they can dramatically reduce anesthetic drug requirements in a dose-dependent manner. When administered alone to healthy patients by a CRI, opioids typically result in a mild reduction in heart rate and blood pressure but have minimal respiratory effects. Despite having some cardiovascular depressant effects, hemodynamic stability is generally improved when opioids are administered to patients under inhalant-based anesthesia, due to the 40–60% reduction in anesthetic requirements. To maximize the hemodynamic benefit of including an opioid CRI during anesthesia, however, the anesthetist must assess the patient's depth of anesthesia and reduce the delivery of inhalant anesthetics. While opioid drugs do not significantly depress ventilation when administered alone, when administered in combination with other CNS depressant agents (i.e., inhalant anesthetics or alpha-2 agonists), respiratory depression can be significant, warranting the close monitoring of ventilation and oxygenation, particularly if the patient is not receiving oxygen supplementation. In general, it is recommended that when starting a CRI, doses in the lower range of those recommended are selected with subsequent adjustments made to achieve the desired level of analgesia.

Q. Which opioid analgesics are typically administered as a CRI in dogs and cats?

A. Fentanyl is commonly administered as a CRI in the dog and cat. When administered intravenously as a bolus, it has a rapid onset of effect (1–2 min) but a relatively short duration (20–30 min). When administering fentanyl as an infusion, the loading dose should ideally be administered as a loading infusion over 5–10 min to avoid pronounced cardiopulmonary changes, particularly if the patient is under general anesthesia. Infusion rates of 5–10 mcg/kg/h generally maintain plasma fentanyl concentrations in the analgesic range, although clinically effective doses may vary. The time to *peak* effect after administration of a dose of fentanyl is approximately 3–4 min. After that time, it is appropriate to assess the degree of analgesia and determine if an increase or decrease in the dose is required. Fentanyl is ideally suited to administration using a syringe pump; however, if this option is not available, it can be diluted in intravenous fluids for delivery. For example, 2.5 mg of fentanyl (50 ml of a 50 mcg/ml fentanyl) can be added to a 500 ml bag of Lactated Ringer's solution, which has had 50 ml of fluid removed. The resulting concentration of fentanyl in the 500 ml solution will be 5 mcg/ml. To deliver fentanyl at 5 mcg/kg/h, the infusion rate can be set at 1 ml/kg/h.

Morphine and hydromorphone are alternative opioids to fentanyl that can be used in the dog, particularly if a prolonged period of analgesia is anticipated and a rapid withdrawal of effect is not required. Due to the potential long-term effects of these agents, they are not recommended for use in the cat. Morphine should only be administered slowly intravenously due to the potential for histamine release; therefore the loading dose should be via a slow intravenous infusion or an intramuscular injection. With both these agents, the time to peak effect is longer than that observed with fentanyl, therefore adjustments in dose should only be done after a 10–15 min interval following a change in delivery rate. Similar to fentanyl, these agents can be administered via a syringe pump, although the concentrations are generally diluted to facilitate administration with a manageable volume. To create a suitable concentration of morphine in Lactated Ringer's solution for infusion with a drip set, a concentration of 0.12 mg/ml morphine is created by adding 60 mg of morphine to a 500 ml bag. A dose of 0.12 mg/kg/h of morphine is provided with a rate of 1 ml/kg/h.

Q. If I gave a premedication of μ agonist opioid like hydromorphone, oxymorphone, or morphine IM, do I still need to do a loading dose before starting my opioid CRI?

A. No! Your IM opioid premedication functions as your loading dose, provided that you are starting your CRI within 30–60 min of giving your premedication. In these instances, starting your CRI after anesthetic induction will maintain effective analgesic levels of the opioid. Depending on which opioid you are using for your CRI, it is important to account for the respective durations of effect. For example, if you premedicated with morphine, which has a relatively long duration of effect, and you plan to use a fentanyl CRI, you may need to start with a lower dose of fentanyl in order to prevent additive, excessive, plasma levels of both drugs. Monitoring of patient anesthetic depth is key.

Q. What are some advantages and disadvantages of administering ketamine as a CRI?

A. Ketamine, an NMDA antagonist, has analgesic properties when used at low doses as well as anesthetic properties at high doses. It has a wide recommended dose range, depending on the objectives of the CRI. When administered as an analgesic in awake patients, it is typically used at low doses (2–3 mcg/kg/min or 0.12–0.18 mg/kg/h). For intra-operative analgesia and an approximately 25% reduction in inhalant dose requirements, a dose of 10 mcg/kg/min is suggested (0.6 mg/kg/h). To further reduce or replace inhalant anesthetics, higher doses can be utilized (see Chapter 14). The duration of recovery from anesthesia may also be increased if high infusion rates are administered for more than a few hours.

Q. What are some advantages and disadvantages of administering lidocaine as a CRI?

A. In addition to opioids and ketamine, lidocaine can be used as an analgesic. In the dog under general anesthesia, lidocaine can lower anesthetic requirements and result in improved hemodynamic stability, although not to the same degree as opioid analgesics or ketamine. Unfortunately, these advantages do not extend to the cat due to this species' sensitivity to lidocaine toxicity. When lidocaine is administered for analgesia in the conscious patient, adverse CNS side effects such as nausea and agitation may manifest if doses higher than 50 mcg/kg/min are used. In the anesthetized patient, the animal should be monitored closely for excessive anesthetic depth when higher doses of lidocaine are provided as a CRI (e.g., 100 mcg/kg/min).

Q. Do I need to administer a loading dose of ketamine or lidocaine?

A. Opinions on this vary. If you have induced anesthesia with a ketamine/benzodiazepine combination, then you have effectively given your loading dose of ketamine. Both ketamine and lidocaine have relatively long half-lives, so if you want to ensure a rapid rise in effective plasma concentrations, then a loading dose of ketamine (0.5 mg/kg) should be given, assuming that you induced anesthesia with a different injectable anesthetic. The loading dose for lidocaine, in the dog, is 1 mg/kg.

Q. What are the advantages and disadvantages of administering a mixture of morphine, lidocaine, and ketamine (MLK)?

A. Several different formulations of a mixture of morphine, lidocaine, and ketamine have been described for use in the dog. Advantages of this combination of agents include analgesia, reduced anesthetic requirements and improved quality of anesthetic recovery. The combination of drugs is not suitable for use in cats and it is more difficult to alter the administration of individual components of the mixture. The reduction in inhalant anesthetic requirements is similar to that achieved with opioids alone, although there may be additional analgesic benefits to the use of a combination [5].

Q. How can I prepare a combination of morphine, lidocaine, and ketamine (MLK)?

A. Several different MLK combinations are reported in the literature that result in slightly different doses of the three drugs. One method of preparing and delivering a combination of MLK is to start with a 500 ml bag of LRS. Add 10 mg morphine (variable volumes depending on concentration of morphine), 150 mg (7.5 ml of 2%) lidocaine and 30 mg (0.3 ml of 10%) ketamine [5]. Remove an equivalent volume from the bag of LRS before adding the drugs. The resulting drug concentrations will be 0.02 mg/ml morphine, 0.3 mg/ml lidocaine, and 0.06 mg/ml ketamine. When the combination is delivered at a rate of 10 ml/kg/h, the patient will receive 0.2 mg/kg/h of morphine, 3 mg/kg/h of lidocaine, and 0.6 mg/kg/h of ketamine. With recent recommendations of a 5 ml/kg/hour fluid rate for maintenance under anesthesia (see Chapter 9), the three drugs can be doubled in amount in the 500 ml bag to achieve the same analgesic doses.

Q. What drugs can be administered as a CRI to provide long-term sedation?

A. Dexmedetomidine, midazolam, and/or propofol may be used either alone or in combination to provide long-term sedation. Dexmedetomidine and midazolam most likely have prolonged context sensitive half-times based on available data, which may result in a prolonged clinical recovery from sedation [6]. While propofol's context-sensitive half-time will be extended with prolonged infusions, clinical recovery is still relatively short, with times under 30 min typically observed with infusions exceeding 6 h. When propofol is used as a CRI for sedation, it must be remembered that this drug is an *anesthetic*, so oxygen supplementation and intubation may be necessary. See Table 22.2 for recommended doses. Any patient receiving a CRI for sedation should be continuously monitored, much like a patient under general anesthesia.

Table 22.2   Recommended intravenous loading and infusion rates of drugs administered to achieve sedation in dogs and cats.

Drug	Loading dose	Infusion dose
Dexmedetomidine	0.5–2 mcg/kg IV	0.5–2 mcg/kg/h
Midazolam	0.1–0.2 mg/kg	0.1–0.4 mg/kg/h
Propofol	To effect	0.1–0.4 mg/kg/min (6–24 mg/kg/h)

References

1 Rowland M, Tozer TN. Constant-rate input. In: Roland M & Tozer TM (eds) *Clinical Pharmacokinetics and Pharmacodynamics. Concepts and Applications*, 4th edn. Lippincott Williams & Wilkins: Philadelphia, PA, 2011:259–292.

2 White PF. Clinical uses of intravenous anesthetic and analgesic infusions. *Anesthesia and Analgesia* 1999; **68**:161–171.

3 Kukanich B, Hogan BK, Krugner-Higby LA, *et al*. Pharmacokinetics of hydromorphone hydrochloride in healthy dogs. *Veterinary Anesthesia and Analgesia* 2008; **35**:256–264.

4 Kennedy MJ, Smith LJ. Anesthesia case of the month. *Journal of the American Veterinary Medical Association* 2014; **245(10)**:1098–1101.

5 Muir WW, Wiese AJ, March PA. Effects of morphine, lidocaine, ketamine and morphine-lidocaine-ketamine drug comination on minimum alveolar concentration in dogs anesthetized with isoflurane. *American Journal of Veterinary Research* 2003; **64**:1155–1160.

6 Johnson KB, Egan TD. Pharmacokinetics and pharmacodynamics that make sense. *ASA Refresher Courses in Anesthesiology* 2008; **36**:45–59.

23 Loco-Regional Anesthesia

Block it out!

Carrie Schroeder

Department of Surgical Sciences, School of Veterinary Medicine, University of Wisconsin, USA

KEY POINTS:

- Regional anesthesia differs from local anesthesia in that a larger field, or region, innervated by branches of a nerve is anesthetized, rather than a small, or local, area. The term loco-regional anesthesia can be used to describe both local and regional anesthesia.

- Loco-regional anesthesia blocks transmission of a painful signal up a peripheral nerve towards the spinal cord.

- Blockade of the radial, ulnar, and median nerves through a four-point block is recommended for cat front paw declaws.

- Epidural anesthesia can be used for a number of procedures. The regions blocked largely depend upon the site of administration and the volume injected.

- The intra-testicular block is a simple technique that can provide loco-regional anesthesia for a castration.

- A Bier block, or intravenous regional anesthesia, can provide regional anesthesia for minor procedures of the distal fore- or hindlimbs for 60–90 min. The Bier block also results in a blood-free surgical field due to the use of a tourniquet.

- The infraorbital block is useful in providing anesthesia to the proximal 1/3rd of the maxilla for procedures such as rhinoscopy.

Q. What is the difference between local and regional anesthesia?

A. Although these two terms are often used interchangeably, there are fundamental differences between providing local and regional anesthesia. In the strictest sense, local anesthesia is simply providing anesthesia to a small area via subcutaneous infiltration of a local anesthetic. An example of this would be blocking a small area around a laceration by infiltration of lidocaine near the peripheral margins of the wound. Regional anesthesia refers to anesthesia of a large region via delivery of local anesthetic to more proximal nerves. An example of this would be a lumbosacral epidural with bupivacaine. A common term that is used to encompass both local and regional anesthesia is loco-regional anesthesia.

Questions and Answers in Small Animal Anesthesia, First Edition. Edited by Lesley J. Smith.
© 2016 John Wiley & Sons, Inc. Published 2016 by John Wiley & Sons, Inc.

Q. What are the components of the pain pathway? What parts of the pain pathway are targeted with loco-regional anesthesia?

A. There are five steps of the nociceptive process [1]:

✓ Transduction: peripheral sensory nerve endings known as nociceptors are activated by a painful stimulus, which is converted into an electrical impulse.

✓ Transmission: the electrical impulse travels up the peripheral nerve towards the dorsal horn of the spinal cord.

✓ Modulation: in the dorsal horn of the spinal cord, endogenous systems either upregulate or downregulate the electrical impulse.

✓ Projection: the electrical stimulus travels through the spinal cord to the brain.

✓ Perception: the painful stimulus is perceived by the brain.

Loco-regional anesthesia targets transduction (e.g., infiltration of lidocaine near the margins of a wound will desensitize nociceptors in the tissue bed), transmission (e.g., injection of a local anesthetic near/on peripheral sensory nerves, as in a sciatic nerve block), and modulation (e.g., epidural administration of a local anesthetic that blocks dorsal root ganglion and dorsal horn sensory neurons that are involved in processing pain from the periphery).

Q. Why is loco-regional anesthesia important if the patient is under anesthesia?

A. When a patient is under general anesthesia, it is generally accepted that they do not "feel" pain as the perception of pain is absent due to the effect of general anesthetics on the cerebral cortex and other brain centers. However, the physiologic responses to painful stimuli are very much present even in the anesthetized state. This is easily observed in the anesthetized patient when painful surgical stimuli result in an increased heart rate, respiratory rate, and blood pressure. While these are the changes easily observed in monitored parameters, there are a whole number of physiologic changes that occur under the surface. These include sympathetic nervous system stimulation resulting in decreased renal blood flow, increased central sensitization to pain ("wind up pain"), sodium and water retention, decreased wound healing, and immune compromise [1]. Furthermore, the painful patient generally requires greater amounts of anesthetic in order to remain adequately anesthetized, often resulting in adverse cardiovascular and respiratory effects.

Loco-regional anesthesia is the most successful element of analgesia in that the pain process is blocked entirely, thus avoiding negative consequences of the physiologic responses to pain. When possible, and applicable to the procedure being performed, incorporation of loco-regional anesthesia is a highly effective multimodal approach to treating pain and will reduce patient requirements for other analgesic drugs such as opioids and NSAIDs. That said, the expected duration of blockade with a loco-regional technique should be considered and other analgesic drugs should be available as soon as it is anticipated that the loco-regional effects are waning.

Table 23.1 Local anesthetic drugs, onset time, duration, and toxic doses.

Drug	Onset	Duration (hours)	Toxic dose (dog)
Lidocaine	Fast	1–3	10 mg/kg (dog) 6 mg/kg (cat)
Mepivacaine	Fast	2–4	>5 mg/kg (dog) >2.5 mg/kg (cat)
Bupivacaine	Moderate	4–12	3 mg/kg (dog) 2 mg/kg (cat)
Ropivacaine	Moderate	5–8	5 mg/kg

Q. What are local anesthetics?

A. Local anesthetics are pharmacologic agents that function primarily to block neuronal transmission. This results in loss of sensory, motor, and autonomic functions of the nerve that has been blocked. The degree of sensory blockade relative to motor and autonomic blockade can depend on the specific local anesthetic used and the dose/route of administration. All of the local anesthetics exert their effects by blocking sodium channels and differ in their onset time and duration of effects.

Q. What are the common local anesthetics used in veterinary medicine? Do they have different durations of effect?

A. The properties of commonly used local anesthetics are listed in Table 23.1. Fast onset refers to nearly immediate effect while moderate onset refers to roughly 15–30 min for effect. Onset time is typically slightly more rapid and duration shorter with epidural or spinal administration versus peripheral nerve blockade.

Q. What are signs of local anesthetic toxicity? What are the toxic doses in dogs and cats?

A. Local anesthetic toxicity may occur in loco-regional anesthesia if inadvertent intravascular injections occur or if dose calculations are incorrect, especially in very small patients. It is important to carefully calculate drug dosages. Dilute local anesthetic agents as necessary and aspirate prior to injection to ensure absence of blood to avoid intravascular injection.

Should local anesthetic toxicity occur, clinical signs include [2]:

✓ nystagmus
✓ muscle twitching
✓ seizures
✓ CNS depression
✓ hypotension
✓ death.

See Table 23.1 for toxic doses in dogs and cats. Individual patient sensitivity can vary and ancillary local anesthetic administration (e.g., lidocaine constant rate infusion) should be factored in when estimating total dose administered to a patient.

Q. What are the side effects of loco-regional anesthesia?

A. That depends upon the nerves that are being blocked by a local anesthetic. It is important to note that nerves do not function solely to transmit sensory information; their functions include providing innervation to muscles and vasculature. Blockade of nerves will not only block sensory function, but motor function and local vasomotor tone. When administering a local infiltrative block, this is of little consequence. However, as more proximal nerves that innervate larger areas are blocked, the clinical consequences of blockade become more significant. For instance, lumbar epidural administration of a local anesthetic provides excellent regional anesthesia for various surgical procedures, but the spinal nerves that provide motor tone to the hind limbs and anal sphincter will also be blocked and the patient will have motor deficits dependent upon the duration of local anesthetic action. These nerves also provide vasomotor tone to the vessels in the blocked region; blockade will result in vasodilation and possible hypotension. It is important to note that somatic nerves are more sensitive to the effects of local anesthetics; sensory blockade may be present without, or with minimal, motor or autonomic blockade [2,3].

Q. How can I provide local anesthesia for a cat declaw?

A. A four-point block can be used for procedures involving the forepaw [4,5]. This technique relies on the deposition of local anesthetic around the nerves that provide sensory innervation to the forepaw: the radial, ulnar, and median nerves. Lidocaine or bupivacaine should be injected in the subcutaneous space at four sites 15–20 min prior to the initial surgical incision. Bupivacaine will provide longer blockade but has a slower onset of effect. In cats, due to their small size, it is important to stay below the toxic dose of these drugs and dilute with saline if necessary to attain the appropriate volume. At all sites, aspirate back to ensure you are not in a vessel before injecting. The four injection sites are described below.

Dorsal side of the paw:

✓ Lateral side: Insert needle directed medially just distal to the carpus so that the needle spans ¾ of the paw width. Inject 0.1 ml of bupivacaine while withdrawing the needle.

  • This blocks dorsal branches of the ulnar and radial nerves.

✓ Medial side: Insert needle directed proximally at the site of articulation between metacarpal I and II on the second digit. Inject 0.1 ml of bupivacaine.

  • This blocks the dorsal digital nerve.

Palmar side of the paw:

✓ Lateral side: Insert the needle just proximal to the carpal pad to the level of the fourth digit. Inject 0.1 ml of bupivacaine while withdrawing the needle.

  • This blocks palmar branches of the ulnar nerve.

✓ Medial side: Insert needle directed laterally just distal to the carpus so that the needle spans ¾ of the paw width. Inject 0.1 ml of bupivacaine while withdrawing the needle.

  • This blocks median nerve and palmar branches of the ulnar nerve.

Q. What regions are anesthetized by a lumbosacral epidural?

A. The pelvic limb is innervated by nerves originating from L3-S1 while the abdomen and peritoneum are innervated by nerves originating from T11-L3 [6]. Innervation to the rectum and perineal area is supplied from sacral segments [6].

Spread of epidural blockade is dependent on a number of factors, most notably volume of injectate. Injection of 0.22 ml/kg in the lumbosacral space provides blockade to regions innervated by spinal nerves L1-L3 [7,8]. This level of blockade is satisfactory for hindlimb procedures and procedures of the caudal abdomen. More cephalad spread of epidural blockade requires either a greater volume of injectate or the advancement of an epidural catheter to more cranial sites [9,10].

Q. How do I perform a lumbosacral epidural?

A. ✓ Position the animal in sternal recumbency with the hindlimbs pulled forward. This opens up the L-S space, but may be painful for dogs with osteoarthritis of the hips.

✓ Clip a generous region overlying the lumbosacral junction and prepare the area as for a sterile procedure.

✓ Using sterile technique (i.e., wearing sterile surgical gloves), palpate the space between L7 and S1 and insert a spinal needle perpendicular to the skin. Advance the needle through the layers of skin, subcutaneous tissue, muscle, and interspinous ligament. Anatomy of this space is shown in Figure 23.1.

✓ Either attach a loss of resistance syringe or fill the hub of the needle with saline to verify placement of the needle tip into the epidural space.

  • Slight resistance or a "pop" will be felt prior to entering the epidural space as the interspinous ligament is penetrated.

  • If bony structures are encountered with advancement, the needle can be withdrawn slightly and gently redirected in the cranial or caudal direction in order to properly locate the epidural space.

  • Do not advance the needle so far that you cause a tail flick. This means you are stimulating the cauda equine and can cause permanent damage.

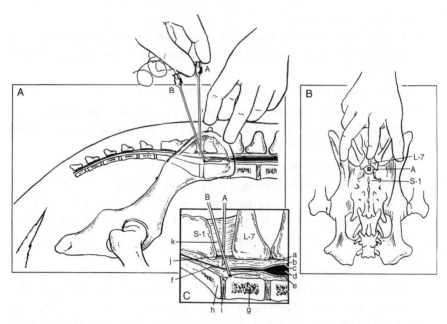

Figure 23.1 Anatomy of the epidural space in the dog. (a) Aseptic needle placement, using sterile surgical gloves, into the lumbosacral epidural space of a dog (**A**) and catheter placement for continuous epidural anesthesia using a local anesthetic and/or analgesia using an opioid (**B**). (b) Dorsal view. Palpation of the dorsal spinous process of the L7 vertebra and dorsoiliac wings. (c) Inset: **a**: epidural space with fat and connective tissue, **b**: dura mater, **c**: arachnoid membrane, **d**: spinal cord, **e**: cerebrospinal fluid, **f**: cauda equine, **g**: seventh lumbar (L7) vertebra, **h**: first sacral (S1) vertebra, **i**: intervertebral disc, **j**: interarcuate ligament (ligamentum flavum), and **k**: interspinous ligament. Skarda RT, Tranquilli WJ. Local and regional anesthetic and analgesic techniques: Dogs. In: WJ Tranquilli, JC Benson, KA Grimm (eds) *Lumb and Jones' Veterinary Anesthesia and Analgesia* 4th edn. Blackwell Publishing: Ames IA, 2007: Figure 20.17, page 575.

✓ Once the epidural space is correctly located, aspiration should be performed to rule out the presence of blood or cerebrospinal fluid. Once this is assured, slow injection (over 1–2 min) of sterile and preservative-free medication can be performed.

Q. How do I know if my needle is in the epidural space?

A. There are a number of possible techniques to determine correct placement into the epidural space. The most common techniques are loss of resistance (LOR) and the hanging drop techniques. With LOR, a specialized loss of resistance syringe containing either a small amount of air or saline is attached to the needle. As the needle is advanced, gentle injection pressure is applied to the syringe; back pressure indicates extradural location, while a loss of resistance to injection indicates needle placement in the epidural space. With the hanging drop technique, the hub of the needle is filled with saline. Correct

Table 23.2 Various drugs or drug combinations used for epidural anesthesia.

Drug	Dose (mg/kg)	Onset(min)	Duration(hours)
Morphine [11]	0.1	30–60	6–24
0.5% Bupivacaine [12]	1.0	10–15	24
Morphine + 0.5% Bupivacaine [13]	0.1 + 1.0	10–15	16–24
Dexmedetomidine + 0.5% Bupivacaine [13]	0.004 + 1.0	10–15	24

placement into the epidural space is confirmed when the hanging drop of saline is "sucked" into the needle.

Q. What drugs should I use for a lumbosacral epidural and what are the doses?

A. Several studies have evaluated different pharmacologic agents administered in the epidural space, including local anesthetics, opioids, alpha-2 agonists, and dissociatives. The most commonly administered agents and their dosages are listed in Table 23.2. It is important to note that pharmacologic agents administered into the epidural space should be free of preservatives. Drug combinations can be diluted to a total volume of 0.22 ml/kg with preservative-free sodium chloride.

Q. I advanced a needle into the lumbosacral space and cerebrospinal fluid (CSF) came out of the needle. What should I do?

A. The presence of CSF fluid in the epidural needle suggests that the dura has been penetrated and the needle tip is in the subarachnoid space. Subarachnoid, or spinal, injection of local anesthetics offers the advantage of more rapid onset and more profound blockade. However, there is a greater potential for more cranial spread as the local anesthetic combines with CSF fluid and the risk of adverse effects is greater as compared to epidural injections. In the event of subarachnoid injection, a volume of 0.05 ml/kg of local anesthetic should be used to prevent untoward effects [10].

Q. What are the contraindications for an epidural?

A. Contraindications may be due to the physical effects of inserting a needle into the epidural space and pharmacologic effects of the injectate. Absolute contraindications are infection at the injection site (e.g., pyoderma), increased intracranial pressure, and uncorrected hypovolemia. Relative contraindications are coagulopathy, thrombocytopenia, spinal or lumbosacral deformities, fractures/luxations of the pelvic structures, and sepsis [10].

Q. Are there any other options for regional anesthesia for orthopedic procedures?

A. A number of more advanced peripheral nerve blocks have been described. These include the brachial plexus block for thoracic limb procedures, paravertebral blocks for thoracic procedures, and femoral, sciatic, and lumbar plexus block for pelvic limb procedures. These regional blocks can be performed under direct visualization with an ultrasound or using indirect nerve localization with electrical stimulation. Loco-regional blocks performed with the aid of ultrasound guidance or nerve stimulation generally require advanced training and additional equipment.

Q. How can I provide local anesthesia for a castration?

A. An intra-testicular block is a fast and simple block that can be incorporated into the anesthetic protocol for castration of dogs and cats. The intra-testicular block provides satisfactory local anesthesia in dogs undergoing castration and should attenuate or eliminate increases in heart rate and blood pressure that accompany exteriorization of the testes and clamping of the spermatic cord. Additional analgesia may be required in the post-operative period, however, as the block may not provide adequate post-operative analgesia [14].

- ✓ Following standard surgical preparation, insert a 23G 1–1.5 in needle 2/3 of the way into the testicle through the caudal pole towards the spermatic cord, along the long axis.
- ✓ Following aspiration free of blood, inject 1/3–1/2 of the total volume of injectate until the testicle feels turgid.
- ✓ Either 0.5% bupivacaine (5 mg/ml; 1 mg/kg total), 2% lidocaine (20 mg/ml; 2 mg/kg total), or a mixture of the two can be used.
- ✓ Repeat the procedure in the second testicle.

Q. What is a Bier block?

A. A Bier block is also known as intravenous regional anesthesia (IVRA). It is used extensively in large animals, but has also been described as an effective regional anesthetic technique in dogs [15–17]. While the Bier block does not provide long-term anesthesia or analgesia, it is extremely useful for quick (<60–90 min) distal limb procedures such as laceration repair or small mass removal in dogs.

- ✓ Place an intravenous catheter in the most distal accessible vein of the limb in question using standard technique.
- ✓ Exsanguinate the limb by wrapping it tightly with an Esmarch bandage.
- ✓ Place a tourniquet proximal to the bandage tightly enough so that arterial pulses distal to the tourniquet become absent.
- ✓ A blood pressure cuff may be used with the cuff inflated to a pressure greatly exceeding arterial pressure (50–100 mmHg higher than systolic arterial pressure) [18].
- ✓ If an elastic tourniquet is used, provide light, smooth padding underneath so as to prevent compression and damage of underlying tissues.
- ✓ Inject 3–4 mg/kg of 0.5% lidocaine (5 mg/ml) into the intravenous catheter.

✓ Regional anesthesia will be effective for procedures distal to the tourniquet in 5–10 min and can be used for up to 90 min.

✓ Following the procedure, *slowly* release the tourniquet to allow blood flow to return.

✓ A "step release" can be utilized to minimize rapid release of local anesthetic into the systemic circulation: release tourniquet for 20–30 s then reapply in the previous manner for 1–2 min; repeat several times over 5–10 min[19].

Q. When can I use an infraorbital block?

A. The infraorbital nerve is a rostral extension of the maxillary branch of the trigeminal nerve that runs through the infraorbital canal and innervates the premolars, canine, and incisor teeth as well as rostral tissues [6]. Blockade of this nerve provides local anesthesia to the maxillary teeth and soft tissues of the maxilla rostral and ipsalateral to where local anesthetic is deposited. This block is of use in dental procedures and procedures of the rostral maxilla on the side on which the block is performed [19–21]. The infraorbital block is often used for rhinoscopy, but bilateral blockade of the maxillary nerve has been found to be superior for this procedure [22].

The infra-orbital foramen, the entrance to the infraorbital canal, can easily be palpated intra-orally and marks the site of injection. In dogs, the infraorbital foramen is located on the lateral maxilla dorsal to the distal root of the third premolar. In cats, it can be palpated at the rostral edge of the bony ridge just ventral to the orbit. There are two different possible approaches: extra-oral, where the needle is inserted percutaneously, and intraoral, where the needle is inserted directly into the gingiva. Due to anatomical variations, the extra-oral approach is recommended in cats, while the intra-oral approach is generally preferred in dogs [21,23].

Once the infra-orbital foramen is located, the block can be performed as follows:

✓ Insert a 23-25G needle into the foramen, directed caudally and parallel to the hard palate, along the long axis of the maxilla.

✓ For cats, using a 27G needle, angle the needle slightly ventro-medially to avoid injuring the closely associated eye.

✓ Attach a syringe containing injectate and aspirate to ensure intravascular injection is not performed.

✓ Slowly inject 0.5% bupivacaine solution (0.2 ml per site in cats and small dogs; 0.5 ml per site in medium to large dogs).

✓ Provide gentle pressure over the injection site for 30–60 s following removal of the needle.

References

1 Muir WW. Physiology and pathophysiology of pain. In: Gaynor JS (ed.) *Handbook of Veterinary Pain Management*, 2nd edn. Mosby Elsevier: Saint Louis, MO, 2009:13–41.

2 Martin-Flores M. Clinical pharmacology and toxicology of local anesthetics and adjuncts. In: Campoy L, Read M (eds) *Small Animal Regional Anesthesia and Analgesia*, Wiley Blackwell Publishing: Ames, IA, 2013:25.

3 Gasser HS, Erlanger J. Role of fiber size in establishment of nerve block by pressure and cocaine. *American Journal of Physiology* 1929; **88**:581–591.

4 Ringwood PB, Smith JA. Anesthesia case of the month. *Journal of the American Veterinary Medical Association* 2000; **217(11)**:1633–1635.

5 Curcio K, Bidwell LA, Bohart GV, *et al.* Evaluation of signs of postoperative pain and complications after forelimb onychectomy in cats receiving buprenorphine alone or with bupivacaine administered as a four-point regional nerve block. *Journal of the American Veterinary Medical Association* 2006; **228(1)**:65–68.

6 Evans HE, de Lahunta A. Spinal nerves. In. Evans HE, de LaHunta A (eds) *Miller's Anatomy of the Dog*, 4th edn. Elsevier: St. Louis, MO, 2013:611–656.

7 Lee I, Yamagishi N, Oboshi K, *et al.* Distribution of new methylene blue injected into the lumbosacral epidural space in cats. *Veterinary Anesthesia and Analgesia* 2004; **31(3)**:190–194.

8 Son WG, Kim J, Seo JP, *et al.* Cranial epidural spread of contrast medium and new methylene blue dye in sternally recumbent anaesthetized dogs. *Veterinary Anaesthesia and Analgesia* 2011; **38(5)**:510–515.

9 Freire CD, Torres MLA, Fantoni DT, *et al.* Bupivacaine 0.25% and methylene blue spread with epidural anesthesia in dog. *Veterinary Anesthesia and Analgesia* 2010; **37**:63–69.

10 Otero PE, Campoy L. 2013. Epidural and spinal anesthesia. In: Campoy L, Read M (eds) *Small Animal Regional Anesthesia and Analgesia*. Wiley Blackwell: Ames, IA, 2013:227–259.

11 Valverde A, Dyson DH, McDonell WN. Epidural morphine reduces halothane MAC in the dog. *Canadian Journal of Anaesthesia* 1989; **36**:629–632.

12 Smith LJ. A comparison of epidural analgesia provided by bupivacaine alone, bupivacaine + morphine, or bupivacaine + dexmedetomidine for pelvic orthopedic surgery in dogs. *Veterinary Anaesthesia and Analgesia*. 2013; **40**:527–536.

13 Kona-Boun JJ, Cuvelliez S, Troncy E. Evaluation of epidural administration of morphine or morphine and bupivacaine for postoperative analgesia after premedication with an opioid analgesic and orthopedic surgery in dogs. *Journal of the American Veterinary Medical Association* 2006; **229**:1103–1112.

14 Huuskonen V, Hughes JM, Estaca Banon E, *et al.* Intratesticular lidocaine reduces the response to surgical castration in dogs. *Veterinary Anesthesia and Analgesia* 2013: **40(1)**:74–82.

15 Webb AA, Cantwell SL, Duke T, *et al.* Intravenous regional anesthesia (Bier block) in a dog. *Canadian Veterinary Journal* 1999: **40(6)**:1132–1136.

16 Macedo GG, DeRossi R, Frazilio FO. Evaluation of two regional anesthetic methods on the front limb of dogs using hyperbaric bupivacaine. *Acta Cirugica Brasilia*. 2010; **25(3)**:298–303.

17 De Marzo C, Crovace A, De Monte V, *et al.* Comparison of intra-operative analgesia provided by intravenous regional anesthesia or brachial plexus block for pancarpal arthrodesis in dogs. *Research in Veterinary Science* 2012; **93(3)**:1493–1497.

18 Staffieri F. Intravenous Regional Anesthesia. In: Campoy L, Read M (eds) *Small Animal Regional Anesthesia and Analgesia*. Wiley Blackwell: Ames, IA, 2013:**261–271**.

19 Davis KJ, McConachie L. Intravenous regional anesthesia. *Current Anesthesia and Critical Care* 1998; **9(5)**:261–264.

20 Gross ME, Pope ER, O'Brien D, *et al.* Regional anesthesia of the infraorbital and inferior alveolar nerves during noninvasive tooth pulp stimulation in halothane-anesthetized dogs. *Journal of the American Veterinary Medical Association* 1997: **211(11)**:1403–1405.

21 Gross ME, Pope ER, Jarboe JM, *et al.* Regional anesthesia of the infraorbital and inferior alveolar nerves during noninvasive tooth pulp stimulation in halothane-anesthetized cats. *American Journal of Veterinary Research* 2000: **61(10)**:1245–1247.

22 Cremer J, Sum SO, Braun C, *et al.* Assessment of maxillary and infraorbital nerve blockade for rhinoscopy in sevoflurane anesthetized dogs. *Veterinary Anasthesia and Analgesia* 2013; **40(4)**:432–439.

23 Gracis M. The Oral Cavity. In: Campoy L, Read M (eds) *Small Animal Regional Anesthesia and Analgesia.* Wiley Blackwell: Ames, IA, 2013:119–140.

24 Troubleshooting Anesthetic Recovery

Time to land!

Andrew Claude

College of Veterinary Medicine, Mississippi State University, USA

KEY POINTS:

- Recovery is a key part of the anesthetic event.
- In small animal patients many complications can occur during anesthetic recovery.
- Dysphoria, emergence delirium, delayed extubation, and hypothermia are common complications associated with anesthetic recovery.
- Veterinary patients recovering from general anesthesia should never be left unattended.
- Human interaction, patient monitoring, and pain assessments are important aspects of patient welfare during anesthetic recovery.
- Patients recovering from major procedures, or with significant severe disease, should be recovered in an environment where they can be continually assessed for 6–24 h.

Q. What is meant by "anesthesia recovery" and why is it important?

A. Anesthesia recovery refers to the interval from the cessation of anesthetic delivery until the patient regains a gag or swallow reflex, is extubated, regains consciousness, remains sternal, and/or regains the ability to walk [1]. The length of time to anesthesia recovery depends on multiple factors, including patient health, body temperature, anesthetic drugs used, and length of anesthesia. Generally speaking, longer recovery times are associated with debilitating diseases, hypothermia, excessive anesthetic depth, and long anesthetic procedures. Serious anesthetic related complications can occur during recovery from general anesthesia. Nearly 50% of canine and greater than 60% of feline deaths occur within 48 h post-operatively [2].

Q. Are there ways to hasten patient recovery from inhalant anesthesia?

A. Elimination of inhalant anesthetic agents follows the opposite pharmacokinetics as agent uptake [3]. During recovery an anesthetized patient will reverse steadily to a conscious state through the planes of anesthesia: eye position returns to normal; reflexes and muscle movements become apparent; and vital signs increase [1]. If the patient is ventilating sufficiently,

---

Questions and Answers in Small Animal Anesthesia, First Edition. Edited by Lesley J. Smith.
© 2016 John Wiley & Sons, Inc. Published 2016 by John Wiley & Sons, Inc.

inhalant anesthetic off-loading can be hastened by shutting off the anesthetic vaporizer, briefly disconnecting the patient from the breathing circuit,
flushing the anesthetic vapors into the scavenging system, and reattaching
the patient to the breathing circuit. A patient breathing 100% oxygen
or room air with no residual inhalant will recover faster than a patient
breathing oxygen on an anesthetic circuit that still contains trace levels of
inhalant agent. The most important point, however, is that the patient must
be ventilating (either spontaneously or with assistance) in order for them
to clear the inhalant from their body, as all modern inhalants are primarily
eliminated via the lungs.

Q. How do I monitor my post-anesthetic patient during recovery?

A. The duties of monitoring the anesthetized patient do not stop when the
anesthetic agent is discontinued. Patient monitoring should continue until
the patient is extubated, sternal, at near-normal body temperature, and able
to ambulate or at least hold up their head without assistance. Important
patient parameters to monitor during the post-anesthetic period include:
cardiovascular status (mucus membrane color and capillary refill times, heart
rate/sounds and blood pressure); ventilation (respiratory rate, lung sounds,
especially in respiratory compromised patients); oxygenation (pulse oximetry, arterial blood gases – especially in patients with respiratory compromise);
level of analgesia (pain scoring and proper modes of pain management); body
temperature (supplemental or heat reduction as needed); patient tolerance
of the endotracheal tube (return of gag reflex and swallowing); and signs
of aversive behaviors (emergence delirium or dysphoria). As the patient
regains consciousness and voluntary control, the degree of monitoring can
be reduced gradually. Monitoring values and drug doses administered during
the post-anesthetic period should be properly chronicled in the patient's
anesthetic record.

Q. What is the difference between emergence delirium and dysphoria?

A. Emergence delirium, also called post-anesthetic excitement, has multiple
potential causes. Pharmacological factors include residual effects of anesthetic
drugs on both divisions of the central nervous system (extrapyramidal and
cerebral). In humans arterial hypoxemia and hypercapnia can contribute to
post-anesthetic agitation and delirium due to functional mental impairment
[4]. Behavioral causes of emergence delirium include post-anesthetic anxiety, confusion and agitation. In many cases of emergence delirium patients
often respond to intervention such as touch and spoken language.
Post-anesthetic opioid dysphoria can clinically resemble emergence delirium,
however the patients do not respond to intervention. Please see below for a
more detailed discussion.

Q. How do I know when to extubate a dog or cat?

A. During recovery the anesthetized patient may shiver, lick, chew, stretch,
and swallow. After the anesthetic has been discontinued, patient extubation

should be anticipated by untying the endotracheal tube from the patient's muzzle or head and deflating the endotracheal tube cuff if the patient is showing imminent signs of a gag reflex. Deflating the endotracheal tube cuff too early in the recovery period can lead to inadvertent aspiration of fluids (water, regurgitant fluid, etc.) that is in the oro-pharynx. Signs of the gag reflex returning are indicated by swallowing and a strong gag-rejection of the endotracheal tube due to physical stimulation of the pharyngeal and laryngeal mucosa. Soon after the gag reflex returns, the patient will show signs of consciousness and will likely chew and paw at the endotracheal tube. It is imperative the endotracheal tube is removed soon after the patient demonstrates a pronounced gag reflex; otherwise, there is a risk the patient could chew through the endotracheal tube while he/she is still intubated. On the other hand, removal of the endotracheal tube before a gag reflex or swallowing occurs could predispose the patient to upper airway obstruction or aspiration pneumonia. Once the patient has demonstrated a gag reflex, the endotracheal tube should be removed gently and inspected immediately for debris, purulent material, or blood. Normally the tube should be clean, with a small amount of saliva and mucus either in the lumen or extra-luminal. If blood, debris, or purulent material is found on or in the tube, the patient should be evaluated for laryngeal or tracheal trauma, regurgitation, aspiration pneumonia, or pulmonary disease.

Due to risk of upper airway obstruction it is advisable to delay extubation in brachycephalic breeds until the patient will not tolerate an endotracheal tube. See Chapter 40 for more discussion of the anesthetic management of brachycephalic breeds.

Cats often recover from anesthesia rather abruptly; therefore, it is important to anticipate endotracheal tube removal to avoid laryngospasm and/or laryngeal trauma. Signs of imminent arousal in cats during recovery include swallowing, active palpebral reflexes, voluntary limb, tail, or head movements. If a cat starts to flick its ears in response to a finger touch, they are often close to arousal and a return of swallow reflex [1].

Q. What should I do if my patient cannot breathe well after anesthesia?

A. Despite demonstrating a gag reflex it is still possible for a patient to have upper airway obstruction after extubation. Causes include re-narcotization, brachycephalic syndrome, surgical inflammation involving the upper airways, and laryngeal collapse or laryngospasm due to direct irritation. Upper airway obstruction should always be anticipated when extubating a patient, thus it is recommended to have an adequate amount of induction agent available to re-induce anesthesia, a laryngoscope, and a clean endotracheal tube of proper size. If signs of upper airway blockade are apparent, the patient should be re-anesthetized, re-intubated, and evaluated for upper airway abnormalities. If the patient is able to move air but exhibits significant inspiratory effort, placing the patient in sternal recumbancy, propping the patient's mouth open, and pulling the tongue rostral from the mouth (if tolerated) may facilitate air movement and ventilation.

Marked expiratory effort and/or poor oxygenation can indicate intrathoracic problems, such as lower airway or pulmonary diseases. The patient should be evaluated for intrathoracic diseases such as lower tracheal obstruction or collapse, bronchial collapse, or aspiration pneumonia. Supplemental oxygen should be employed.

Q. Should I always give my recovering patient supplemental O_2?

A. Generally speaking, anesthetic patients benefit from supplemental oxygen administered during the immediate recovery phase. In healthy patients anesthetized for less than 15–30 min, oxygen supplementation may be considered optional [5]. Positional atelectasis is an expected outcome with anesthetic procedures that exceed 15–30 min. For any procedure longer than 30 min, with obese or pregnant patients, and in patients with known pulmonary disease or ventilation abnormalities, oxygen supplementation and assessment of oxygenation are recommended [5].

Q. What are some other important factors to consider for my patient during anesthetic recovery?

A. Patient welfare should be an important consideration during all aspects of the surgical procedure, including anesthesia. Analgesia is an integral aspect of patient welfare. Preventive analgesia includes pre-emptive, intro-operative, and post-operative nociceptive/pain management strategies [6]. Recovering patients that undergo surgery, or any procedure involving noxious stimuli, should be evaluated for pain post-operatively. Chapters 25 and 26 review pain assessment methods for dogs and cats, respectively.

Q. I administered analgesics post-operatively but my patient still seems painful. What do I do?

A. In dogs and cats there are three post-operative conditions that may appear clinically similar; emergence delirium, μ agonist opioid dysphoria, and pain. In all three conditions dogs can vocalize, demonstrate controlled/uncontrolled muscle movements, and appear anxious or disoriented. Emergence delirium can be related to either a conscious behavior (extreme anxiety) or unconscious muscle movements (stage 2 anesthesia). Administering a tranquilizer (acepromazine, dexmedetomidine) will often help relieve post-anesthetic anxiety and emergence delirium but may not relieve pain or dysphoria. Diagnosing μ agonist opioid dysphoria requires administering an opioid antagonist (naloxone) or mixed agonist/antagonist (butorphanol), which reverses the dysphoria; however, this will also reverse the analgesia [7]. With dogs, if you suspect "dysphoric" behavior is actually due to pain, administer a μ agonist first and then monitor results. If the dog appears more comfortable your suspicion was correct; however, if the dog becomes more anxious, and does not respond to his/her name or spoken commands, then opioid dysphoria is likely the problem. Intravenous diluted

(1 ml: 9 ml saline [0.04 mg/ml]) naloxone can be titrated at 1 ml/30 s to the point at which the dysphoria begins to improve. Butorphanol is another good option for addressing μ opioid related dysphoria and does retain some minimal analgesia. Dexmedetomidine can also be helpful because alpha-2 agonist drugs have some analgesic properties. Other conditions that can cause post-anesthetic anxiety in dogs are urgency to defecate, a full urinary bladder, and/or hunger [7].

In cats, opioid dysphoria may lead to hyperthermia, both of which can be reversed with naloxone [8].

Q. What are other common problems seen during small animal anesthetic recovery?

A. ✓ hypothermia
   ✓ regurgitation
   ✓ hypoventilation and hypercapnia.

In veterinary medicine hypothermia is a frequent problem encountered during general anesthesia, especially in small animals. Hypothermia can significantly delay recovery and should be addressed intra-operatively as well as post-operatively with supplemental warming. Causes of hypothermia and its treatment are covered in more detail in Chapter 20.

Vomiting and regurgitation are most common during anesthetic pre-medication and induction; however, regurgitation can occur intra- and post-operatively as well. Regurgitation early during the recovery phase can lead to esophagitis and aspiration pneumonitis or pneumonia, especially if the endotracheal tube cuff is deflated prematurely. Maintaining proper endotracheal tube cuff pressures are paramount to help avoid stomach contents from passing into the trachea. Regurgitated material should be swabbed or suctioned from the mouth and esophagus. The adage "dilution is the solution to pollution" describes the ideal method of treating regurgitated material within the mouth and esophagus. After thoroughly clearing the mouth and esophagus, warm tap-water can be syringed into the esophagus followed again by suctioning. This procedure is repeated until the suctioned material is clear. Aggressive suctioning should be avoided (i.e., high negative pressures) as this can damage the esophageal mucosa and increases the risk of esophagitis or strictures. Vomiting or regurgitation after extubation is more troublesome because the decision to re-anesthetize and re-intubate is imperative. If the patient has good gag and swallow reflexes, more than likely the airway is protected. On the other hand if the patient is still markedly sedate, it may be necessary to re-intubate, suction, flush, and assess for aspirated material.

Residual respiratory depressant effects of general anesthetics can cause hypoventilation in the recovery period. If hypoventilation is severe enough, arterial PCO_2 tensions can rise to the point that they are anesthetic themselves (e.g., $P_aCO_2 > 90$ mmHg) [9]. If a patient is having a delayed recovery, the end-tidal CO_2 should be checked with a capnometer and, if high, the patient's ventilation should be increased with assistance using an Ambu bag or an anesthetic circuit, O_2, and rebreathing bag. Once the arterial CO_2 tension has been decreased, the patient should begin to wake up.

Q. What about recovering neonatal/pediatric patients?

A. Neonatal and pediatric patients are uniquely challenging throughout the entire anesthetic event, including recovery. Because their cardiovascular, autonomic, and thermoregulatory systems are not yet fully developed, puppies and kittens under 12 weeks old are susceptible to bradycardia, hypotension, delayed sympathetic responses, and hypothermia. In addition, younger patients lack glycogen storage and are susceptible to hypoglycemia. Managing body temperature, heart rate, and blood glucose is essential to optimize recovery such that the neonatal/pediatric patient can nurse/eat post-anesthesia.

Q. What about recovering known aggressive small animal patients?

A. It is safe to assume patients that are truly aggressive or fractious pre-operatively will likely be so post-operatively. The goal of IM/IV drug administration in aggressive dogs and cats is to facilitate safe handling pre- and post-operatively. If possible, it is ideal to recover aggressive dogs inside a well-padded cage. It may be necessary to place a basket muzzle on the dog immediately after extubation when the patient is able to swallow and protect his/her airway. For recovery, aggressive cats can be placed inside a carrier with the head toward the opening. As soon as the patient is extubated, close the carrier door.

Monitoring aggressive patients during recovery is a balance between patient and personnel safety. It may be necessary to remove the IV catheter directly after extubation to avoid handling the patient when they are fully awake. It may be necessary to have potent sedative drugs available post-operatively with aggressive dogs and cats, such as dexmedetomidine.

References

1 Flecknell P, Hollingshead WK, McKelvey D. Canine and feline anesthesia. In: Thomas JA, Lerche P (eds) *Anesthesia and Analgesia for Veterinary Technicians*, 4th edn. Mosby Inc: St Louis, MO. 2011:253–256.

2 Brodbelt DC, Pfeiffer DU, Young LE, *et al.* Results of the confidential enquiry into perioperative small animal fatalities regarding risk factors for anesthetic-related deaths in dogs. *Journal of the American Veterinary Medical Association* 2008; **233(7)**:1096–1104.

3 Steffey EP, Mama KR. Inhalation anesthetics. In: Tranquilli WJ, Thurmon JC, Grimm KA (eds) *Lumb & Jones Veterinary Anesthesia and Anagesia*, 4th edn. Blackwell Publishing: Ames, IA. 2007:369.

4 Burns S. Delirium during emergence from anesthesia: A case study. *Critical Care Nurse* 2003, **23(1)**:66–69.

5 Bednarski RM. Anesthesia management of dogs and cats. In: Grimm KA, Tranquilli WJ, Lamont LA (eds) *Essentials of Small Animal Anesthesia*, 2nd edn. John Wiley & Sons, Inc. 2011:286–288.

6 Gurney MA. Pharmacological options for intra-operative and early postoperative analgesia: an update. *Journal of Small Animal Practice* 2012; **53**:377–386.

7 Hofmeister EH, Herrington JL, Massaferro EM, Opioid dysphoria in three dogs. *Journal of Veterinary Emergency and Critical Care* 2006; **16(1)**:44–49.

8 Robertson SA, Wegner K, Antinociceptive and side-effects of hydromorphone after subcutaneous administration in cats. *Journal of Feline Medicine and Surgery* 2009; **11(2)**:76–81.

9 Johnson RA, de Morais HA. Respiratory acid-base disorders. In: DiBartola SP (ed.) *Fluid, Electrolyte, and Acid-Base Disorders*, 4th edn. Elsevier: St. Louis, 2012:293–298.

25 Recognition and Assessment of Pain in Dogs

How do I know if they hurt?

Jo Murrell

School of Veterinary Sciences, University of Bristol, UK

KEY POINTS:

- Pain assessment is a prerequisite to adequate pain management in all animals; it helps to avoid both under- and over- treatment of pain.

- Altered behavior is the most reliable sign of pain in dogs.

- The Glasgow Composite Pain Scale has been validated as a tool to quantify acute pain in dogs.

- Recognizing chronic pain is challenging in dogs because signs of pain vary over time and may not be apparent in the consulting room.

- With education, owners are probably best placed to recognize signs of chronic pain in their pet.

- Owner questionnaires have been developed to quantify pain in dogs with chronic pain conditions.

Q. Why is it important to recognize and assess pain in dogs?

A. Recognition and assessment of pain is pivotal to effective pain management. Unless pain is accurately assessed there is the danger that either pain will go unrecognized and inadequately treated, or that dogs will receive too much analgesia and drug side effects as a result of over treatment of pain will occur. Only with assessment of pain can analgesic administration be titrated to meet requirements for analgesia, ensuring optimal patient wellbeing.

Q. How is pain recognized in dogs?

A. Changes in behavior are currently considered to be the most reliable indicator of pain in dogs. Assessment of behavior can inform about both the sensory component of pain (where does it hurt and how much does it hurt?) and the emotional/affective component of pain (fear, anxiety, pain unpleasantness) and it is important that both of these aspects are considered when carrying out

---

Questions and Answers in Small Animal Anesthesia, First Edition. Edited by Lesley J. Smith.
© 2016 John Wiley & Sons, Inc. Published 2016 by John Wiley & Sons, Inc.

pain assessment in an individual patient. Changes in behavior associated with pain may either comprise the expression of "new" pain related behaviors, or the absence of "normal" behaviors, for example reduced interaction with the owner. Therefore a reduction or change in an animal's normal behavioral repertoire must not be overlooked as it could be a sign of pain.

Q. What is the main difference between acute pain and chronic pain?

A. Acute pain is typically pain of short duration that does not outlast the period of tissue healing. Chronic pain is commonly defined as pain that persists for longer than three months. Chronic pain may be associated with ongoing tissue injury, for example in the case of osteoarthritis, but chronic pain may also continue despite healing of the original injury that initiated the pain. It is maladaptive and serves no useful evolutionary purpose to the animal [1].

Q. What are typical behavioral signs of acute pain in dogs?

A. It is difficult to be prescriptive about changes in behavior associated with pain in dogs because there is a large amount of individual variability. Table 25.1 lists some behaviors that are commonly associated with acute pain in dogs and the types of circumstances in which they occur.

Q. How can I improve my ability to recognize behavioral signs of acute pain in dogs?

Table 25.1 Typical behavioral signs of acute pain in dogs.

Behavioral change	Notes
Unwillingness to interact with people	
Postural changes	Abnormal posture, or lying in an abnormal position, inability to rest easily, hunched up position or guarding of the abdomen or another body part
Adoption of the "praying position"	This describes a standing position of the dog with the head down, abdomen stretched and the hindlimbs extended. It is typically adopted in dogs with cranial abdominal pain
Sitting at the back of the cage	
Aggression	Dogs that are not normally aggressive can show signs of aggression when in pain, which abate when pain is adequately managed
Exaggerated pain response to palpation of a wound or painful area	This phenomenon is described as hyperalgesia and accompanies upregulation of pain pathways
Painful response to stimuli that are not normally painful such as touch	This phenomenon is described as allodynia and accompanies upregulation of pain pathways
Unwillingness to move	
Vocalization	Some animals may be silent, others whine, scream, whimper, bark (more or less) growl, attempt to bite
Absence of normal behaviors	Failure to do normal things such as stretch out, less vigorous shaking etc, less playful/curious, appetite changes

A. There are a number of key factors that will increase your ability to recognize behavioral signs of pain in dogs as follows:

✓ Know what is "normal" behavior for an individual patient.

✓ Try to untangle behavioral changes due to anxiety and hospitalization from behavioral changes associated with pain.

✓ Be aware of changes in behavior throughout the day, particularly in response to analgesic drug administration.

✓ When patients are hospitalized, listen to veterinary technicians and animal care staff. They spend a lot of time interacting and caring for patients and therefore are very experienced in recognizing behavioral changes that may be associated with pain.

Q. Are physiological changes a reliable indicator of acute pain in dogs?

A. Changes in heart and respiratory rate and blood pressure are generally accepted to be insensitive indicators of pain in dogs. Do not rely on them and consider that physiological changes may occur for many reasons (e.g., stress, cardiovascular disease, residual anesthetic effects).

Q. Why pain scoring tools are helpful in acute pain management?

A. In addition to aid in recognizing pain, it is advantageous to quantify pain using a pain scoring tool. This allows tracking of changes in pain level using a numerical indicator which aids decision-making about requirement for analgesic drug administration and provides a robust means to confirm that analgesic treatment has been effective.

Q. What pain scoring tool would you recommend for acute pain in dogs and why?

A. The Glasgow Composite Pain Scale is widely used to assess acute pain in dogs and is recommended as the best currently available tool for acute pain assessment in dogs [2]. It is a composite scale that measures both the sensory and emotional component of pain. It can be freely downloaded and has the following advantages:

✓ It is simple to use and quick to complete.

✓ It is robust in a hospital setting where multiple people may be carrying out pain assessments on the same patient.

Q. How does the Glasgow Composite Pain Scale work?

A. The Glasgow Composite Pain Scale comprises a series of questions relating to the dog that take a stepwise approach to assessment [3,4]. The dog is first appraised from outside of the kennel, followed by assessment of responses to interaction with the evaluator and then responses to palpation of a wound or presumptive painful area are noted. For each question there is a selection of 4–5 possible answers to which one is ticked. The different responses are attributed a score, and the scores from all responses are summed to give an overall score which can be out of 24 (if the dog can be walked outside) or 20 (if the dog cannot be walked).

Q. How long does it take to assess pain using the Glasgow Composite Pain Scale?

A. It takes approximately 5 min to assess a patient using the Glasgow Composite Pain Scale, which is easily achievable in veterinary practice.

Q. What do I need to watch out for when using the Glasgow Composite Pain Scale?

A. The scale differentiates poorly between patients that are very sedate and patients that are very painful, therefore when you use the tool apply your common sense! At the end of the assessment you will have come to a conclusion about whether you think the dog is painful or not, irrespective of the assigned score. Therefore if a dog scores highly because it is sedated, but your "gut feeling" is that the dog is comfortable, don't automatically give additional analgesia.

Q. How do I know when more analgesia is needed using the Glasgow Composite Pain Scale?

A. Intervention scores have been developed for the Glasgow Composite Pain Scale, that is the score at which further analgesia is indicated. These scores are $\geq 5/20$ or $\geq 6/24$ dependent on total possible score (i.e., whether the dog can be walked outside or not). Dogs attributed these scores likely require rescue analgesia.

Q. Let us move on to chronic pain. Why is assessment of chronic pain in dogs challenging?

A. Recognizing chronic pain is more difficult than recognizing acute pain in dogs:
   ✓ Behavioral changes associated with chronic pain may be very subtle.
   ✓ Chronic pain may wax and wane over time, therefore changes in behavior are not always consistent.
   ✓ Chronic pain caused by some conditions (e.g., degenerative joint disease) is more common in older dogs and it can be difficult to discriminate between behavioral changes caused by aging and changes due to pain.

Q. How can recognition of behavioral changes caused by chronic pain be improved?

A. ✓ Question the owner carefully in the consultation about changes in behavior; that is appearance of new behaviors or a reduction in behavioral repertoire.
   ✓ Ask questions that relate to the emotional component of pain and quality of life (e.g., questions about activities that the dog normally enjoys and whether these behaviors have changed).
   ✓ Try to gain a sense of how behavior changes day to day and week to week to detect whether pain levels are variable through time.
   ✓ Allow sufficient time (at least 20 min in the first instance) for history taking and a thorough clinical examination. Follow-up appointments to engage the owner with pain assessment may require more time.

Table 25.2   Typical behavioral signs of chronic pain in dogs.

Behavioral change	Notes
Mobility changes	Altered mobility commonly accompanies chronic pain, particularly pain associated with degenerative joint disease. May manifest as difficulty walking, jumping (e.g., into the car), getting up and down stairs
Decreased enjoyment of life	Question the owner about activities that the dog has previously enjoyed e.g., swimming, going for walks, getting up and greeting the owner when they arrive home
Changes in grooming behavior	Poor coat condition may be associated with decreased grooming either because the dog is unable to groom due to impaired mobility or is less motivated to do so
Chewing, licking, biting at parts of the body	Abnormal sensations (or dysaesthesias) can accompany neuropathic pain. This can lead to excessive attention being paid to one part of the body that may lead to self-trauma
Decreased behavioral repertoire	A loss of normal behaviors expressed by an individual dog can be a cardinal sign of chronic pain, particularly associated with decreased quality of life

Q. What sort of behavioral changes can I expect in dogs with chronic pain?

A. See Table 25.2 for typical changes in behavior associated with different types of chronic pain.

Q. Are there any scoring systems developed to quantify chronic pain in dogs?

A. There are no scoring tools that have been specifically designed for veterinarians to quantify chronic pain in dogs; however a number of different owner questionnaires have been developed [5–7]. With education, owners are very capable of recognizing and quantifying chronic pain in their own pet, and due to the amount of time that they spend with the animal are probably best placed to do this. Table 25.3 details some useful scoring systems that have been developed for owners, their relative advantages and where they can be accessed.

Q. How can owner scoring tools be incorporated into clinical patient care?

A. The aims of using owner based scoring systems to assess chronic pain in dogs are to (i) provide information on requirement for analgesia and adequacy of analgesic treatment regimens that supplements "snap shot" clinical assessments made in a veterinary consultation; (ii) inform the owner about the progression of pain and quality of life, which can be helpful when discussing ongoing treatment or time of euthanasia; (iii) involving the owner in monitoring pain can be a key driver of maintaining good compliance with respect to analgesic medication. Pivotal to the success of these scoring systems is prior education of owners about how to use them and their importance in the holistic care of their pet. Frequency of their completion depends on the stability of the pain condition and analgesic medication; for example completing

Table 25.3 Examples of owner-based questionnaires used to quantify chronic pain in dogs.

Questionnaire	Where can it be accessed? (accessed on May 11, 2014) & Notes
Helsinki Chronic Pain Index	http://www.vetmed.helsinki.fi/english/animalpain/hcpi/ Designed to measure pain caused by osteoarthritis in dogs. Quick to fill out, easy to understand by owners
Canine Brief Pain Inventory	http://research.vet.upenn.edu/PennChart/AvailableTools/tabid/1969/Default.aspx Designed to measure pain caused by bone cancer, but can be applied to other forms of chronic pain including osteoarthritis. Allows good tracking of changes in pain level over time. Quick and easy to complete
Client-specific outcome measures	Together with the owner, key behaviors and activities are identified that the dog now has difficulties with. Changes in these behaviors and activities are tracked over time. For a further description see [8] Behaviors and activities are tailored to the individual animal. Quick and easy to complete

a questionnaire every one to two weeks may be appropriate in animals with stable, well managed pain, but more frequent completion, such as every week or twice weekly, might be helpful at the start of analgesic treatment or when adjustments to analgesic medication are made. It is useful to ask for a questionnaire to be completed immediately prior to a veterinary consultation to provide an up to date assessment of pain level.

References

1 Greene SA. Chronic pain: pathophysiology and treatment implications. *Topics in Companion Animal Medicine* 2010: **25**:5–9.

2 University of Glasgow, School of Veterinary Medicine. Short Form Pain Questionnaire. http://www.gla.ac.uk/schoools/vet/research/painandwelfare/downloadacutepainquestionnaire/ (accessed January 9, 2015).

3 Holton L, Reid J, Scott EM, *et al.* Development of a behavior-based scale to measure acute pain in dogs. *Veterinary Record* 2001; **148**:525–531.

4 Holton LL, Scott EM, Nolan AM, *et al.* Relationship between physiological factors and clinical pain in dogs scored using a numerical rating scale. *Journal of Small Animal Practice* 1998; **39**:469–474.

5 Brown DC, Boston R, Coyne JC, *et al.* A novel approach to the use of animals in studies of pain: validation of the canine brief pain inventory in canine bone cancer. *Pain Medicine* 2009; **10**:133–142.

6 Brown DC, Boston RC, Coyne JC, *et al.* Ability of the canine brief pain inventory to detect response to treatment in dogs with osteoarthritis. *Journal American Veterinary Medical Association* 2008; **233**:1278–1283.

7 Mölsä SH, Hielm-Björkman AK, Laitinen-Vapaavuori OM. Use of an owner questionnaire to evaluate long-term surgical outcome and chronic pain after cranial cruciate ligament repair in dogs: 253 cases (2004-2006). *Journal American Veterinary Medical Association* 2013; **243**:689–695.

8 Lascelles BDX, Gaynor JS, Smith ES, *et al.* Amantadine in a multimodal analgesic regimen for alleviation of refractory osteoarthritis in dogs. *Journal of Veterinary Internal Medicine* 2008; **22(1)**:53–59.

26 Recognition and Assessment of Pain in Cats

It is possible!

Beatriz Monteiro[1] and Paulo Steagall[2]

[1] *Département de Biomédecine Vétérinaire, Faculté de Médecine Vétérinaire, Université de Montréal, Canada*
[2] *Département de Sciences Cliniques, Faculté de Médecine Vétérinaire, Université de Montréal, Canada*

KEY POINTS:

- Acute pain is commonly caused by tissue injury, trauma, and inflammation. Assessment of acute pain is an observational, dynamic, and interactive process with palpation of the surgical incision or area of tissue injury in the clinical setting.

- Subjective changes in behavior and facial expressions are used for the recognition and assessment of pain in cats. Physiological and neuroendocrine changes are not reliable indicators of acute pain in this species.

- The UNESP-Botucatu multidimensional composite pain scale (MCPS) is a validated, reliable and consistent method for the assessment of post-operative pain in cats. The MCPS involves pain expression, psychomotor changes, and physiological variables. It can be incorporated as a valuable tool in feline pain assessment in practice.

- Chronic pain has a negative impact on quality of life and animal welfare, causing depression and reduced activity and mobility.

- The assessment of chronic pain is challenging in feline patients. It is based mostly in the assessment of behavior changes.

- Owners play a crucial role in the assessment and treatment-effect outcome in feline chronic pain.

- Degenerative joint disease (DJD) is a very common cause of chronic pain, especially in geriatric cats. Therefore, this population should always be evaluated for chronic pain.

Q. Why is it important to recognize and treat pain in cats?

A. Pain negatively affects quality of life, delays recovery, induces behavioral changes that affect owner–companion animal bond, and causes unnecessary fear, anxiety, and stress. It may lead to sympathetic nervous system activation, and alter food intake and metabolism. In that sense, veterinary caretakers have a moral and ethical responsibility to mitigate animal suffering to the

Questions and Answers in Small Animal Anesthesia, First Edition. Edited by Lesley J. Smith.
© 2016 John Wiley & Sons, Inc. Published 2016 by John Wiley & Sons, Inc.

best of their ability [1]. Pain is now considered to be the fourth vital sign, and its assessment should be incorporated into the clinical evaluation of all patients.

Q. What is the difference between acute (adaptive) and chronic (maladaptive) pain?

A. Acute pain is also known as *adaptive pain* where inflammation and nociception prevail (i.e., post-operative pain). It is generally associated with potential or actual tissue damage and serves to avoid or minimize damage during healing. It is usually self-limiting [1].

Chronic pain is also known as *maladaptive pain* and is characterized by neuropathic or functional pain, such that the degree of pain does not necessarily correlate with the pathology observed or perceived by the individual. It is not associated with healing. It persists beyond the expected course of an acute disease process and it has no clear end-point [2].

In some cases, acute pain can persist and become pathologic and maladaptive especially when neuropathic pain (e.g., limb amputation) is involved or pain was not addressed properly at the time of initial injury.

Acute Pain

The website www.animalpain.com.br provides multilanguage, free and extensive training in the recognition and assessment of acute pain in cats.

Q. What are the causes of acute pain in cats?

A. Acute pain is commonly caused by tissue injury, trauma, and inflammation. Examples may include orthopedic and soft tissue surgery (amputations, abdominal surgery, fractures, etc.), trauma ("hit by car"), dental extractions, incision and drainage of abscesses, and so on. The intensity and duration are related directly to the severity and duration of tissue injury. Some medical and infectious conditions may cause severe acute pain in cats. These include idiopathic cystitis, pancreatitis, lymphocytic-plasmacytic gingivitis and stomatitis, chronic inflammatory bowel disease, ocular ulcers, and so on.

Q. What is the approach for assessment of acute pain in cats in the clinical setting?

A. In the clinical setting, cats are first examined without being removed from their cages and without being disturbed. Then the cat is approached, spoken to, and the cage door opened while observing its reactions and behaviors (aggression, posture, hiding, abnormal gait, etc.). The cat is gently handled, petted, encouraged to interact with the observer, to walk, and to move around. The incision site or area of tissue injury and surrounding skin are gently touched and palpated and the reaction to palpation is evaluated. Individual variability in response to analgesic therapy and palpation is important. In addition, the cat's normal behavior (according to the owners or before surgery) should be taken in consideration. Analgesic treatment (supplemental or interventional analgesic administration) is given when the cat presents pain-related behaviors (see below) and/or overreacts (flinching, vocalizing, etc.) to palpation of the area of tissue injury. Analgesic treatment can also be a diagnostic tool in evaluating pain – if the cat's behavior improves then it is likely that pain was contributing to the abnormal behaviors observed.

Q. What are the behavior changes associated with acute pain in cats?

A. Assessment of pain is an important part of the clinical examination (temperature, pulse, and respiration). Some behaviors may help in this process:

✓ Non-painful cats will continue grooming and using the litter box. Cats that are sleeping, resting, or curling up are usually comfortable and should not be disturbed in the post-operative period. Of importance, bandages may induce agitation in cats that is not necessarily pain-induced.

✓ The cat's normal behavior should be known and owners can provide useful information in this regard. The presence of new behaviors in the post-operative period may guide the clinician in identifying pain and discomfort. For example, a friendly cat becomes aggressive, or it tries to hide or escape during physical examination.

✓ Abdominal tension, hunched-up position, vocalization, and/or escape reaction are indicators of pain after abdominal surgery [3]. In this case, cats will have a low "hung head" and their elbows drawn back. Some cats will demonstrate excessive licking of the painful area.

✓ Abnormal gait or shifting of weight (i.e., after declawing), and sitting or lying in abnormal positions may reflect discomfort and protection of an injured area [1].

✓ An immobile cat and reluctance to move can be signs of severe pain after surgery.

✓ Other non-specific behaviors may include reduced activity and demeanor, aggression, depression, loss of appetite, quietness, hissing, growling, and tail flicking.

✓ *Declawing* may induce licking, shaking and chewing of the feet. The cat appears to be walking as if on "hot coals." The cat may not tolerate their feet being touched and may spontaneously vocalize for no apparent reason, or have periods of suddenly sitting still, or periods of aggression [4].

Q. Are facial expressions important in the recognition of acute pain in cats?

A. Changes in facial expressions have been shown to be a reliable and highly accurate measure of pain in different species. They have been used to quantify the severity and intensity of post-operative pain, and monitor analgesic therapy. A recent study evaluating facial expression in acute pain in cats identified specific features in the areas of the orbit (eyes), ears, and mouth that differed between painful and pain-free cats. Facial scoring scales were designed describing the changes in the ear position and the nose/muzzle shape [5].

Clinical experience shows that cats experiencing pain will have furrowed brow, orbital squeezing (squinted eyes), and a hanging head (head down).

Q. Are physiological and neuroendocrine changes reliable indicators of acute pain in cats?

A. For most of the physiological and neuroendocrine changes, the answer is NO! Thus, heart rate, pupil size, and respiratory rate will not help the clinician in identifying acute pain in cats. A lack of appetite has been shown to be a reliable indicator of pain and can be almost intuitive to the clinician. In the research setting, neuroendocrine assays measuring plasma concentrations of β-endorphin, catecholamines, and cortisol have been correlated with acute pain in cats, however these assays are not clinically applicable and stress, anxiety, fear, general anesthesia, and some drugs will influence these variables [6,7]. Blood pressure has been used in combination with subjective assessment of pain (i.e., behavior changes), however it is usually not practical to evaluate blood pressure in a painful cat [8].

Q. Pain scoring systems can be a valuable tool in the assessment of acute pain in the clinical setting. Is there a validated scoring system for use in cats?

A. Currently, the UNESP-Botucatu multidimensional composite pain scale (MCPS) is the only validated, reliable, consistent, and sensitive pain scoring system for assessing acute pain in cats undergoing abdominal surgery [8]. This instrument combines pain expression (reaction to palpation), psychomotor changes (posture, comfort, activity, and attitude), and physiological variables (arterial blood pressure and appetite) for global pain assessment. When used consistently, this scoring system is an effective clinical decision-making means of evaluating pain in the clinical setting. When a cut-off score is used, the MCPS may provide clinical guidance for analgesic therapy. The instrument is available to download online and free of charge (http://www.biomedcentral.com/1746-6148/9/143). However, this particular scale has some limitations in clinical practice. It may require some time to be completed which could be an issue in a busy clinical practice. In addition, it has not been tested for other types of acute pain besides ovariohysterectomy.

Recently, an acute pain scale to be used in a broad range of clinical conditions called CPMS-feline (CMPS-F) has been proposed. This scale was based on the Glasgow Composite Measure Pain Scale (CMPS), which was developed for routine clinical use where the emphasis was on ease of use and speed of completion [9].

Q. How does one assess and recognize pain in aggressive and feral cats?

A. Assessment of pain is challenging in truly feral cats. Pre-emptive (preventative) analgesic administration is recommended based on the severity and duration of the proposed surgical procedure. Some cats may become "less feral" when sick or after trauma, which may allow better assessment and treatment of pain. In any case, analgesic regimens are extrapolated from a non-feral population of cats that would be undergoing the same surgical procedure.

Q. How can sedation affect pain assessment and recognition in cats?

A. Sedation may affect the cat's level of consciousness, which can inevitably affect pain assessment. Of interest, clinical trials have shown that a stress-free and pain-free recovery from anesthesia are associated with higher levels of sedation (scores) in animals receiving analgesics. In the authors' experience, cats will normally have a calm anesthetic recovery when appropriate analgesic regimens are administered. Opioid overdosing may cause dysphoria. On the other hand, a painful cat may be given acepromazine due to excessive agitation and continuous activity; however, pain-induced behavior changes will not be "treated" and signs of pain may only get worse. In the research setting, statistical models have shown that sedation with dexmedetomidine does not affect pain thresholds [10].

Q. How does one differentiate post-operative emergence delirium, dysphoria, and pain in cats?

A. This is a real challenge to the clinician. Cats may thrash and growl after extubation. These signs could be related to pain, emergence delirium, or dysphoria.

  ✓ Dysphoria is commonly induced by high doses of opioid analgesics or ketamine, and can be controlled with the administration of sedatives such as acepromazine or dexmedetomidine. Opioid reversal with naloxone is a treatment option but analgesia will also be reversed. Clinical experience shows that dysphoria may also be induced by hyperthermia in cats.

  ✓ Emergence delirium is usually restricted to the early post-operative period and is also controlled with the administration of sedatives. In addition, if the delirium is "acceptable," the cat may only require some minutes to eliminate the inhalant anesthetic and regain full consciousness. In some occasions, physical restraint will only induce more agitation and activity. The cat may be better off left alone in a quiet, warm, and dark environment.

  ✓ Pain can usually be elicited by gentle palpation of the wound which will induce changes in behavior. For example, response to palpation is exacerbated and the cat becomes more aggressive or agitated with growling (vocalization). In this case, an "analgesic challenge" (administration of an analgesic drug) is given. If the cat returns to its normal behavior, behavior changes were probably pain induced. Otherwise, worsening of behavior changes may reflect opioid-induced dysphoria. With the latter, sedatives are administered.

Chronic Pain

Q. What are the implications of chronic pain on the quality of life (QoL) of cats?

A. The physiological and psychological consequences of chronic pain in cats have not been thoroughly described. However, clinical experience shows that chronic pain causes suffering, anxiety, impaired mobility, depression, and isolation, among other negative consequences. Chronic pain has a negative impact on the QoL, which becomes a welfare issue [4,11].

Q. What are the causes of chronic pain in cats?

A. The most common causes of feline chronic painful conditions include:

- ✓ Osteoarthritis, DJD.
- ✓ Periodontal disease.
- ✓ Some neoplasias.
- ✓ Skin conditions (e.g., otitis, severe pruritus, burns, chronic wounds).
- ✓ Oral conditions (e.g., gingivitis, stomatitis, feline oral resorptive lesions).
- ✓ Ocular conditions (e.g., corneal disease and ulcers).
- ✓ Gastrointestinal conditions (e.g., megacolon, constipation, inflammatory bowel disease).
- ✓ Urogenital conditions (e.g., interstitial cystitis).
- ✓ Neuropathic pain after onychectomy, limb or tail amputation, among others.

Q. What are the clinical signs and behavioral changes associated with chronic pain in cats?

A. Recognizing chronic pain in cats is more difficult than in dogs. The spectrum of when, how, where, and why there was a change in behavior is most important to evaluate. In that sense, owners become crucial in describing the cat's behavior at home and in reporting treatment/effect. At the clinic, the cat will likely not exhibit chronic pain-induced behaviors that were expressed at home. The cat's responses to painful stimuli will be affected by where and with whom they are.

The clinical signs and behavior changes associated with chronic pain in cats may be subtle and unspecific. They can be inconsistent as signs can improve and/or deteriorate over time.

- ✓ decreased mobility;
- ✓ owner–cat or other pet–cat bond is reduced;
- ✓ depression and isolation;
- ✓ irritation or vocalization when handled;
- ✓ aggression;
- ✓ decreased grooming;
- ✓ increased or decreased appetite;
- ✓ inappropriate (or lack of) use of litter box.

Q. Client communication is crucial in the diagnosis of chronic pain in cats. What questions should be asked during the first clinical assessment of the patient?

Table 26.1   Broad categories used for assessment of quality of life in cats with chronic pain.

Category	Examples
General mobility	Ease of movement, fluidity of movement
Performing activity	Playing, hunting, jumping, using a litter-box
General body functions	Eating, drinking
Specific behaviors	Grooming, scratching
Resting, observing, relaxing	How well these activities can be enjoyed by the cat
Social activities	Involving people and other pets
Temperament	Whether it has changed

Adapted from Mathews K, Kronen PW, Lascelles D, *et al*. Guidelines for recognition, assessment and treatment of pain: WSAVA Global Pain Council members and co-authors of this document. *Journal of Small Animal Practice* 2014; 55(6):E10-68.

A. The first clinical consultation of a cat with possible chronic pain is usually time-consuming since client communication is important for the diagnosis and assessment of the cat's quality of life (QoL). A general assessment of QoL has been recommended by a panel of experts [1]. See Table 26.1.
Suggested questions:

✓ How easy is for your cat to move around? Does the movement seem fluid as it used to be in the past? Do you notice that it is difficult for your cat to get up or to move after a long rest?

✓ Is your cat able to perform routine activities such as playing with toys, hunting, or jumping up and down?

✓ How does your cat get in and out of his litter box? Is it easy for him/her? Have you noticed any inappropriate urination/defecation around the house?

✓ Does he/she eat and drink normally?

✓ Is your cat grooming and using his/her scratch posts normally?

✓ Does your cat interact with you, family, and other pets as it used to?

✓ Have you noticed any change in temperament/demeanour such as sadness, irritation, aggressiveness? Does your cat complain/vocalize/growl when you pick him up?

Q. Let us be practical. What is the step-wise approach for recognition of chronic pain in cats in the clinical setting?

A. ✓ Low-stress physical examination is the first step. A thorough evaluation of the body condition, oral cavity, eyes, ears, skin and fur, paws (whether claws are present), and genitals. Thoracic auscultation and abdominal palpation may reveal abnormalities and/or pain. Close monitoring of the cat's body language and facial expressions is important during assessment. The cat's temperament and resistance to manipulation should also be noted.

✓ Response to pain will normally induce one or more of the following behaviors:
  - tenses the body, resists manipulation;
  - vocalization (hiss, growl, howl);
  - attempt to escape (avoidance);
  - aggression (bite and/or scratch).

✓ An orthopedic examination should follow, especially in geriatric cats that can be affected by DJD. Few cats will be willing to walk around the examination room and even so, lameness is unlikely to be observed. Palpation of all joints and long bones is performed. Passive movements of joints for range of motion and crepitation may or may not give a hint of where it hurts.

✓ Neurologic examination may help to identify cases of neoplasia and neuropathic pain. It may reveal spinal conditions, which are not common in cats but could be a source of chronic pain.

✓ Laboratory bloodwork is of limited usefulness.

✓ Radiographs may reveal DJD or neoplasia. It can be a useful tool when combined with physical examination and patient history.

✓ Other advanced imaging or laboratory evaluations may be useful depending on the clinical case.

An "analgesic challenge" is considered when chronic pain is suspected but not clear. Analgesics are prescribed and a decrease or resolution of the aforementioned clinical signs may confirm the diagnosis of chronic pain. Age-induced behavioral changes may overlap with chronic pain and it is important to differentiate between the two with a rigorous and thorough examination of the cat. Chronic pain must be ruled out before assuming that behavior changes are age-related only. One must consider that geriatric cats are very likely to present with DJD.

Q. What scoring systems are used in the assessment of chronic pain in cats?

A. Currently there are no validated scoring systems to access chronic pain in cats.

Q. DJD/Osteoarthritis (OA) has been lately recognized as one of the main sources of chronic pain in geriatric cats. What is the prevalence and how do I specifically access it in the clinical setting?

A. The prevalence of DJD can be as high as 61% in cats that are six years or older [12]. In cats that are older than 12 years, however, it can be as high as 90% and commonly affects the elbows and the coxofemoral joints [13]. In the clinical setting, cats have a remarkable ability to compensate for orthopedic-induced changes due to their low body weight, superior flexibility, and frequent bilateral disease. Lameness does *not* seem to be a clinical sign in a large proportion of cats with DJD. Instead, behavioral changes will prevail and include:

✓ Decreased mobility (including less jumping, decreased height of obstacles, stiffness, and problems walking up and down stairs).

✓ Less grooming.

✓ Increased urination and/or defecation directly over the edge of the litter box [12].

Radiographs may confirm the diagnosis of DJD when combined with history and physical examination; however, radiographic signs of DJD do not necessarily correlate with clinical signs or signs of pain. Owners may provide a reliable perspective of the cat's everyday behavior. Although there are no validated scales, several owner-based questionnaires have been recently developed specifically to evaluate DJD in cats [14–18]. This assessment will help to evaluate the degree of pain affecting the cat, as well as to evaluate treatment response, which ultimately will guide the choice of the appropriate therapeutic protocol.

Q. How does one monitor efficacy of treatment (reassessment) in cases of chronic pain?

A. Monitoring of treatment efficacy is based on routine assessment of owner-observed behavior and lifestyle changes as previously discussed. Treatment of chronic pain should improve activity, mobility and wellbeing. The same tools used to assess chronic pain in the first visit will be used to monitor the progression of clinical signs and the cat's quality of life as a result of treatment.

Monitoring and evaluation of analgesic drug-induced adverse effects should also be performed.

References

1 Mathews K, Kronen PW, Lascelles D, *et al.* Guidelines for recognition, assessment and treatment of pain: WSAVA Global Pain Council members and co-authors of this document. *Journal of Small Animal Practice* 2014; **55(6)**:E10-68.

2 Sparkes AH, Heiene R, Lascelles BDX, *et al.* ISFM and AAFP Consensus Guidelines. Long-term use of NSAIDs in cats. *Journal of Feline Medicine and Surgery* 2010; **12**:521–538.

3 Waran N, Best L, Williams V, *et al.* A preliminary study of behaviour-based indicators of pain in cats. *Animal Welfare* 2007; **16**:105–108.

4 Robertson S, Lascelles D. Long-term pain in cats - How much do we know about this important welfare issue. *Journal of Feline Medicine and Surgery* 2010; **12(3)**:188–199.

5 Holden E, Calvo G, Collins M, *et al.* Evaluation of facial expression in acute pain in cats. *Journal of Small Animal Practice* 2014; **55(12)**:615–621.

6 Cambridge AJ, Tobias KM, Newberry RC, *et al.* Subjective and objective measurements of postoperative pain in cats. *Journal of the American Veterinary Medical Association* 2000; **217(5)**:685–690.

7 Smith JD, Allen SW, Quandt JE. Changes in cortisol concentration in response to stress and postoperative pain in client-owned cats and correlation with objective clinical variables. *American Journal of Veterinary Research* 1999; **60(4)**:432–436.

8 Brondani JT, Mama KR, Luna SP, *et al.* Validation of the English version of the UNESP-Botucatu multidimensional composite pain scale for assessing postoperative pain in cats. *BMC Veterinary Research* 2013; **9**:143.

9 Calvo G, Holden E, Reid J, *et al.* Development of a behaviour-based measurement tool with defined intervention level for assessing acute pain in cats. *Journal of Small Animal Practice.* 2014; **55(12):**622–629.

10 Slingsby LS, Taylor PM. Thermal antinociception after dexmedetomidine administration in cats: a dose-finding study. *Journal of Veterinary Pharmacology and Therapeutics* 2008; **31(2):**135–142.

11 Bennett D, Ariffin SMZ, Johnston P. Osteoarthritis in the Cat. 1. How common is it and how easy to recognise? *Journal of Feline Medicine and Surgery* 2012; **14:**65–75.

12 Slingerland LI, Hazewinkel HA, Meij BP, *et al.* Cross sectional study of the prevalence and clinical features of osteoarthritis in 100 cats. *Veterinary Journal* 2011; **187(3):**304–309.

13 Hardie EM, Roe SC, Martin FR. Radiographic evidence of degenerative joint disease in geriatric cats: 100 cases (1994–1997). *Journal of the American Veterinary Medical Association* 2002; **220:**628–632.

14 Lascelles BDX, Hansen BD, Roe S, *et al.* Evaluation of client-specific outcome measures and activity monitoring to measure pain relief in cats with osteoarthritis. *Journal of Veterinary Internal Medicine* 2007; **21:**410–416.

15 Bennett D, Morton C. A study of owner observed behavioural and lifestyle changes in cats with musculoskeletal disease before and after analgesic therapy. *Journal of Feline Medicine and Surgery* 2009; **11:**997–1004.

16 Zamprogno H, Hansen BD, Bondell HD, *et al.* Item generation and design testing of a questionnaire to assess degenerative joint disease-associated pain in cats. *American Journal of Veterinary Research* 2010; **71(12):**1417–1424.

17 Klinck MP, Frank D, Guillot M, *et al.* Owner-perceived signs and veterinary diagnosis in 50 cases of feline osteoarthritis. *Canadian Veterinary Journal* 2012; **53(11):**1181–1186.

18 Benito J, Hansen B, DePuy V, *et al.* Feline musculoskeletal pain index: responsiveness and testing of criterion validity. *Journal of Veterinary Internal Medicine* 2013; **27:**474–482.

27 Post-Operative Analgesia – Approaches and Options

So many choices!

Erin Wendt-Hornickle

Department of Veterinary Clinical Sciences, College of Veterinary Medicine, University of Minnesota, USA

KEY POINTS:

- Any procedure deemed painful to people should be considered painful in dogs and cats.

- Multimodal analgesia is the best approach to post-operative pain control.

- Unless there is a contraindication, every patient should receive a nonsteroidal anti-inflammatory drug, even if after surgery.

- Every patient expected to experience moderate to severe pain should receive a μ agonist opioid.

- Limited evidence for the use of adjunctive therapies exists, but they still may be useful in the management of pain when paired with typical analgesics such as nonsteroidal anti-inflammatory drugs or opioids.

Q. What are the benefits of providing analgesia to my post-operative patients?

A. Any injurious event (i.e., surgery) will not only cause changes in the sensory nervous system and produce pain, but will also cause changes in the autonomic nervous system, endocrine and immune systems. In addition, inflammatory substances such as cytokines, prostaglandins, and bradykinins that are released locally can have an effect on subsequent neural processing of pain if not treated promptly and appropriately. When analgesia is provided to patients peri-operatively, these deleterious interactions between body systems are avoided and patients recover faster with a lower rate of complications.

Q. What is the best approach in the treatment of post-operative pain?

A. In the last several decades, there have been major advances in the knowledge and understanding of acute pain physiology. For instance, we know that there are several biological processes that occur prior to a patient perceiving

---

Questions and Answers in Small Animal Anesthesia, First Edition. Edited by Lesley J. Smith.
© 2016 John Wiley & Sons, Inc. Published 2016 by John Wiley & Sons, Inc.

pain. This is called nociception and consists of the transduction, transmission, modulation, and perception of pain. Each of these processes can be broken down further and targeted separately with analgesics of different classes. This is termed multimodal analgesia and is the most complete approach to pain management.

Though controversial, the timing of analgesic administration may also be important. Most evidence suggests that analgesia given at some point prior to recovery and return of consciousness is best. Frequently assessing patients for the presence of pain and continuing treatment when necessary provides more effective pain management.

Q. Which drugs should I choose to treat post-operative pain?

A. There are four major groups of analgesics: nonsteroidal anti-inflammatory drugs (NSAIDs), local anesthetics, opioids, and other adjuncts. Recognizing that pain is a fairly complex physiologic process, a combination of these analgesics is usually best.

Q. Why and how should I choose a NSAID?

A. NSAIDs are extremely useful in the treatment of post-operative pain that is inflammatory in origin, and should be included unless there is a contraindication. Since each of the well-known COX enzymes (COX 1 and COX 2) also serves very important positive physiologic functions such as gastric mucosal defense and healing, modulation of vascular tone in the kidney and proper functioning of platelets, one must choose NSAIDs carefully. It is advantageous to choose an NSAID that has limited inhibition of COX-1 to decrease the gastrointestinal side effects related to administration of these drugs. NSAID approval for use in certain species varies by country. For more information about NSAID use in veterinary medicine, see Chapter 6.

Q. Should I include a local anesthetic as part of my protocol?

A. Yes! Local anesthetics reversibly block impulse conduction through sodium channels, thus preventing membrane depolarization and action potential formation of sensory afferent neurons. These drugs vary in their potency, onset, and duration. Many types of post-operative pain can be managed, in part, by performing local or regional anesthetic techniques prior to surgery. Topical, infiltrative, and regional techniques are valuable in cats and dogs with acute pain. For more information about specific local anesthetic drugs and techniques, see Chapters 24 and 28.

Lidocaine can also be used as an intravenous constant rate infusion (CRI) to provide peri-operative analgesia. If used intra-operatively, it can be continued into the post-operative period at rates of 25–50 mcg/kg/min in dogs [1,2]. If the lidocaine infusion is not started until the post-operative period, a loading dose of 1–2 mg/kg in dogs should precede infusion [1]. It is imperative to use a fluid pump or syringe pump for accurate lidocaine delivery and avoidance of toxicity. For more details regarding lidocaine CRI, see Chapter 22.

A transdermal lidocaine patch is available (LIDODERM, Endo Pharmaceuticals; LidoPAIN SP, EpiCept Corporation) as another option in the treatment of post-operative pain. Originally developed for the treatment of neuropathic pain induced by shingles in humans, lidocaine patches can be safely used on skin incisions for 3–5 days in dogs [3]. They can be cut to fit the size of the patient or shape of the incision without affecting the integrity of the patch [3]. Plasma concentrations of lidocaine are low for the duration of adherence, suggesting very local effects rather than systemic uptake [4,5]. Clinical studies proving their effectiveness are lacking.

Q. Can I give opioids to my patient post-operatively?

A. Yes and you definitely should give them post-operatively in all patients with moderate to severe pain! Opioids, specifically µ agonists, remain the most effective analgesics in controlling moderate to severe acute pain, especially as part of a multimodal regime [6]. There are many different potential routes of administration, including injectable, oral transmucosal, transdermal/topical, and oral.

Q. What opioids can I give via injection?

A. Several full and partial µ agonists are available in an injectable formulation given as bolus injections and also as constant rate infusions. Morphine, hydromorphone, oxymorphone, fentanyl, meperidine, methadone, and buprenorphine are the most commonly used injectable opioids in veterinary medicine. Though these drugs are similar in action, their pharmacokinetic profiles differ considerably. For more detailed information on specific opioids and their analgesic uses, see Chapter 6.

Q. Is there something injectable that lasts longer than 8 h?

A. Simbadol™ (buprenorphine injection; Abbott Laboratories, IL, USA) is the first FDA approved long-lasting injectable analgesic for use in cats. It is administered subcutaneously every 24 h for a maximum of 3 days at a dosage of 0.24 mg/kg. Analgesic effects of Simbadol™ begin 1 h from injection; it is recommended to administer it 1 h prior to surgery. This formulation showed analgesic efficacy in both orthopedic (onychectomy) and soft tissue surgeries, though 39 and 29% of cats, respectively, required additional analgesia [7].

There is also a sustained release formulation of buprenorphine (ZooPharm, CO, USA) that provides analgesia for up to 72 h when given subcutaneously. Limited studies suggest that it provides similar analgesia and has a similar side effect profile to OTM buprenorphine when used prior to ovariohysterectomy in dogs and cats [8]. Clinical experience has found that some patients develop a local skin reaction at the site of injection. Since some patients often object to medication, these longer-acting options have a definite advantage for treating mild to moderate post-operative pain.

Q. What if I have a patient that will not tolerate injections?

A. Some opioids can be given via the oral transmucosal route (OTM). This route of opioid administration is most commonly associated with cats due to their small dosage requirements and basic (high pH) mouths. There are two opioids that have been administered most often via this route: methadone and buprenorphine.

Methadone can be administered OTM in cats and has adequate bioavailability and analgesic qualities when given by this route. The antinociceptive effects of OTM methadone may last longer than intravenous administration; though plasma levels are lower [9]. Euphoric effects (kneading, purring, rubbing against objects) are commonly seen along with mydriasis; however, dysphoric effects (excitement, anxiety, restlessness) are not common [9–12].

Buprenorphine, a partial μ agonist, is almost 100% bioavailable when given to cats via the OTM route at doses of 0.02 mg/kg [13]. It is very well tolerated by feline patients. Studies of its efficacy at providing analgesia by this route are contradictory, but may be related to the doses used (i.e., 0.02 mg/kg is more effective than 0.01 mg/kg) [14–16]. Because of buprenorphine's partial agonist actions, it is best suited for treating mild to moderate pain.

Q. Can I give an oral opioid for post-operative pain?

A. Despite limited evidence-based information of the analgesic efficacy of opioids given orally in veterinary patients, this route is used for the treatment of post-operative analgesia.

Codeine alone, or in combination with acetaminophen, has been used in dogs for the management of mild to moderate pain on an outpatient basis. Similar to other oral opioids, this drug has limited bioavailability (4%) and a short half-life when given orally. Plasma levels of one of its metabolites, codeine-6-glucuronide, remain high and may provide analgesia [17]. The acetaminophen may also contribute to the apparent analgesic effects.

The pharmacokinetics of hydrocodone with and without acetaminophen in dogs has also been described [18,19]. At clinically relevant doses, plasma concentrations of hydrocodone and its active metabolite, hydromorphone, are above the level thought to provide analgesia for dogs [20].

Other oral opioids have been examined (morphine, oxycodone, methadone) but they have low oral bioavailability, low plasma concentrations, and short half-lives, suggesting limited clinical effect [21]. The evidence for using any of these drugs for the treatment of post-operative pain is very low. It is important to remember that many formulations of these opioids are in combination products with acetaminophen, which is highly toxic to cats and may not be tolerated by some dogs. The bottom line: more studies need to be done to establish the analgesic efficacy of these drugs given orally for veterinary patients.

Q. What about tramadol, isn't that an opioid?

A. Tramadol, though considered a weak mu opioid, also inhibits serotonin and norepinephrine reuptake within the central nervous system and may have other actions as well. Dogs do not metabolize tramadol in the same way that humans do, and therefore do not experience substantial opioid effects of this drug [22,23]. Yet, it is still effective in treating post-operative pain in some circumstances [24]. Tramadol is probably most effective at treating acute pain when given in combination with an NSAID [25].

Cats, on the other hand, metabolize tramadol similarly to people and therefore may experience prominent opioid effects after tramadol administration [26,27]. Like dogs, tramadol seems to be most effective post-operatively when given concurrently with an NSAID [28].

Q. What about placing a patch or giving something topically?

A. There are currently two opioids used via the transdermal patch route, fentanyl and buprenorphine, and one opioid available in a topical formulation (fentanyl).

Fentanyl patches can successfully provide post-operative analgesia in both dogs and cats [29,30]. There is a lot of individual variation in the level of analgesia between patients, so it remains important to continue to assess these patients for pain and administer additional analgesics if necessary. Recommended dosages are 2–5 mcg/kg/h in dogs and 25 mcg/cat. In cats < 5 kg, a 25 mcg patch may provide excessive doses of fentanyl. In these smaller patients, a 12.5 mcg/h patch should be used.

Buprenorphine patches have been used in dogs for post-operative analgesia as well. Similar to fentanyl when given via this route, individual variation in the uptake of buprenorphine makes pain assessment essential in order to determine the need for additional analgesics [31,32]. Unfortunately buprenorphine via this route does not seem to be clinically useful in cats, as evidence suggests that it may not provide effective analgesia [33].

There is also a new formulation of fentanyl available: a 50 mg/ml transdermal fentanyl solution (Recuvyra, Elanco Animal Health, IN, USA) for the treatment of post-operative pain in dogs. This product dries rapidly, is applied in similar fashion to topical flea and tick products, and offers distinct advantages over intravenous and transdermal patch routes. The patient does not need to have an intravenous catheter, the drug levels stay constant over a minimum of 4 days [34] and the veterinarian does not have to worry about patch adherence. This transdermal fentanyl solution effectively provides post-operative analgesia in dogs [35,36], but should not be administered to cats. This formulation can result in profound sedation in some canine patients and should not be used in any patient that historically does not do well with μ opioid administration or in any situation where the patient cannot be monitored closely. In addition, since this solution is extremely concentrated, it is important to follow the manufacturer's guidelines regarding administration and care of the patient.

Q. Is there anything else I can add to my regime that does not fall into the categories mentioned?

A. Yes! There are many drugs that have other analgesic effects and may be beneficial as adjuncts in the treatment of post-operative pain. Most drugs that fall into this category, however, have limited clinical evidence in regards to their use in post-operative pain management.

Tapentadol is a μ opioid that, like tramadol, also inhibits norepinephrine reuptake within the central nervous system. In contrast to tramadol, it does not require metabolism to active metabolites [37]. Tapentadol's clinical use in veterinary patients has not been reported; however, one experimental antinociception model in dogs showed promising results [37]. In this study, tapentadol had antinociceptive qualities similar to morphine. While more studies testing the clinical applications of this drug need to be performed, it seems tapentadol may be an option in the treatment of post-operative pain in dogs in the near future. The ideal dose of tapentadol for dogs and cats has not yet been established.

Amantadine is an antiviral drug, but also increases dopamine concentration in the central nervous system and acts as an NMDA antagonist. Because of its mechanism of action on NMDA receptors, it is likely only effective at treating pain when central sensitization has occurred, as in patients with chronic pain or ongoing acute pain. It is effective in dogs with refractory hindlimb osteoarthritis pain when used with meloxicam and has been effective in the treatment of neuropathic pain as well [38,39]. Amantadine may be considered part of a post-operative plan if a patient has had longstanding pain prior to the procedure. Recommended dosages for dogs and cats are 2–5 mg/kg every 12–24 h [21,39,40].

Gabapentin is an anticonvulsant that is also used as an analgesic in veterinary patients. It is a structural analog of gamma-aminobutyric acid (GABA), but does not bind to GABA receptors. Instead, it binds to the alpha-2 delta subunit of calcium channels to decrease the ascending transmission of neuronal impulses (including pain) within the central nervous system. It also increases the amount of GABA available within the central nervous system. Even though alpha-2 delta expression changes have not been reported in inflammatory pain states, gabapentin does inhibit inflammatory pain in experimental models, suggesting there are other mechanisms of action [41]. Although the current evidence supporting use of gabapentin for post-operative pain in dogs and cats is low, pharmacokinetic studies suggest that dosages of 10–20 mg/kg every 8 h are necessary to achieve effects [42,43]. Most case reports documenting the use of gabapentin have used inappropriately low dosages; therefore more studies need to be done to assess its use as a post-operative analgesic.

Pregabalin is also an anticonvulsant with mechanisms similar to gabapentin that has been used as an analgesic in veterinary patients. Although the pharmacokinetics have been described in dogs and a dosage of 4 mg/kg every 12 h is suggested [44], evidence for analgesic efficacy is lacking. Pregabalin is a controlled drug (DEA CV) and is currently quite expensive.

Q. When can I discontinue post-operative analgesia?

A. The most effective way to know if you can discontinue analgesia is to regularly assess your patient for pain. Acute pain, by definition, will subside once tissues have healed, and it is likely that most patients will not need additional analgesia beyond 1–2 weeks after surgery. If a patient has experienced chronic pain or has had a procedure that may predispose them to developing chronic pain, the administration of analgesics may need to be continued for longer periods.

Q. Are there non-pharmaceutical methods to aid in the treatment of post-operative pain?

A. There are several non-pharmaceutical methods available. Acupuncture, rehabilitation (physical therapy), and low-level laser therapy (LLLT) are a few examples. The specifics of these therapies are beyond the scope of this chapter; however, they are most often used in conjunction with pharmaceutical methods and may be very useful in the management of post-operative pain in some patients.

Q. What is an example of a reasonable post-operative analgesia plan for a healthy dog that has undergone a fracture repair for which a local anesthetic technique is not an option? How long should I continue analgesia?

A. This is a patient who would benefit from multimodal analgesia. The dog should receive a μ opioid agonist (i.e., morphine, hydromorphone, oxymorphone) prior to surgery. Intra-operatively, a constant rate infusion of morphine (0.24 mg/kg/h), lidocaine (25–100 mcg/kg/min), and ketamine (2–10 mcg/kg/min) would be appropriate*. All of these drugs provide inhalant minimum alveolar concentration (MAC) reduction and analgesia. Post-operatively, this patient can remain on the CRI for 12–48 h depending on the severity of pain and level of analgesia required. After discontinuation of the CRI, the patient should receive a parenteral μ agonist as needed for pain; this may be required for up to 3 days post-operatively. Alternatively, a fentanyl patch could be placed prior to discontinuation of the CRI. In addition, unless there is a contraindication, this patient should receive an appropriate NSAID for anti-inflammatory and analgesic effects. The NSAID can be continued for 7–14 days. Oral analgesics, including tramadol and an NSAID, are appropriate choices for continuation beyond discharge. As always, it is important during recovery to frequently assess the patient for pain to determine the need for additional analgesia.

*If a fluid pump is not available, do not include the lidocaine as it may lead to inadvertent overdose with subtle changes in fluid administration rates.

Q. What is an example of a reasonable post-operative analgesic plan for a cat that has had an exploratory laparotomy for a linear foreign body? How long should I continue analgesia?

A. This patient should receive a μ agonist prior to surgery (i.e., morphine, hydromorphone, oxymorphone). Intra-operatively, an opioid CRI (i.e., fentanyl 5–10 mcg/kg/h) could be considered; however, depending on the duration of the procedure and the cat's level of pain, it may not be necessary. Post-operatively, opioids should be continued for a minimum of 24 h. Buprenorphine is a reasonable choice for mild to moderate post-operative pain in cats. If the patient is experiencing severe pain, a µ agonist is a better choice. Depending on the level of surgical intervention and the current health of the gastrointestinal tract, an appropriate NSAID may also be considered. As always, it is important during recovery to frequently assess the patient for pain to determine the need for additional analgesia.

References

1 Dyson DH. Perioperative pain management in veterinary patients. *Veterinary Clinics of North America: Small Animal Practice* 2008; **38**:1309–1327.
2 Gaynor JS, Muir WW. *Handbook of Veterinary Pain Management*. 2nd edn. Mosby: St. Louis, 2002.
3 Weil AB, Ko J, Inoue T. The use of lidocaine patches. *Compendium of Veterinary Continuing Education* 2007; **29**:208–216.
4 Ko J, Weil A, Maxwell L, *et al*. Plasma concentrations of lidocaine in dogs following lidocaine patch application. *Journal of the American Animal Hospital Association* 2007; **43**: 280–283.
5 Ko JC, Maxwell LK, Abbo LA, *et al*. Pharmacokinetics of lidocaine following the application of 5% lidocaine patches to cats. *Journal of Veterinary Pharmacology and Therapeutics* 2008; **31**:359–367.
6 Hunt JR, Attenburrow PM, Slingsby LS, *et al*. Comparison of premedication with buprenorphine or methadone with meloxicam for postoperative analgesia in dogs undergoing orthopaedic surgery. *Journal of Small Animal Practice* 2013; **54**:418–424.
7 Simbadol™ manufacturer insert; Abbott Laboratories, Abbott Park, IL, USA.
8 Catbagan DL, Quimby JM, Mama KR, *et al*. Comparison of the efficacy and adverse effects of sustained-release buprenorphine hydrochloride following subcutaneous administration and buprenorphine hydrochloride following oral transmucosal administration in cats undergoing ovariohysterectomy. *American Journal of Veterinary Research* 2011; **72**:461–466.
9 Ferreira TH, Rezende ML, Mama KR, *et al*. Plasma concentrations and behavioral, antinociceptive, and physiologic effects of methadone after intravenous and oral transmucosal administration in cats. *American Journal of Veterinary Research* 2011; **72**:764–771.
10 Dobromylskyj P. Assessment of methadone as an anaesthetic premedicant in cats. *Journal of Small Animal Practice* 1993; **34**:604–608.
11 Rohrer Bley C, Neiger-Aeschbacher G, Busato A, *et al*. Comparison of perioperative racemic methadone, levo-methadone and dextromoramide in cats using indicators of post-operative pain. *Veterinary Anaesthesia and Analgesia* 2004; **31**:175–182.
12 Steagall, PVM, Carnicelli P, Taylor PM, *et al*. Effects of subcutaneous methadone, morphine, buprenorphine or saline on thermal and pressure thresholds in cats. *Journal of Veterinary Pharmacology and Therapeutics* 2006; **29**:531–537.
13 Robertson SA, Taylor PM, Sear JW. Systemic uptake of buprenorphine by cats after oral mucosal administration. *Veterinary Record* 2003; **152**:675–678.
14 Robertson SA, Lascelles BD, Taylor PM, *et al*. PK-PD modeling of buprenorphine in cats: intravenous and oral transmucosal administration. *Journal of Veterinary Pharmacology and Therapeutics* 2005; **28**:453–460.

15 Giordano T, Steagall PV, Ferreira TH *et al*. Postoperative analgesic effects of intravenous, intramuscular, subcutaneous or oral transmucosal buprenorphine administered to cats undergoing ovariohysterectomy. *Veterinary Anaesthesia and Analgesia* 2010; **37**:357–366.

16 Porters N, Bosmans T, Debille M, *et al*. Sedative and antinociceptive effects of dexmedetomidine and burprenorphine after oral transmucosal or intramuscular administration in cats. *Veterinary Anaesthesia and Analgesia* 2014; **41**:90–96.

17 Kukanich B. Pharmacokinetics of acetaminophen, codeine and the codeine metabolites morphine and codeine-6-glucuronide in healthy Greyhound dogs. *Journal of Veterinary Pharmacology and Therapeutics* 2010; **33**:15–21.

18 Findley JW, Jones EC, Welch RM. Radioimmunoassay deterimination of the absolute oral bioavailabilies and O-demethylation of codeine and hydrocodone in the dog. *Drug Metabolism and Disposition* 1979; **7**:310–314.

19 KuKanich B, Spade J. Pharmacokinetics of hydrocodone and hydromorphone after oral hydrocodone in healthy Greyhounds dogs. *Veterinary Journal* 2013; **196**:266–268.

20 Guedes AG, Papich MG, Rude EP, *et al*. Pharmacokinetics and physiologic effects of intravenous hydromorphone in conscious dogs. *Journal of Veterinary Pharmacology and Therapeutics* 2008; **31**:334–343.

21 Kukanich B. Outpatient oral analgesics in dogs and cats beyond nonsteoridal anti-inflammatory drugs: an evidence=based approach. *Veterinary Clinics of North America: Small Animal Practice* 2013; **43**:1109–1125.

22 Kukanich B, Papich MG. Pharmacokinetics of tramadol and the metabolite O-desmethyltramadol in dogs. *Journal of Veterinary Pharmacology and Therapeutics* 2004;**27**: 239–246.

23 Kukanich B, Papich MG. Pharmacokinetics and antinociceptive effects of oral tramadol hydrochloride administration in Greyhounds. *American Journal of Veterinary Research* 2011; **72**:256–262.

24 Teixeira RC, Moneiro ER, Campagnol D, *et al*. Effects of tramadol alone, in combination with meloxicam or dipyrone, on postoperative pain and the analgesic requirement in dogs undergoing unilateral mastectomy with or without ovariohysterectomy. *Veterinary Anaesthesia and Analgesia* 2013; **40**:641–649.

25 Davila D, Keeshen TP, Evans RB, *et al*. Comparison of the analgesic efficacy of perioperartive firocoxib and tramadol administration in dogs undergoing tibial plateau leveling osteotomy. *Journal of the American Veterinary Medical Association* 2013; **243**:224–231.

26 Pypendop BH, Ilkiw JE. Pharmacokinetics of tramadol, and its metabolite O-desmethyltramadol, in cats. *Journal of Veterinary Pharmacology and Therapeutics* 2008; **31**:52–59.

27 Cagnardi P, Villa R, Zonca A, *et al*. Pharmacokinetics, intraoperative effect and postoperative analgesia of tramadol in cats. *Research in Veterinary Science* 2011; **90**:503–509.

28 Brondani J, Loureiro Luna SP, Beier SL, *et al*. Analgesic efficiacy of perioperative use of vedaprofen, tramadol or their acombination in cats undergoing ovariohysterectomy. *Journal of Feline Medicine and Surgery* 2009; **11**:420–429.

29 Franks JN, Boothe JW, Taylor L, *et al*. Evaluation of transdermal fentanyl patches for analgesia in cats undergoing onychectomy. *Journal of the American Veterinary Medical Association* 2000; **217**:1013–1020.

30 Bellei E, Roncada P, Pisoni L, *et al*. The use of fentanyl-patch in dogs undergoing spinal surgery: plasma concentration and analgesic efficacy. *Journal of Veterinary Pharmacology and Therapeutics* 2011; **34**:437–441.

31 Pieper K, Schuster T, Levionnois O, *et al*. Antinociceptive efficacy and plasma concentrations of transdermal buprenorphine in dogs. *Veterinary Journal* 2011; **187**:335–341.

32 Moll X, Fresno L, Garcia F, *et al*. Comparison of subcutaneous and transdermal administration of buprenorphine for pre-emptive analgesia in dogs undergoing elective ovariohysterectomy. *Veterinary Journal* 2011; **187**:124–128.

33 Murrell JC, Robertson SA, Taylor PM, *et al.* Use of a transdermal matrix patch of buprenorphine in cats: preliminary pharmacokinetic and pharmacodynamic data. *Veterinary Record* 2007; **160**:578–583.

34 Freise KJ, Savides MC, Riggs KL, *et al.* Pharmacokinetics and dose selection of a novel, long-acting transdermal fentanyl solution in healthy laboratory Beagles. *Journal of Veterinary Pharmacology and Therapeutics* 2012; **35**:21–26.

35 Linton DD, Wilson MG, Newbound GC, *et al.* The effectiveness of a long-acting transdermal fentanyl solution compared to buprenorphine for the control of postoperative pain in dogs in a randomized, multicentered clinical study. *Journal of Veterinary Pharmacology and Therapeutics* 2012; **35**:53–64.

36 Martinez SA, Wilson MG, Linton DD, *et al.* The safety and effectiveness of a long-acting transdermal fentanyl solution compared with oxymorphone for the control of postoperative pain in dogs: a randomized, multicentered clinical study. *Journal of Veterinary Pharmacology and Therapeutics* 2013; Dec 18. doi: 10.1111/jvp.12096. [Epub ahead of print].

37 Kogel B, Terlinden R, Schneider J. Characterization of tramadol, morphine and tapentadol in an acute pain model in Beagle dogs. *Veterinary Anesthesia and Analgesia* 2014; **41**:297–304.

38 Madden M, Gurney M, Bright S. Amantadine, an N-Methyl-D-Aspartate antagonist, for the treatment of chronic neuropathic pain in a dog. *Veterinary Anesthesia and Analgesia* 2014; doi: 10.1111/vaa.12141. [Epub ahead of print].

39 Lascelles BD, Gaynor JS, Smith ES, *et al.* Amantadine in a multimodal analgesic regimen for the alleviation of refractory osteoarthritis pain in dogs. *Journal of Veterinary Internal Medicine* 2008; **22**:53–59.

40 Siao KT, Pypendop BH, Stanley SD, *et al.* Pharmacokinetics of amantadine in cats. *Journal of Veterinary Pharmacology and Therapeutics* 2011; **34**:599–604.

41 Yoon MH, Yaksh TL. The effect of intrathecal gabapentin on pain befavior and hemodynamics on the formalin test in the rat. *Anesthesia and Analgesia* 1999; **89**:434–439.

42 Siao KT, Pypendop BH, Ilkiw JE. Pharmacokinetics of gabapentin in cats. *American Journal of Veterinary Research* 2010; **71**:17–21.

43 Kukanich B, Cohen RL. Pharmacokinetics of oral gabapentin in greyhound dogs. *Veterinary Journal* 2011; **187**:133–135.

44 Salazar V, Dewey CW, Schwark W, *et al.* Pharmacokinetics of a single-dose oral pregabalin administration in normal dogs. *Veterinary Anaesthesia and Analgesia* 2009; **36**:574–580.

28 Anesthetic Considerations for Dental Prophylaxis and Oral Surgery

From bad breath to pearly whites

Jason W. Soukup and Lesley J. Smith

Department of Surgical Sciences, School of Veterinary Medicine, University of Wisconsin, USA

KEY POINTS:

- Many dental patients are geriatric, therefore a thorough physical exam, pre-operative blood work, and close anesthetic monitoring are imperative.

- Because of the use of water coolant for dental instruments, particular attention to airway security and prevention of aspiration is required.

- Tracheal trauma in cats occurs due to over-inflation of the endotracheal tube cuff and movement of the patient with the circuit connected to the endotracheal tube. The use of spring-loaded mouth gags can lead to cortical blindness in cats.

- Loco-regional blocks are commonly employed to minimize anesthetic requirements and to provide post-operative analgesia.

- The addition of buprenorphine to local anesthetics may improve the duration of action of the loco-regional technique.

- Local anesthetics should be avoided in areas of neoplastic tissue and significant inflammation/infection.

- Jaw fractures and oral tumor surgeries require alternative intubation techniques.

Q. Who is my "typical" patient presenting for a dental prophylaxis?

A. The most common patients that require dental cleanings are middle-aged to geriatric dogs and cats who have achieved their owner's attention because they have significant halitosis or have demonstrated a reduction in appetite or a change in chewing behavior. Because many of these patients are of a more "advanced" age, co-morbidities associated with aging should be considered. These patients should receive a thorough physical examination and bloodwork as indicated based on breed, history, physical exam findings, concurrent medications, and so on.

Questions and Answers in Small Animal Anesthesia, First Edition. Edited by Lesley J. Smith.
© 2016 John Wiley & Sons, Inc. Published 2016 by John Wiley & Sons, Inc.

In general, geriatric patients have reduced organ "reserve," which means that they tolerate the physiologic insults of general anesthesia more poorly than young robust patients. Close attention to monitoring of blood pressure, heart rate, oxygenation, ventilation, and temperature are imperative in order to ensure a successful outcome and recovery from anesthesia.

Q. What are special airway management concerns for dentistry patients?

A. Many dentistry and oral surgery patients are positioned in dorsal recumbency to improve the operator's view of the entire oral cavity. This demands special consideration for airway protection. Dorsal recumbency will cause fluid from ultrasonic scalers and high-speed hand pieces to accumulate in the pharynx. Therefore, patients should be intubated with an appropriately sized endotracheal tube and the cuff should be checked multiple times during the procedure for possible leaks. In addition, suction placed in the pharyngeal region is recommended to collect fluid. Alternatively, the pharynx can be packed with sponges. If this method is chosen, the sponges should be replaced regularly as they become saturated. Additionally, measures should be instituted to insure the sponges are removed at the end of the procedure. Such methods may include a long strip of tape attached to the sponges that hangs out of the mouth or a piece of tape in a conspicuous location such as an ear or the muzzle that would serve as a reminder. Tracheal tears in cats have been shown to be significantly associated with dental procedures [1,2]. This association seems to be linked to over-inflation of the endotracheal tube cuff rather than with the dental procedure themselves or with re-positioning the patients. That said, it is advisable to disconnect the endotracheal tube from the anesthetic circuit when repositioning cats because the "drag" on the cuff/tube can cause further damage during repositioning if not disconnected. Over-inflation of the cuff most likely occurs because of an overzealous effort to maintain a protected airway. The appropriate volume of air for cats has been shown to be in the 1–2 ml range [1].

Q. Why is the use of spring-loaded mouth gags not advisable in cats?

A. When a spring-loaded mouth gag forces the cat's mandible open the result is potential compromise of perfusion of blood to the cortical regions of the brain. This is because the anatomy of cerebral blood flow in cats is unique. Branches of the mandibular artery are the sole supply of oxygenated blood to the cortex. When the jaw is held open, soft tissues in the caudal pharynx compress the manibular artery, limiting flow of arterial blood. With concurrent hypotension, flow is even more compromised. Cats may demonstrate significant central neurologic defects, particularly blindness, upon recovery.

Q. If the endotracheal tube is in the way, are there any alternatives to traditional orotracheal intubation?

A. In some cases orotracheal intubation is impracticable or even not possible. Pharyngotomy intubation is an alternative intubation technique when the oral cavity must be bypassed. However, iatrogenic complications associated with damage to the neurovascular structures of the region (external carotid artery, jugular vein, linguo-facial vein, maxillary vein, hypoglossal nerve, vago-sympathetic trunk of the recurrent laryngeal nerve) are possible. Alternatively, a transmylohyoid orotracheal intubation can be utilized. Because of its relatively simple approach the transmylohyoid technique decreases the risk of iatrogenic complications when compared to pharyngotomy intubation. This technique utilizes a surgical approach through the skin and mylohyoid muscles in the intermandibular region [3].

Fortunately, there are only a few rare oral diseases that may lead to complete trismus (masticatory myositis, cranio-mandibular osteopathy, temporo-mandibular apparatus dysplasia/trauma/neoplasia, salivary gland disease, post-radiation fibrosis). In these cases the oral cavity cannot be opened far enough to intubate orally. Thus, when presented with these cases, the anesthetist should be prepared for endoscopic intubation of the trachea or a tracheostomy.

Q. What are the common local anesthetic techniques used for dental procedures and where do they block?

A. There are five commonly used local nerve blocks in veterinary dentistry and oral surgery. See Figures 28.1, 28.2, and 28.3.

  ✓ *Caudal Maxillary Block*: This block would target both the infraorbital nerve and the major palatine nerve, which requires the needle to be advanced through the infraorbital canal and into the pterygopalatine fossa so that both nerves can be anesthetized. In small-to medium-sized dogs and in

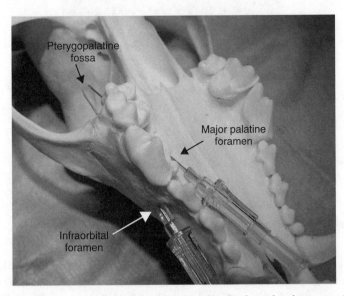

Figure 28.1 Ventral view of a dog skull showing the infraorbital canal and pterygopalatine fossa.

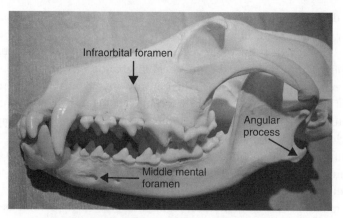

Figure 28.2 Lateral view of a dog skull showing the infraorbital canal. The middle mental foramen is also depicted in this figure.

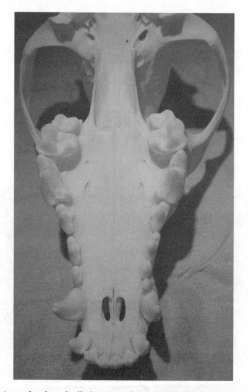

Figure 28.3 Ventral view of a dog skull showing the major palatine foramen.

cats, this block should desensitize the hard and soft palate and the molar teeth. In larger dogs, the inability to reach the pterygopalatine fossa with the needle lengths available in standard hypodermic needles will prevent proper anesthesia of the hard and soft palate and will diminish the ability to anesthetize the molar teeth. Therefore, a 3-in spinal needle may be required in large breed dogs. In many dogs it may be more appropriate to deliver an infraorbital and a major palatine block separately.

✓ *Infraorbital Block:* With this block the anesthetic is delivered just within the infraorbital canal immediately caudal to the infraorbital foramen. Placement of local anesthetic in this location will not anesthetize the palatal mucosa and the fourth premolar tooth may not be anesthetized. The infraorbital block, when administered properly, can anesthetize the third premolar rostrally to include the first incisor and the upper lip from the infraorbital canal to the philtrum.

✓ *Major Palatine Block*: The major palatine nerve innervates half of the palatal mucosa and this block is often used in conjunction with the infraorbital block in larger dogs or simply to better ensure anesthesia to the palatal soft tissues when extracting teeth rostral to the major palatine foramen. The major palatine foramen is located on a line midway between the palatal midline and the palatal aspect of the maxillary dentition and intersects a point along a line somewhere between the mesial aspect of the first molar and mesial aspect of the fourth premolar. The local anesthetic should be delivered at the mesial aspect of these landmarks to insure the anesthetic is injected rostral to the foramen.

✓ *Inferior Alveolar (Caudal Mandibular) Block*: The mandibular branch of the trigeminal nerve enters the mandibular canal through the mandibular foramen on the lingual aspect of the caudal mandible and continues as the inferior alveolar nerve. The nerve exits the mandibular canal at the caudal, middle, and rostral mental foramina. In dogs and cats, the mandibular foramen is located on the lingual aspect of the mandibular ramus approximately halfway between the mandibular third molar and the angular process. There is an intra- and extra-oral approach to the mandibular foramen. The intra-oral approach is described here with the animal in dorsal recumbency as this author believes this to be the most accurate approach. The index finger should be placed on the angular process outside of the mouth while simultaneously using the thumb to open the lower jaw. The needle tip should be placed onto the mucosa immediately lingual to the last molar tooth. The needle should be directed along the periosteum and toward the angular process. Local anesthetic should be deposited half the distance between the point of needle entry and the angular process. When successfully delivered, this nerve block should anesthetize all mandibular teeth ipsilateral to the block up to the first incisor, and the lower lip from the caudal mental foramen rostral. If larger volumes of anesthetic are used, the tongue may also be anesthetized.

✓ *Middle Mental Block*: This block should anesthetize the teeth and lip from the middle mental foramen forward to the ipsilateral first incisor. The middle mental foramen is located ventral to the mesial root of the second premolar. The needle bevel should be placed at the level of the middle mental foramen. However, the needle should not be threading into the foramen as this practice may cause traumatic nerve damage. See Figure 28.2.

Q. Is one local anesthetic better than the other?

A. Commonly reported local anesthetics used for nerve blocks in small animals include lidocaine, bupivacaine, mepivacaine, and lidocaine/bupivacaine combinations. Some variability exists regarding the reported time to onset and duration of activity of the commonly used anesthetics depending on species and the specific block in question. However, lidocaine can be considered a fast-acting anesthetic with a short duration of activity. Bupivicaine is considered to be slow-acting with a longer duration of activity when compared to lidocaine. Bupivacaine's onset of action is 6–10 min when used for dental loco-regional blocks, which is considered intermediate. If proper planning is done, this longer onset is not a concern. For example, the anesthetic can be delivered prior to surgical preparation or polishing so that it has time to take effect before the painful procedure is begun. The duration of action of bupivicaine is considered to be 4–6 h. However, the effects may last up to 6–8 h when placed in a foramen. Some clinicians believe that in some cases an anesthetic with a long duration of action is undesirable. It is thought that completely anesthetized tissues may encourage increased manipulation of the surgical site by the patient with tongue thrusting. Thus, when suture breakdown may result in significant complications, such as maxillectomies or other palatal defect repairs, use of a shorter acting local anesthetic (lidocaine) followed by aggressive post-operative pain management with systemically delivered analgesics may be preferred. Therefore, one local anesthetic is not better than the other. However, certain local anesthetics may be better suited for some surgical procedures and post-operative pain management goals.

Q. Can an opioid be added to increase the effectiveness of local anesthetics?

A. Humans studies have shown a prolonged analgesic effect of at least 28 h when buprenorphine is added to bupivacaine [4]. Additionally, 75% of patients required no rescue medication due to uncontrolled pain when buprenorphine had been added to the local anesthetic. To date, there is no proof that the addition of opioids to local anesthetics provides any benefit to veterinary patients. Proving similar synergistic effects in dogs and cats may be challenging. However, the addition of buprenorphine (at 15 mcg per patient) to bupivacaine is routine in this author's practice.

Q. What dosages are appropriate?

A. Toxic or maximum doses should always be considered when deciding how much local anesthetic to administer. The appropriate dosages in the dog and cat for lidocaine are 5 mg/kg (dog) and 1 mg/kg (cat). Bupivicaine can be given at 2 mg/kg for dogs and 1 mg/kg for cats.

Q. Are there any complications or contraindications to the use of local anesthetics?

A. Prolonged paresthesia or paralysis of the jaws after administration of a local anesthetic have a reported prevalence of 0.00013–0.01% in humans [5]. It is reasonable to assume that these complications may also occur in animals with a similar prevalence. However, the diagnosis of such complications is extremely difficult, if not impossible. Additionally, the consequences of such a complication in animals are unknown. Care should be taken when performing local nerve blocks in areas of a potential neoplasia because of the risk of tumor seeding with the introduction of a needle into the area. If there is any chance the lesion is neoplastic, the risk/benefit ratio of local anesthetics favors their avoidance and the reliance on other means of multimodal pain management. Any area of infection or significant inflammation will result in a lower local tissue pH, which diminishes the effect of local anesthetics. In order to combat the effects of inflammation the clinician should deliver the anesthetic away from the area of inflammation. Second, a larger volume of anesthetic can be delivered as long as the total dosage remains less than the toxic dose for that species.

References

1 Hardie EM, Spodnick GJ, Gilson SD, *et al.* Tracheal rupture in cats: 6 cases (1983-1998). *Journal of the American Veterinary Medical Association* 1999; **214(4)**:508–512.

2 Mitchell SL, McCarthy R, Rudloff E, *et al.* Tracheal rupture associated with intubation in cats: 20 cases (1996-1998). *Journal of the American Veterinary Medical Association* 2000; **216(10)**:1592–1595.

3 Soukup JW, Snyder CJ. Transmylohyoid orotracheal intubation in surgical management canine maxillofacial fractures: An alternative to pharyngotomy endotracheal intubation. Veterinary Surgery 2014; Jan 22. Epub ahead of print.

4 Modi M, Rastogi S, Kumar A. Buprenorphine with bupivacaine for intraoral nerve blocks to provide postoperative analgesia in outpatients after minor oral surgery. *Journal of Oral and Maxillofacial Surgery* 2009; **67(12)**:2571–2576.

5 Hillerup S, Jensen R. Nerve injury caused by mandibular block analgesia. *International Journal of Oral and Maxillofacial Surgery* 2006; **35**:437–443

29 Anesthetic Considerations for Neurologic Disease

Doc, I'm feeling dizzy

Stephen A. Greene

Department of Veterinary Clinical Sciences, College of Veterinary Medicine, Washington State University, USA

KEY POINTS:

- Intracranial disease accompanied by raised intracranial pressure is associated with increased anesthetic morbidity/mortality.
- Avoid high doses of ketamine and Telazol® in patients with a seizure history.
- Elevated carbon dioxide tension and inhaled anesthetics disrupt autoregulation of cerebral blood flow and lead to raised intracranial pressure.
- Controlled ventilation to maintain normocapnia can prevent raised intracranial pressure associated with anesthesia in patients with intracranial disease.

Q. What are some common clinical conditions in dogs and cats that may lead to raised intracranial pressure (ICP)?

A. ✓ head trauma
   ✓ space occupying intracranial masses
   ✓ hydrocephalus
   ✓ inflammatory brain diseases.

Q. What are common anesthetic-related complications in patients with intracranial disease?

A. Common complications include seizures, altered mentation, lethargy, altered gait, and altered sensation [1]. During general anesthesia, respiratory depression or apnea is common due to the effects of many anesthetics on respiratory drive. Respiratory depression that leads to hypercapnia will exacerbate neurologic signs because intracranial pressure (ICP) rises in direct correlation to arterial CO_2 tension. Many anesthetics impair cerebral autoregulation of blood flow which may also lead to raised ICP.

Q. Which anesthetics are commonly associated with seizure activity?

A. In normal animals, administration of ketamine and Telazol® may be associated with seizure activity. The injectable anesthetic, etomidate, has been

---

Questions and Answers in Small Animal Anesthesia, First Edition. Edited by Lesley J. Smith.
© 2016 John Wiley & Sons, Inc. Published 2016 by John Wiley & Sons, Inc.

associated with increased myoclonic activity and induction of epileptic elec-troencephalographic (EEG) activity in patients known to have epilepsy. How-ever, in patients not previously diagnosed with epilepsy, etomidate is used to control refractory status epilepticus.

Q. Will administration of acepromazine cause seizures in patients with intracra-nial disease?

A. Sedation with acepromazine may not be indicated in patients that are obtunded or lethargic secondary to intracranial disease. Some patients, however, may need light sedation with acepromazine if they have altered mentation or are generally excitable despite their neurologic diagnosis. While high doses of acepromazine have been anecdotally reported to lower the seizure threshold in dogs with seizure disorders, it is commonly believed that the benefits of using acepromazine for long-lasting tranquilization in patients with intracranial disease outweigh the risks. Retrospective studies have examined the incidence of seizure activity in dogs with a seizure history after use of acepromazine and found no correlation between its administration and the recurrence of seizure activity during hospitalization [2,3]. A prospective study on use of acepromazine as a premedication in dogs undergoing myelography showed no difference in the incidence of seizures compared to dogs that did not receive acepromazine [4].

Q. What physiologic mechanisms control ICP?

A. Intracranial pressure is directly related to the volume within the cranial vault. Increases in cerebral blood flow (CBF) or cerebrospinal fluid (CSF) produc-tion, obstruction of CSF flow, intracranial hemorrhage, or growth of intracra-nial masses may lead to increased volume within the cranium. In adult animals, there is essentially no elasticity of the cranium such that increased volume within the bony structure will lead to increased pressure. Depending on the duration of the increased ICP, neurologic damage may occur due to lack of perfusion and oxygenation. The primary mechanism of physiologic control over the ICP is known as CBF autoregulation.

Q. How is ICP measured?

A. Intracranial pressure can be measured using invasive techniques that involve placement of a pressure transducer into intraventricular, subarachnoid, or epidural sites. The intraventricular placement of a probe using a strain-gauge transducer requires perforation of brain tissue. Subarachnoid devices avoid insertion through the brain and only require drilling a burr hole in the skull. For subarachnoid and epidural placement, there are fiberoptic and pneumatic transducers available. Normal canine values for ICP range between 8 and 20 mmHg [5].

Q. Where is CSF produced?

A. Cerebrospinal fluid originates from the choroid plexus with some contribu-tion from transependymal diffusion via brain interstitium into the cerebral ventricles. Flow of CSF from the lateral ventricles enters the third ventricle via the foramen of Monro. Passing through the aqueduct of Sylvius, the CSF enters the fourth ventricle and subsequently enters the subarachnoid space via the foramen of Magendie and the foramina of Luschka. Thus, communication with the subarachnoid space allows CSF to also bathe the spinal cord. Resorption of CSF occurs in the dural venous sinuses.

Q. What are signs of raised ICP in awake animals?

A. Altered mentation, lethargy, change in breathing pattern, hypertension with bradycardia (referred to as the Cushings response), and abnormal pupillary responses are associated with raised ICP.

Q. Why does the Cushings response occur?

A. This is a physiologic response to raised ICP in which the systemic arterial pressure increases in order to maintain adequate cerebral perfusion pressure (cerebral perfusion pressure = mean arterial blood pressure − ICP). Often, there will be reflex bradycardia associated with the hypertension.

Q. What is the relationship between cerebral metabolic rate of oxygen consumption and CBF?

A. Generally, CBF is coupled to the cerebral metabolic rate of oxygen consumption such that increased oxygen demand leads to increased blood flow. Because most anesthetics decrease the cerebral metabolic rate of oxygen consumption, their administration is consequently associated with decreased CBF (note the exceptions discussed below).

Q. What variables are associated with CBF autoregulation?

A. Autoregulation of cerebral blood flow maintains relatively constant CBF and ICP over a range of mean arterial blood pressure between 50 and 150 mmHg. Physiologic variables that interfere with autoregulation include intracranial space occupying masses, hypoxia (P_aO_2 < 60 mmHg) and altered carbon dioxide tension in either direction from a normal P_aCO_2 ~ 40 mmHg. Pharmacologic agents that disrupt autoregulation include inhaled anesthetics and some injectable anesthetics.

Q. What is meant by "chemical regulation" of CBF?

A. The chemical regulation of CBF is through carbon dioxide and oxygen. Arterial carbon dioxide levels between 25–40 mmHg will tend to decrease CBF and ICP, while carbon dioxide levels > 40, as well as oxygen tensions <60 mmHg, will tend to increase CBF and ICP.

Q. Which anesthetics are associated with raised ICP?

A. Although inhaled anesthetics decrease the cerebral metabolic rate of oxygen consumption, they are associated with an increase in CBF. Expect raised ICP when using greater than 1 MAC of halogenated inhaled anesthetics (e.g., isoflurane, sevoflurane, desflurane). The injectable dissociative anesthetics (e.g., ketamine, tiletamine) increase both the cerebral metabolic rate of oxygen consumption and the CBF leading to raised ICP when administered alone. In healthy normocapnic animals, there may be only a transient mild increase in ICP associated with these anesthetics. In healthy animals without a pre-existing elevation in ICP, hypoxia and hypercapnia will cause some increase in ICP.

Q. Are there anesthetics that lower CBF and ICP?

A. Yes, most injectable anesthetics (except ketamine) lower the CBF and the ICP. Propofol, etomidate, alfaxalone, and thiobarbiturates are associated with decreased CBF and ICP. A caveat to this statement is that etomidate can cause retching and gagging, particularly when used alone as an induction agent in unpremedicated patients. Retching and gagging will increase ICP.

Q. Does nitrous oxide affect CBF?

A. It depends on which co-administered anesthetics are used. When administered alone, nitrous oxide is associated with the most significant increase in CBF. When co-administered with isoflurane, a milder increase in CBF is observed. When co-administered with propofol, only a slight increase in CBF occurs [6].

Q. How can the effects of inhaled anesthetics on ICP be mitigated?

A. Patients with neurologic disease can be safely maintained on inhaled anesthetics by controlling ventilation such that arterial carbon dioxide tensions are normal or slightly below normal.

Q. Can ketamine's effect on ICP be tempered by using co-induction agents?

A. Yes. Evidence indicates minimal increases or no clinically significant effects on ICP when ketamine is co-administered with diazepam or midazolam for induction of general anesthesia. In addition (as with inhalant anesthetics), maintenance of normocapnia by controlling ventilation is associated with minimal increases in ICP [7–9]. A recent meta-analysis of the use of ketamine in human patients presented for emergency procedures suggests that ICP, cerebral perfusion pressure, neurologic outcome, and mortality are not adversely affected compared to other IV induction agents [10].

Q. What are the effects of opioids on ICP?

A. Direct effects of opioids on CBF and ICP appear to be negligible. While respiratory depression caused by opioids may lead to disruption of autoregulation, clinical experience in dogs and cats with neurologic disease indicates that the degree of respiratory depression from commonly used doses of opioids does not warrant elimination of opioids from the anesthetic protocol.

Q. What are the effects of sedatives and tranquilizers on CBF and ICP?

A. The alpha-2 agonists (e.g., xylazine, medetomidine, dexmedetomidine) have generally been associated with no change or mild decreases in ICP. However, use of atipamezole to antagonize effects of alpha-2 agonists has been associated with a transient increase in ICP. Tranquilizers (e.g., acepromazine, diazepam, and midazolam) also decrease CBF and ICP.

Q. How important is it to maintain good blood pressure in patients with intracranial disease?

A. In normal animals with variations in blood pressure there will be little effect on CBF and ICP due to autoregulation. During anesthesia of patients with intracranial disease, autoregulation is likely to be dysfunctional. In these patients, arterial blood pressure must be maintained within a normal range (e.g., a mean arterial pressure between 70–80 mmHg) in order to provide adequate cerebral perfusion pressure; controlled ventilation is required to maintain normocapnia.

Q. What is the consequence of excessively high ICP?

A. With very high ICP, as might be caused by tumors or exacerbated by anesthesia, hypoxia, or hypercapnia, the likely consequences are decreased cerebral perfusion pressure resulting in cerebral hypoxia and, in extreme elevations, herniation of the brainstem through the foramen magnum. While brainstem herniation may not immediately cause death, there will be irreversible damage to the brainstem respiratory centers. Some of these patients will not spontaneously breathe after an incident like this or fail to regain consciousness. Euthanasia is the eventual outcome.

Q. How can anesthetic monitoring improve outcome for anesthetized patients with intracranial disease?

A. Attention to arterial blood pressure and capnometry values during anesthesia can lead to favorable outcomes in patients with intracranial disease. Maintenance of mean arterial blood pressure between 70 and 80 mmHg will optimize cerebral perfusion pressure while use of capnography will guide judicious ventilation to maintain normocapnia or mild hypocapnia. Excessive hypocapnia (P_aCO_2 or $P_{et}CO_2$ < 30 mmHg) in patients with intracranial disease has been associated with poor neurologic outcomes due to reduced cerebral perfusion pressure. Ideally, the P_aCO_2 or $P_{et}CO_2$ will be maintained between 35 and 40 mmHg (normally, these values are similar, with $P_{et}CO_2$ expected to be slightly less than P_aCO_2).

Q. Has elevated serum lactate been associated with intracranial disease?

A. Yes. A retrospective study of 85 dogs presented for primary neurologic disease identified hyperlactatemia (>2.5 mmol/l) in dogs with meningioma [11]. Administration of prednisone has also been associated with mild elevations (>2.5 mmol/l) in serum lactate [12].

Q. Describe an anesthetic protocol suitable for a patient with intracranial disease undergoing diagnostic imaging or surgery.

A. Intramuscular premedication may be accomplished using an opioid (e.g., hydromorphone, 0.1 mg/kg) or an opioid in combination with either acepromazine (0.01–0.05 mg/kg) or dexmedetomidine (2–10 mcg/kg) or midazolam (0.1–0.2 mg/kg). Wait for sedation and induce anesthesia using propofol (3–5 mg/kg, IV, given to effect). Transition to an inhalant anesthetic such as sevoflurane or isoflurane and use controlled ventilation to maintain normocapnia. Cerebral perfusion pressure may be better maintained with sevoflurane compared to isoflurane [5]. Supplemental analgesic (e.g., fentanyl continuous infusion, 2–10 mcg/kg/h, IV) administration can aid in lowering the inhalant anesthetic requirement to better preserve autoregulation of

CBF. Alternatively, a propofol infusion (0.2 to 0.6 mg/kg/min, IV) may be useful for maintenance of anesthesia at MRI facilities not equipped for inhalant administration. Monitor arterial blood pressure and expired carbon dioxide as described above.

Q. Are there any special precautions I should take if anesthetizing a patient for a CSF tap?

A. Beside consideration of the underlying disease, overall health status, physical exam findings and blood work abnormalities, anesthetic management of these patients is fairly routine. It is advisable, if possible, to intubate using a wire-reinforced or "guarded" tube, to prevent the tube from kinking if the head is positioned "chin on chest" for a cisternal tap.

Q. What anesthetic concerns are there for patients undergoing a myelogram?

A. These are often patients presenting for suspected disk herniation or a fibro-cartilagenous embolus. They are usually fairly healthy dogs that are paretic or non-ambulatory. The anesthetic risk lies in the actual myelogram procedure itself. Seizures are common after myelography. To help prevent seizures, IV fluid administration should be generous (e.g., 5–10 ml/kg/h) to help with diuresis and remove contrast from the system. If possible, the head and neck should be elevated at about a 30° angle during recovery to encourage contrast to drain away from the brain via CSF. During the actual injection of contrast, the anesthetist should be vigilant to sudden changes in breathing pattern, blood pressure, or heart rate. The addition of a volume of contrast into the CSF can cause pressure changes that affect the brainstem and can lead to dramatic and sudden physiologic changes. Should these changes begin to occur, the contrast injection should be stopped immediately and appropriate interventions instituted to address the complication (e.g., assist ventilation).

References

1 Hicks JA, Kennedy MJ, Patterson EE. Perianesthetic complications in dogs undergoing magnetic resonance imaging of the brain for suspected intracranial disease. *Journal of the American Veterinary Medical Association* 2013; **243(9)**:1310–1315.

2 Tobias KM, Marioni-Henry K, Wagner R. A retrospective study on the use of acepromazine maleate in dogs with seizures. *Journal of the American Animal Hospital Association* 2006; **42**:283–289.

3 McConnell J, Kirby R, Rudloff E. Administration of acepromazine maleate to 31 dogs with a history of seizures. *Journal of Veterinary Emergency and Critical Care* 2007; **17(3)**:262–267.

4 Drynan EA, Gray P, Raisis AL. Incidence of seizures associated with the use of acepromazine in dogs undergoing myelography. *Journal of Veterinary Emergency and Critical Care* 2012; **22**:262–266.

5 Chohan AS, Greene SA, Keegan RD, *et al.* Intracranial pressure and cardiopulmonary variables during isoflurane or sevoflurane anesthesia at various minimal alveolar concentration multiples in normocapnic dogs. *American Journal of Veterinary Research* 2013; **74**:369–374.

6 Patel PM, Drummond JC. Cerebral physiology and the effects of anesthetics and techniques. In: Miller RD (ed.) *Miller's Anesthesia*, 6th edn. Elsevier Churchill Livingstone: Philadelphia, 2005:813–857.

7 Artru AA, Katz RA. Cerebral blood volume and CSF pressure following administration of ketamine in dogs; modification by pre- or post-treatment with hypocapnia or diazepam. *Journal of Neurosurgical Anesthesiology* 1989; **1(1)**:8–15.

8 Nimkoff L, Quinn C, Silver P, *et al.* The effects of intravenous anesthetics on intracranial pressure and cerebral perfusion pressure in two feline models of brain edema. *Journal of Critical Care* 1997; **12(3)**:132–136.

9 Himmelseher S, Durieux ME. Revising a dogma: ketamine for patients with neurological injury? *Anesthesia and Analgesia* 2005; **101**:524–534.

10 Cohen L, Athaide V, Wickham ME, *et al.* The effect of ketamine on intracranial and cerebral perfusion pressure and health outcomes: A systematic review. *Annals of Emergency Medicine* 2015; **65**:43–51.

11 Sullivan LA, Campbell VL, Klopp LS, *et al.* Blood lactate concentrations in anesthetized dogs with intracranial disease. *Journal of Veterinary Internal Medicine* 2009; **23(3)**:488–492.

12 Boysen SR, Bozzetti M, Rose L, *et al.* Effects of prednisone on blood lactate concentrations in healthy dogs. *Journal of Veterinary Internal Medicine* 2009; **23**:1123–1125.

30 Anesthetic Considerations for Ocular Disease

An eye for the details

Lesley J. Smith

Department of Surgical Sciences, School of Veterinary Medicine, University of Wisconsin, USA

KEY POINTS:

- Increased intraocular pressure should be avoided in patients with corneal ulcers, descemetocele, glaucoma, and cataracts.

- Maintaining normocapnia and avoiding drugs that cause vomition/retching helps to keep intraocular pressure normal.

- Avoid patient struggling or excessive restraint at induction and recovery.

- Ensure appropriate analgesia to smooth recovery and minimize the risk of trauma to the eye.

- Anesthetic management *per se* will be dictated largely by the patient's underlying health status.

- Reinforced endotracheal tubes prevent tracheal obstruction when the head is positioned "chin on chest."

- Non-depolarizing neuromuscular blocking agents are necessary to maintain a centrally positioned pupil for cataract surgery. Mechanical or assisted ventilation is *essential* when these drugs are used.

Q. What are some common reasons that animals present needing ocular surgery?

A. Common reasons that dogs and cats present for ocular surgery include trauma, corneal ulcers, glaucoma or orbital cancer, cataracts (dogs), eyelid masses, entropion, and ectopic cilia. Depending on the disease state, the patient may be geriatric or quite young and healthy. Dogs with cataracts maybe be young with congenital cataracts or older with acquired cataracts due to diabetes or age. The underlying health status of the patient will largely dictate most details of its anesthetic management.

Q. What are some common themes to be aware of when planning anesthesia for patients needing surgery of the eye?

Questions and Answers in Small Animal Anesthesia, First Edition. Edited by Lesley J. Smith.
© 2016 John Wiley & Sons, Inc. Published 2016 by John Wiley & Sons, Inc.

A. Some common themes will be dependent on the underlying ocular condition, but general considerations are to avoid struggling at induction and/or aggressive restraint during premedication or catheter placement, as these will increase intraocular pressure. Similarly, you want recovery to be smooth, with no thrashing or self-induced trauma to the post-operative eye. If surgical manipulation is likely to put pressure on the globe, then the anesthetist should be aware of the possibility of an oculocardiac reflex, i.e., increased vagal tone, and a sudden drop in heart rate. This usually resolves quickly with an IV dose of atropine or glycopyrrolate. In cases where an increase in intraocular pressure can be devastating (e.g., a descemetocele, deep corneal ulcer, corneal laceration), try to avoid drugs that can induce vomiting such as IM administration of pure μ agonist opioids. Some patients presenting for ocular surgery are geriatric, so underlying disease associated with old age should be considered and screened for. Acquired cataracts are often the result of chronic diabetes, so these patients require careful monitoring of blood glucose levels and judicious administration of insulin. Chapter 37 provides detailed discussion of the anesthetic management for diabetic patients.

Q. Are there any concerns with positioning for eye surgery?

A. Often, for ideal placement of the eye for surgery, the patient is positioned in dorsal recumbency with "chin on chest." Standard commercially available endotracheal tubes can kink inside the trachea in this position. The anesthetist may notice a sudden decrease in chest compliance, or elevations in end-tidal CO_2 or decreases in S_pO_2. The resultant hypoxia or hypercapnia can be severe and life-threatening! To avoid this complication, intubate the patient at induction with a reinforced or "guarded" tube. These are commercially available and have a wire reinforced wall that prevents the tube from kinking even when bent to > 120°.

Q. What should I be aware of for enucleation surgery?

A. Enucleation is most often required for alleviation of pain associated with intractable glaucoma, devastating eye trauma, or orbital neoplasia. Because the eye is being removed, elevations in intraocular pressure are not a huge concern. Premedication should include a pure μ agonist opioid such as hydromorphone. NSAIDs should be included if they are not contra-indicated due to renal disease, hypotension, GI disease, or concurrent therapy with glucocorticoids. One study demonstrated that NSAIDs (specifically carprofen) were much more effective than tramadol in providing post-operative analgesia for dogs undergoing enucleation [1]. Another very effective pain management option for enucleation surgery is the retrobulbar block. This block can be applied to almost any case except, possibly, infection or orbital neoplasia, where there is a risk of seeding neoplastic cells into the systemic circulation. The block involves insertion of a slightly curved spinal needle over the orbital

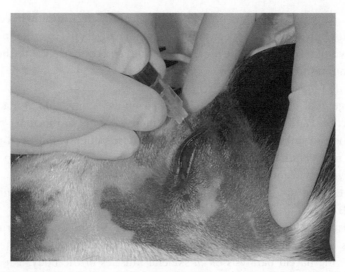

Figure 30.1 Retrobulbar injection of 5% bupivacaine in an anesthetized dog. The slightly bent 2.5-in spinal needle is inserted over the orbital rim ventral to the eye. Aspirate before injection to confirm the absence of blood. Inject slowly. Slight protrusion of the globe will occur as local anesthetic is injected. Pupillary dilation will occur as the local anesthetic begins to take effect.

rim and infiltration of 2–3 ml of 5% (not exceeding 2 mg/kg total) bupivacaine into the retrobulbar space [2]. Figure 30.1 depicts the retrobulbar block in a dog.

Q. Are there any special considerations for patients having surgery for lid masses, entropion, ectopic cilia, and so on?

A. These procedures are all extra-ocular and, other than ensuring a smooth recovery with good analgesia, +/− sedation if needed, there is no specific anesthetic concern for these patients.

Q. Anything special with anesthesia for eye trauma, corneal ulcers, descemetocele?

A. Patients with corneal trauma, corneal ulcers, or descemetocoeles all have a risk of globe rupture if they are heavily restrained or have an increase in intraocular pressure due to vomiting, gagging, or jugular occlusion from a neck leash. Avoid vomiting by administering pure μ agonist opioids IV, with sedation using IM drugs if needed to minimize patient struggling during catheter placement. For example, a dog could be premedicated with IM acepromazine or dexmedetomidine, a catheter placed, and then IV hydromorphone could be given prior to anesthetic induction. For induction, ensure a deep enough plane prior to intubation that the patient does not cough or gag with laryngeal stimulation. Some clinicians advocate a low IV dose of lidocaine (1 mg/kg) prior to intubation to help minimize the gag reflex. These patients may also need sedation and additional analgesia at recovery to keep them calm and minimize ocular trauma that will negatively impact the surgical repair.

Some patients, depending on where the corneal defect is, may need paralysis with non-depolarizing neuromuscular blocking agents in order to position the eye/pupil centrally. The use of these drugs and concurrent anesthetic considerations is covered below.

Q. How do I manage cataract surgery?

A. The general considerations as discussed above apply: aim for a smooth induction and recovery, minimize increases in intraocular pressure, and use a reinforced endotracheal tube. These patients will need paralysis with non-depolarizing neuromuscular blocking agents in order to position the eye/pupil centrally during the phacoemulsification.

Q. OK, tell me about the non-depolarizing neuromuscular blocking agents (NMBAs)?

A. This is a very brief overview of this class of drugs. In the simplest terms, these drugs block acetylcholine at the skeletal muscle neuromuscular junctions, rendering flaccid paralysis of *all* skeletal muscles of the body. The muscles of ocular movement are quite sensitive to the paralytic effects of these drugs, so the eye will rapidly rotate from its typical ventromedial rotation at a surgical depth of anesthesia into a central position with dilated pupil. However, it is very important to recognize that *all* muscles of the body are at least somewhat paralyzed by these drugs. What this means is that the patient *must* be mechanically or hand-ventilated to maintain a normal end-tidal CO_2. It also means that the animal cannot respond to surgical stimulation with gross purposeful movement, therefore the anesthetist must rely on autonomic signs of anesthetic depth such as increases/decreases in blood pressure and heart rate. The anesthetist also must ensure that the effect of these drugs has worn off by the time the inhalant is discontinued and the animal recovered, otherwise it will not be able to breathe adequately and will succumb to life-threatening hypoxia and hypercapnia.

Q. These NMBAs sound scary! How do I use them without a huge risk to my patient?

A. The key is to be ready to ventilate and to monitor the blockade and track the recovery of normal muscular function. Get the patient set up in the OR, with appropriate monitoring in place. Establish (ideally) mechanical ventilation or have a person dedicated to *just* the job of hand-ventilating the patient. Capnography is essential for monitoring whether the ventilation (either mechanical or by hand) is appropriate. See Chapter 31 for guidelines on mechanical ventilation.

Once you are prepared to ventilate, or have the patient on a ventilator, you can attach a commercially available nerve stimulator sold for monitoring neuromuscular blockade (e.g., Halyard peripheral nerve stimulator) to any peripheral nerve (the ulnar and peroneal are commonly used). The positive lead should be positioned proximal on the nerve with the negative lead more distal. Wet the leads with alcohol, turn on the nerve stimulator, and increase the mA to ~ 20 mA. Push the "TOF" (train of four) button on the nerve stimulator and, if your leads are properly placed, you should see four equally sized twitches of the foot over 2 s. If the size of your last twitch appears equal to that of your first twitch, you have a "train of four" ratio of 100%. This is the baseline, non-paralyzed, state.

Now that your baseline TOF is established, you can administer your NMBA. Common drugs that are commercially available today are atracurium, pancuronium, and vecuronium. All of these drugs are chemically related to curare and will cause flaccid paralysis of all skeletal muscles. They differ somewhat in their expected duration of action and their metabolic pathway. Atracurium is broken down in plasma by a process called "Hoffman elimination" that depends on normal blood pH and temperature. Vecuronium and pancuronium are metabolized by the liver. Table 30.1 lists drug doses and anticipated duration of action of these drugs. These drugs are administered IV via slow bolus. Tachycardia is an occasional side effect when these drugs are given. The eye will become paralyzed soon afterwards and the TOF will change: specifically, the fourth twitch will become much smaller or non-existent, and the first, second, and third twitches may also decrease or become absent. Sequential monitoring of the TOF during the remaining anesthetic time will allow you to see the TOF returning to near 100%, but remember to re-wet the leads with alcohol to maintain electrical contact, otherwise your TOF will always look like 0%! To the naked eye, a TOF that appears to be 100% may actually only be 50–75%, so it is also important to watch the clock and estimate the anticipated waning of neuromuscular blockade based on the expected duration. Only when you have what appears to be a TOF = 100% and the expected duration of blockade has been reached is it safe to turn off the inhalant and allow the patient to return to spontaneous ventilation. Watch end-tidal CO_2 once the patient begins to breathe spontaneously to ensure that they can generate a big enough tidal volume to maintain normocapnia.

Q. Is there any way to reverse the NMBAs?

A. Yes. You can use drugs that inhibit acetylcholinesterase, so that acetylcholine levels build up at the neuromuscular junction and compete with the NMBA.

Table 30.1 NMBA drug doses and durations, and reversal agents.

Drug	Dose (mg/kg)	Duration
atracurium	0.1–0.2	20–40 min
vecuronium	0.05 [cat] 0.1 [dog]	30 min
pancuronium	0.07	40–60 min
edrophonium	0.25	reversal
neostigmine	0.04	reversal

Such drugs are edrophonium and neostigmine. See Table 30.1 for dosages. Unfortunately, acetylcholine also accumulates at autonomic synapses, so a dramatic decrease in heart rate should be expected when these drugs are given. It is advisable to pre-treat the patient with atropine just before giving edrophonium or neostigmine. Generally a better approach is to monitor TOF, watch the clock, and allow the NMBA to wear off, rather than reversing it.

References

1 Delgado C, Bentley E, Hetzel S, Smith LJ. Carprofen provides better analgesia than tramadol in dogs for post-operative pain after enucleation: a randomized, double-masked clinical trial. *Journal of the American Veterinary Medical Association* 2014; **245(12)**:1375–1381.
2 Myrna KE, Bentley E, Smith LJ. Local anesthetic retrobulbar block reduces postoperative pain following enucleation of canine eyes: a randomized, placebo controlled, double-masked clinical trial. *Journal of the American Veterinary Medical Association* 2010; **237(2)**:174–177.

31 Anesthetic Considerations for Upper and Lower Respiratory Disease

Take a deep breath!

Rebecca A. Johnson

Department of Surgical Sciences, School of Veterinary Medicine, University of Wisconsin, USA

KEY POINTS:

- Stabilization of the patient with respiratory disease prior to anesthesia is preferred.
- Many premedications, including opioids, cause at least some degree of respiratory depression. These effects are likely to be enhanced in patients with respiratory disease.
- Inhalant anesthetics are profoundly respiratory depressant in veterinary patients.
- Monitoring of oxygenation and ventilation during anesthesia/sedation is essential.
- Mechanical ventilation, including techniques such as positive end-expiratory pressure (PEEP), may be required in these patients.
- Alternatives to orotracheal intubation include tracheotomy, pharyngotomy, and transmylohyoid intubation.

Q. What are the pre-anesthetic considerations for patients with respiratory disease?

A. The main purpose of pre-anesthetic assessment of patients with respiratory disease (or any other disease) is to identify those at risk for peri-anesthetic complications so that appropriate therapy can be instituted in a timely manner. As such, patient morbidity and even mortality will be reduced. Many general anesthetics and analgesics have profound effects on the respiratory system in normal patients and these effects will be amplified in one with respiratory disease. Therefore, a complete physical exam focusing on cardiothoracic auscultation is highly recommended. If respiratory disease is suspected then thoracic radiographs, pulse oximetry +/− capnometry, and arterial blood gas analyses are warranted.

Unless respiratory disease is severe, physical exam findings may be subtle and non-specific. Tachypnea may be present; however, that will not indicate that the animal is normoxic or normocapnic; respiratory frequency *cannot* be used

---

Questions and Answers in Small Animal Anesthesia, First Edition. Edited by Lesley J. Smith.
© 2016 John Wiley & Sons, Inc. Published 2016 by John Wiley & Sons, Inc.

to determine adequacy of ventilation since ventilatory deficiencies mainly manifest as impaired respiratory volumes (i.e., tidal volume, functional residual capacity, etc.). If disease is more severe, dyspnea may be present. Mucous membranes may be cyanotic (from hypoxia), bright red/flushed (from hypercapnia), or normal pink in color. Abnormal lung sounds may or may not be present, depending on the disease process, and may include crackles or wheezes. Severe cases can present with collapse and hyper- or hypothermia. Since these signs are variable, further diagnostics including radiographs will aid in the diagnosis of respiratory disease. Pulse oximetry should be viewed as a screening tool only for patient oxygenation (see Chapter 18). Capnometry is warranted if disorders concerning CO_2 production or elimination (ventilation) are suspected. However, accurate readings require endotracheal intubation. Thus, arterial blood gas analyses are required to definitively identify and quantify the severity of hypoxia, hypo-, or hypercapnia and additional acid-base derangements associated with respiratory disease.

Q. How can patients with respiratory disease be classified prior to general anesthesia?

A. The American Society of Anesthesiologists (ASA) physical status classification system is a system for assessing patient condition prior to anesthesia and consists of five classes from healthy/normal to moribund. In patients with respiratory disease, this system can be adapted as follows:

  I. Normal, healthy patient.

  II. Patient showing dyspnea with moderate exertion.

  III. Patient showing dyspnea with mild exertion.

  IV. Patient with dyspnea at rest, constant threat to life.

  V. Terminal pulmonary disease, not expected to survive with or without intervention.

It is important to note that this classification system may not be appropriate for every patient with respiratory disease, nor is it a "risk assessment." It simply allows the anesthetist to evaluate and classify the patient's condition before anesthesia.

Q. Why does the patient with respiratory disease present unique challenges with regards to general anesthesia?

A. Patients with respiratory disease commonly have physiological abnormalities such as hypoventilation, ventilation-perfusion abnormalities, and ineffective gas exchange mechanisms. These impairments further compound the issues that patients with no respiratory disease encounter during general anesthesia since both CO_2 elimination (via ventilation) and oxygenation are impaired in many normal anesthetized patients.

For example, current techniques in veterinary anesthesia commonly center on inhalant-based anesthetic procedures. If patients cannot exchange oxygen (O_2) and/or remove carbon dioxide (CO_2) efficiently, transfer of inhalants into the lungs might also be impaired. Inhalants are unique among pharmacologic agents as their uptake and elimination depend almost solely on normal respiratory function, with minimal metabolism in the body.

In addition, general anesthesia itself has profound effects on respiratory function. Patients routinely become hypoxemic if enriched oxygen mixtures are not used (inspired fraction of O_2 at least 0.3–0.4). Moreover, the resting lung volume or functional residual capacity is reduced during anesthesia [1], lung compliance is reduced [2], and overall pulmonary system resistance increases considerably [2].

Significant atelectasis has long been associated with general anesthesia, contributing to anesthesia-associated hypoxemia [3]. The dead space to tidal volume ratio (V_D/V_T) is also increased during anesthesia (to ~50% or more) [4]. Thus, ventilation-perfusion mismatching leading to hypoxemia is also extremely common. In addition, many drugs such as inhalant anesthetics and opioids depress minute ventilation in a dose-dependent manner, shifting the CO_2-response curve to the right and reducing the slope (see Chapter 19). Altogether, these effects are further amplified in patients with ventilatory impairment.

Q. What are some common ventilatory disorders in patients requiring anesthesia?

A. Common upper and lower airway diseases/conditions that affect normal ventilation are listed in Table 31.1.

Q. What are the effects of sedatives on ventilation in dogs and cats?

A. Sedatives and tranquilizers such as the phenothiazines (acepromazine) [5,6], alpha-2 agonists (dexmedetomidine) [7–9] and the benzodiazepines (diazepam, midazolam) [10] have at least some respiratory depressant effects in dogs and cats, although the clinical significance is minimal when each

Table 31.1 Common causes of ventilatory dysfunction.

Upper airway	Lower airway	Other causes of respiratory compromise
Laryngeal paralysis	Acute respiratory distress syndrome	CNS depression (drugs, neurologic disease)
Tracheal collapse		
Brachycephalic syndrome	Chronic obstructive pulmonary disease	Neuromuscular disease (myasthenia gravis, tetanus, electrolyte abnormalities)
Feline upper respiratory disease complex	Asthma	
Canine infectious respiratory disease complex	Severe pulmonary edema	Restrictive extrapulmonary disorders
	Pulmonary thromboemboli	
Space-occupying mass (hematoma, neoplasia, foreign body)	Pneumonia	Marked obesity
	Fibrosis	

sedative is used alone. For example, medetomidine in dogs decreases respiratory frequency and increases P_aCO_2 but has no effect on P_aO_2. However, these mild respiratory depressant effects are likely to be exaggerated which used in combination with other anesthetic/analgesic agents and in patients with pre-existing respiratory disease [11].

Q. What are the effects of opioids on ventilation in dogs and cats?

A. Many pure µ opioid agonist analgesics depress minute ventilation via mechanistic effects near or within the brainstem. They depress respiratory frequency, tidal volume or both [12]. The respiratory depression is less pronounced when mixed agonists–antagonists or partial agonists are used [6,13]. In fact, mixed agonists–antagonists such as butorphanol may be used to reverse, at least in part, the respiratory depression seen with pure µ-agonists (e.g., oxymorphone) [6,14,15].

Q. What are the effects of injectable and inhalant anesthetics on ventilation in dogs and cats?

A. Similar to opioid agonists, injectable (i.e., propofol) and inhalant (i.e., sevoflurane, isoflurane) anesthetics produce respiratory depression. Propofol decreases P_aO_2 and increases P_aCO_2 [16]. Ketamine appears to be somewhat less depressant, although its exact effects on ventilation remain controversial and may be dose dependent [17]. All inhalants shift the CO_2-response curve to the right and reduce the slope in a dose-dependent manner [18,19].

Q. How is respiratory function monitored during anesthesia?

A. Patients with respiratory disease should be closely monitored for hypoxemia and ventilatory insufficiency (i.e., hypercapnia) during anesthesia and treated accordingly (see Chapters 18 and 19). Following premedication, especially with combinations of sedatives and opioids, a pulse oximeter should be placed (e.g., on the tail base, lip, digit, etc.) to observe the patient for hypoxemia. Once general anesthesia is induced, a capnometer should be placed between the endotracheal tube and respiratory circuit to monitor the patient for hypo- or hypercapnia. Although pulse oximetry and capnometry are non-invasive, relatively inexpensive, and easy to use, blood gas analyses should be performed to obtain a definitive diagnosis of respiratory impairment and to determine the severity of the acid-base changes associated with the underlying disease. Normal arterial blood gas values for dogs and cats are reported in Chapter 18. *Respiratory function cannot be determined simply by evaluating respiratory frequency or "watching the bag."*

Q. What is an appropriate anesthetic protocol to use in patients with respiratory disease?

A. Usually, the specific choice of anesthetic/analgesic agents is not as important as the case management in a patient with underlying respiratory disease. A critical consideration is to reduce the peri-anesthetic stress and anxiety in order to minimize unnecessary O_2 consumption from struggling or undue hyperactivity. Accordingly, proper administration of sedatives and analgesics and patient pre-oxygenation are important components of the anesthetic plan in respiratory compromised patients (see below). Be mindful of the relative respiratory depressant effects of the sedatives and opioids. Thus, rapid airway control with intensive respiratory monitoring and ventilatory support (with assisted or controlled ventilation as necessary) should be used as soon as possible in these patients. Following the procedure, extreme vigilance should be used during the post-anesthetic period since: (i) residual respiratory depressant effects of the anesthetic agents may still be present; (ii) post-anesthetic shivering and muscle activity increase O_2 consumption and may further deplete O_2 stores; and (iii) patients will usually transition from inhalant anesthesia with enriched O_2 levels (usually approaching 100%) to room air (~20.9% O_2) which can result in hypoxia. As the inspired O_2 decreases when the animal begins to breathe room air, the alveolar, and thereby the arterial O_2 level will also decrease; supplemental O_2 may be required during this transitional period. In addition, long-lasting sedatives should be avoided (i.e., acepromazine) so patients can remain in sternal recumbency if possible and maintain the ability to protect their airway from foreign material such as vomitus or regurgitation during the immediate post-anesthetic period. Sternal recumbency may improve pulmonary atelectasis and reduce the incidence of aspiration, which is especially common following upper airway surgery but is also associated with general anesthesia itself [20,21,22].

Q. How is respiratory depression/hypoventilation associated with general anesthesia in dogs and cats treated?

A. Respiratory depression associated with hypoventilation and increased P_aCO_2 is common in patients undergoing general anesthesia, especially when inhalants and opioids are used. The initial treatment goal is to remove the inciting cause by: (i) minimizing the inhalant vaporizer setting; (ii) using multimodal anesthetic techniques to minimize the respiratory depressant effects of each agent and to reduce inhalant requirement as much as possible; and (iii) reversing any respiratory depressant agents (i.e., opioids) if the procedure allows for it. However, reversal of pharmacologic agents may not be feasible due to the nature of the procedure requiring anesthesia. For example, opioid analgesics should never be withheld from a painful surgical procedure simply because of their respiratory depressant properties.

If the previous techniques do not improve P_aCO_2 levels, assisted or controlled ventilation techniques using positive-pressure ventilation are needed to maintain normal acid-base status throughout an anesthetic procedure.

Q. If the patient cannot be orotracheally intubated, what are some alternative ways to provide assisted or controlled ventilation?

A. At times, specific circumstances preclude orotracheal intubation of the patient. For example, orotracheal intubation may not be possible in patients with orofacial fractures, significant oral neoplasia or other soft tissue disorders, palatal surgery, and some orthodontic procedures. If orotracheal intubation is not possible, and assisted or controlled ventilation is required, other techniques are available to the practitioner. Classically, tracheotomy was used to bypass the oral cavity; however, this technique may result in significant morbidity [23]. In addition, pharyngotomy endotracheal intubation has also been used. However, a new technique of transmylohyoid orotracheal intubation is becoming more popular due to: (i) a shorter intubation time with a simpler surgical approach and (ii) a lower inherent risk of iatrogenic complications [24]. Nasotracheal intubation is also used in rabbits and large animals, but is not frequently performed in dogs and cats [25,26].

Q. What are common complications associated with positive-pressure mechanical ventilation?

A. Mechanical ventilation is used in cases to improve patient hypoxemia as well as to address or prevent hypercapnia. Positive-end expiratory pressure (PEEP) can aid in stabilizing lung units, thereby increasing functional residual capacity, reducing shunt fraction, and increasing P_aO_2. Mechanical ventilation also decreases or negates the work of breathing and facilitates inhalant anesthesia by improving gas exchange [12]. However, positive airway pressure mechanical ventilation can also result in: (i) decreased cardiac output via decreased venous return and compression of cardiac chambers; (ii) barotrauma from increased transpulmonary pressures; (iii) volutrauma from increased alveolar-capillary permeability; (iv) atelectrauma from repeated opening and closing of lung units; and (v) biotrauma from activation of inflammatory cytokines by ventilation of diseased pulmonary tissue [12]. Thus, extreme care should be taken when the decision to use mechanical ventilation is made and the patient should be diligently monitored throughout.

Q. What are the types of mechanical ventilators used in veterinary medicine?

A. Mechanical ventilators are mainly categorized into two groups, based on the major control variable: *volume* or *pressure-limited*. Volume-limited ventilators have a preset rate and tidal volume; when the set tidal volume is reached, the inspiration stops, despite the peak inspiratory pressure reached. In contrast, the pressure-limited ventilator is set to a predetermined peak inspiratory pressure after which the inspiration stops, and is generally regarded to be somewhat "safer" to use since excessive airway pressures should not be reached [12].

Q. What are common ventilator settings employed in dogs and cats?

A. The general guidelines for positive pressure mechanical ventilation of dogs and cats with relatively normal lungs are: (i) a peak airway pressure of 10 to 20 cm of H_2O; (ii) a tidal volume of 10–15 ml/kg; (iii) an inspiratory to expiratory time ratio of 1 : 2 or greater (i.e., 1 : 3, 1 : 4, etc.) to allow for full inspiration as well as expiration; (iv) a respiratory frequency of 10–15 times per min; and (v) 0–2 cm H_2O of PEEP [27]. Remember that these are just guidelines – and need to be adjusted on an individual patient basis, especially in one with respiratory disease where the lungs may be less compliant than normal lungs. Ventilator settings should be adjusted to maintain P_aCO_2 and P_aO_2 within the target ranges ($\sim P_aCO_2$: 35–50 mmHg and P_aO_2: > 80–100 mmHg).

Q. What is the purpose of pre-oxygenation (or post-procedural oxygenation) and how do we apply it to our patients?

A. Many patients with respiratory disease will benefit from pre-anesthetic O_2 supplementation or supplementation of O_2 following the procedure. Criteria include patients that are marginally able or unable to maintain normoxia while breathing room air; frequently these patients are cyanotic (~ 5 g/dl of deoxygenated Hb). Oxygen is frequently administered via face mask, O_2 chamber, or nasal cannulas. However, inspired levels do not reach 100%. For example, nasal insufflation with 100% O_2 frequently results in less than 60% inspired O_2 levels (dependent on insufflation and respiratory rates and tidal volume) [28]. Pre-oxygenation should not be applied to patients if the process causes excessive stress or anxiety due to increased patient O_2 demands associated with struggling. However, the benefit to pre-oxygenation is that it provides a longer time before a patient becomes hypoxemic during an apneic period, for example following induction [29,30]. Pre-oxygenation with enriched O_2 mixtures theoretically fills the alveolus with a higher than normal O_2 concentration, which is then available to the pulmonary blood when apnea occurs. However, to effectively wash out other pulmonary gases and replace them with high levels of O_2 takes many minutes of pre-oxygenation and any break in the supplemental O_2 delivery will require restarting of the oxygenation procedure [29]. Ideally a patient with respiratory compromise of any kind should be pre-oxygenated for at least 5 min before induction of anesthesia.

References

1 Wahba RWM. Perioperative functional residual capacity. *Canadian Journal of Anaesthesia* 1991; **38**:384–400.

2 Don H. The mechanical properties of the respiratory system during anesthesia. *International Anesthesiology Clinics* 1977; **15**:113–126.

3 Bendixen HH, Hedleywhite J, Laver MB. Impaired oxygenation in surgical patients during general anesthesia with controlled ventilation – a concept of atelectasis. *New England Journal of Medicine* 1963; **269**:991–996.

4 McDonell WN. *Ventilation and acid-base equilibrium with methoxyflurane anesthesia in dogs.* MSc Thesis. Guelph, University of Guelph, 1969.

5 Farver TB, Haskins SC, Patz JD. Cardiopulmonary effects of acepromazine and of the subsequent administration of ketamine in the dog. *American Journal of Veterinary Research* 1986; **47(3)**:631–635.

6 Talavera J, Kirschvink N, Schuller S, *et al.* Evaluation of respiratory function by barometric whole-body plethysmography in healthy dogs. *Veterinary Journal* 2006; **172(1)**:67–77.

7 Sabbe MB, Penning JP, Ozaki GT, *et al.* Spinal and systemic action of the alpha 2 receptor agonist dexmedetomidine in dogs. *Antinociception and carbon dioxide response. Anesthesiology* 1994; **80(5)**:1057–1072.

8 Lamont LA, Bulmer BJ, Grimm KA, *et al.* Cardiopulmonary evaluation of the use of medetomidine hydrochloride in cats. *American Journal of Veterinary Research* 2001; **62(11)**:1745–1749.

9 Selmi AL, Mendes GM, Lins BT, *et al.* Evaluation of the sedative and cardiorespiratory effects of dexmedetomidine, dexmedetomidine-butorphanol, and dexmedetomidine-ketamine in cats. *Journal of the American Veterinary Medical Association* 2003; **222(1)**:37–41.

10 Haskins SC, Farver TB, Patz JD. Cardiovascular changes in dogs given diazepam and diazepam-ketamine. *American Journal of Veterinary Research* 1986; **47(4)**:795–798.

11 Sinclair MD. A review of the physiological effects of α2-agonists related to the clinical use of medetomidine in small animal practice. *Canadian Veterinary Journal* 2003; **44(11)**:885–897.

12 Kerr CL, McDonell WN. Oxygen supplementation and ventilator support. In: Muir WW, Hubbell JAE (eds) *Equine Anesthesia*, 2nd edn. Saunders: St. Louis, 2009:332–352.

13 Ko JC, Bailey JE, Pablo LS, *et al.* Comparison of sedative and cardiorespiratory effects of medetomidine and medetomidine-butorphanol combination in dogs. *American Journal of Veterinary Research* 1996; **57(4)**:535–540.

14 McCrackin MA, Harvey RC, Sackman JE, *et al.* Butorphanol tartrate for partial reversal of oxymorphone-induced postoperative respiratory depression in the dog. *Veterinary Surgery* 1994; **23(1)**:67–74.

15 Bragg P, Zwass MS, Lau M, *et al.* Opioid pharmacodynamics in neonatal dogs: differences between morphine and fentanyl. *Journal of Applied Physiology* 1995; **79(5)**:1519–1524.

16 Maney JK, Shepard MK, Braun C, *et al.* A comparison of cardiopulmonary and anesthetic effects of an induction dose of alfaxalone or propofol in dogs. *Veterinary Anaesthesia and Analgesia* 2013; **40(3)**:237–244.

17 Boscan P, Pypendop BH, Solano AM, *et al.* Cardiovascular and respiratory effects of ketamine infusions in isoflurane-anesthetized dogs before and during noxious stimulation. *American Journal of Veterinary Research* 2005; **(12)**:2122–2129.

18 Munson ES, Larson CP Jr, Babad AA, *et al.* The effects of halothane, fluroxene, and cyclopropane on ventilation: a comparative study in man. *Anesthesiology* 1966; **27**:716–728.

19 Mutoh T, Nishimura R, Kim HY, *et al.* Cardiopulmonary effects of sevoflurane, compared with halothane, enflurane, and isoflurane, in dogs. *American Journal of Veterinary Research* 1997; **58(8)**:885–890.

20 Mercurio A. Complications of upper airway surgery in companion animals. *Veterinary Clinics of North America Small Animal Practice* 2011; **41**: 969–980.

21 Wilson DV, Evans AT, Miller R. Effects of preanesthetic administration of morphine on gastroesophageal reflux and regurgitation during anesthesia in dogs. *American Journal of Veterinary Research* 2005; **66**:386–390.

22 Wilson DV, Boruta DT, Evans AT. Influence of halothane, isoflurane, and sevoflurane on gastroesophageal reflux during anesthesia in dogs. *American Journal of Veterinary Research* 2006; **67**:1821–1825.

23 Nicholson I, Baines S. Complications associated with temporary tracheostomy tubes in 42 dogs (1998–2007). *Journal of Small Animal Practice* 2012; **53**:108–115.

24 Soukup JW, Snyder CJ. Transmylohyoid orotracheal intubation in surgical management of canine maxillofacial fractures: an alternative to pharyngotomy endotracheal intubation. *Veterinary Surgery* 2014; 1–5 [Epub ahead of print].

25 Stephens Devalle JM. Successful management of rabbit anesthesia through the use of nasotracheal intubation. *Journal of the American Association of Laboratory Animal Science* 2009; **48**:166–170.

26 Riebold TW, Engel HN, Grubb TL, *et al.* Orotracheal and nasotracheal intubation in llamas. *Journal of the American Veterinary Medical Association* 1994; **204**:779–783.

27 Haskins S. CanWest Veterinary Conference. Proceedings. http//canadawestvets.com/symposium2011/ (accessed May 6, 2014).

28 Zimmerman ME, Hodgson DS, Bello NM. Effects of oxygen insufflation rate, respiratory rate, and tidal volume on fraction of inspired oxygen in cadaveric canine heads attached to a lung model. *American Journal of Veterinary Research* 2013; **74(9)**:1247–1251.

29 McNally EM, Robertson SA, Pablo LS. Comparison of time to desaturation between preoxygenated and nonpreoxygenated dogs following sedation with acepromazine maleate and morphine and induction of anesthesia with propofol. *American Journal of Veterinary Research* 2009; **70(11)**:1333–1338.

30 Sirian R, Wills J. Physiology of apnoea and the benefits of preoxygenation. *Continuing Education in Anaesthesia, Critical Care and Pain* 2009; **9(4)**:105–108.

32 Anesthetic Considerations for Cardiovascular Disease

Does this make your heart skip a beat?

Andre C. Shih

College of Veterinary Medicine, University of Florida, USA

KEY POINTS:

- There is no perfect anesthetic for cardiac disease patients. Most anesthetic agents depress contractility and cause hypotension.

- Therapeutic interventions routinely used during anesthesia, like crystalloid fluid boluses and use of inotropes, may be contraindicated in some cardiac diseases.

- Etomidate may be one of the preferred injectable induction anesthetics for patients with cardiac disease, but it is not without side effects.

- Balanced anesthesia, that is adding opioids and benzodiazepines to the protocol, allows reduction of the total amount of drugs necessary to maintain anesthesia and therefore decreases negative cardiovascular side effects.

- The use of constant rate infusions during anesthesia further serves to provide balanced anesthesia and reduces inhalant requirement, thereby minimizing negative cardiovascular effects of the inhalants in patients with cardiac disease.

Q. When performing a pre-anesthetic evaluation on a patient suspected of having cardiac disease, are there any special considerations?

A. As with any patient undergoing general anesthesia, a complete physical exam should be performed in a manner that does not stress the already compromised patient. A complete history with a complete list of currently prescribed drugs is also important. Due to ongoing medications, cardiac disease patients are prone to hypotension, hyponatremia, hypokalemia, and azotemia. The pre-anesthetic work up should include, in addition to the physical exam, a CBC, serum chemistry (specifically a renal panel), non-invasive

---

Questions and Answers in Small Animal Anesthesia, First Edition. Edited by Lesley J. Smith.
© 2016 John Wiley & Sons, Inc. Published 2016 by John Wiley & Sons, Inc.

blood pressure (BP), echocardiogram (Echo), electrocardiogram (ECG), and thoracic radiographs.

Cardiac patients have a lower cardiac vital reserve capacity; human error that leads to anesthetic drug calculation errors, delays in intubation, provision of oxygen, monitoring, and supportive care can be devastating in a patient with cardiac disease. Before the patient is brought to the induction area, ensure that the anesthesia machine and all monitoring equipment are working properly. The number of drugs required during a cardiac procedure can be intimidating; printing a table with the pre-calculated doses of any emergency agents will save time and decrease morbidity. An example of this table can be found in Table 32.1. Additionally, creating a printed table with a checklist (Box 32.1) would ensure that equipment malfunction is detected before the procedure, avoiding unnecessary delays and complications.

Table 32.1   Examples of different drugs and recommended doses to have available when anesthetizing a patient with cardiac disease.

Drugs	Dose	Volume	Route
Vasoactives and Inotropes:			
Epinephrine	0.01–0.1 mg/kg		IV
Dopamine	2–10 ug/kg/min		IV infusion
Dobutamine	1–10 ug/kg/min		IV infusion
Ephedrine	0.1 mg/kg		IV
Isoproterenol	0.1–0.3 ug/kg/min		IV slow
Vasodilators:			
Nitroprussate	1–2 ug/kg/min		IV infusion
Nitroglycerine			Dermal
Antiarrhythmic:			
Lidocaine	1–2 mg/kg		IV
Procainamide	0.5 mg/kg		IV
Esmolol	0.5 ug/kg or CRI of 100–200 ug/kg/min		IV
Atropine	0.04 mg/kg		IV
Glycopyrrolate	0.02 mg/kg		IV
Amiodorone	5 mg/kg		IV slow
Magnesium sulfate	20 mg/kg		IV
Others:			
Hypertonic saline	1–4 ml/kg		IV
Hetastarch	1–10 ml/kg		IV
Furosemide	0.1–2 mg/kg		IV
Nitric oxide	Inhalant		Inhalant
Albuterol spray	Inhalant		Inhalant

Box 32.1 Checklist before any cardiac anesthetic procedure

PRE-OPERATIVE CHECKLIST:

[–] / NA: Oxygen source operational

[–] / NA: Anesthesia machine pressure tested

[–] / NA: Endotracheal tube and laryngoscope

[–] / NA: Monitoring equipment operational

[–] / NA: Infusion pump/fluid set up ready

[–] / NA: Heat blankets ready

[–] / NA: Pre-operative drugs and antibiotics

[–] / NA: Drug cart stocked and updated

[–] / NA: Crash cart stocked and updated

[–] / NA: Patient has IV catheter. Surgical area is pre-clipped

[–] / NA: Patient cross-matched and blood bank ready, when applicable

Q. Which anesthetic drug is the safest for cardiac patients?

A. Unfortunately, no anesthetic drug is safest. The complexity of the patho-physiologic changes with cardiac disease and the specific types of cardiac disease make it impossible for one anesthetic drug to be safe for all cardiac patients. For example, patients with mitral regurgitation (MR) may benefit from drugs that increase basal heart rate and cause mild vasodilation. On the other hand, a patient with hypertrophic cardiomyopathy (HCM) would not do well with a drug that causes tachycardia and vasodilation because of the increased myocardial oxygen demand of tachycardia. Most general anesthetic agents (inhalants and induction drugs) depress contractility and cause hypotension. In order to choose a good anesthetic protocol it is important to understand how anesthetic drugs affect the cardiovascular system.

✓ Inhalant anesthetics (i.e., isoflurane, sevoflurane): The overall effect of inhalant anesthetics is a reduction in blood pressure and cardiac contractility. To alleviate those negative cardiovascular effects, the concomitant use of sedatives/local anesthetics and opioids reduce required concentrations of inhalants (MAC sparing effect). Mask or chamber induction without proper sedation causes extreme stress and should *not* be considered an appropriate method to induce anesthesia.

✓ Etomidate: This is one of the preferred injectable induction anesthetics for patients with heart disease. Etomidate provides a very stable heart rate and rhythm, minimal myocardial depression, and minimal change to stroke volume. It can cause dose-dependent hypotension due to moderate systemic vasodilation [1].

This drug is not without side effects. Use of etomidate in an unsedated patient is not recommended as it can lead to excitation, myoclonus, and muscle fasciculation. Current etomidate formulations that are available in the USA contain propylene glycol that, at high doses, can lead to vasodilation and myocardial depression. Etomidate also leads to severe depression of the adreno-cortical axis and should not be used in patients with risk of sepsis or vasodilatory shock [2]. The adrenal suppressive effects of etomidate, after a single induction dose, can last hours up to 12 h [3].

✓ Propofol: Propofol causes a dose-dependent decrease in blood pressure due to a reduction in systemic vascular resistance (vasodilation) and myocardial contractility [4,5]. Its effects are very short lived and hemodynamic parameters return to normal in 15–30 min. Propofol is also a potent respiratory depressant leading to hypercapnia and apnea. If propofol is being used, the patient should be intubated, provided 100% O_2, and ventilation assisted [4]. Adding opioids and benzodiazepines to the induction protocol allows reduction of the total amount of propofol necessary and therefore fewer negative side effects.

✓ Alfaxalone: Alfaxolone was introduced in the 1970s (Saffan) and at that time was composed of a mixture of two neurosteroids (alfaxolone and alfadolone acetate). Its vehicle composition (Cremophor EL) caused severe histamine release, making it unsuitable for cardiac patients. A novel formulation of Alfaxolone (using cyclodextrin technology) does not cause histamine release in dogs and cats. Alfaxalone, when used for induction, causes minimal cardiovascular and respiratory depression. Even at high doses, alfaxolone only causes a moderate drop in cardiac output and blood pressure. With the use of opioids as premedication, this induction drug is a good option for patients with moderate mitral regurgitation [6]. Alfaxolone has an extra advantage of being well tolerated as TIVA (total intravenous infusion) to maintain anesthesia in patients where inhalant anesthesia could be deleterious [7]. This drug has been used for some time with good success in Australia, Canada and Europe, and has recently been introduced to the USA.

✓ Ketamine and tiletamine (telazol): Ketamine and tiletamine increase sympathetic nervous system activity, leading to an indirect increase in blood pressure, heart rate, stroke volume, and cardiac output. Its cardiovascular effects are short lived and increased blood pressure usually returns to normal in the first 15–30 min. Ketamine alters systolic contraction and increases myocardial oxygen consumption. Ketamine should be used with caution in hypertensive patients, in patients with tachyarrhythmias and patients with hypertrophic cardiomyopathy. *In vitro*, ketamine can cause severe cardiac depression, emphasizing the importance of an intact sympathetic system for cardiac stimulation.

✓ Alpha-2 agonists (dexmedetomidine and medetomidine): These drugs are excellent analgesics and sedatives, however they cause an increase in systemic vascular resistance and severe reflex bradyarrhythmias. Alpha-2 agonists classically cause hypertension initially followed by a period of hypotension [8]. Due to severe effects on cardiovascular function, alpha-2 agonists are usually contraindicated in most cardiac patients.

✓ Opioids: These drugs are very effective analgesics and sedatives, and represent a mainstay of the balanced anesthetic approach required for patients with cardiac disease. At appropriate doses, opioids do not cause significant myocardial depression; however, most opioids lead to dose-dependent bradycardia. Opioids produce their cardiovascular effect by decreasing sympathetic tone and increasing parasympathetic tone.
Opioids are one of the most useful classes of drugs used during anesthesia or sedation of cardiac patients. Opioid pure μ agonists (fentanyl, hydromorphone, morphine, oxymorphone, and methadone) produce the most reliable analgesia and sedation. If needed, opioid effects can be easily reversed with the use of naloxone. See Chapter 6 for a complete discussion of opioids.

✓ Phenothiazines (acepromazine): This is an alpha and dopamine receptor antagonist. Because of acepromazine's effects on blood pressure (i.e., decrease due to vasodilation) it is contraindicated for most cardiac patients. Acepromazine, at low doses, might be a sedative option in some cardiac diseases where systemic vasodilation or a decrease in afterload is desired (e.g., severe mitral regurgitation). Acepromazine also has some anti-arrhythmic effects. Acepromazine does not have an antagonist reversal drug.

✓ Benzodiazepines (midazolam, diazepam): These sedatives cause minimal changes in contractility, minimal myocardial depression, and very little effect on the vascular system. Used in combination with opioids, these can be a very good sedative choice for patients with cardiac disease. Benzodiazepines should not be used as a sole sedative agent as they can lead to excitation and euphoria. Although rarely needed in dogs and cats, the reversal agent for benzodiazepines is flumazenil.

Q. How should I change my anesthetic protocol when dealing with a cardiac disease patient?

A. As a general rule, before induction, the patient will benefit from pre-clipping of the affected area, placement of basic monitoring, and pre-oxygenation with a face-mask before anesthetic induction. Fluid therapy should be used with care because most cardiac patients will not tolerate a rapid increase in preload and may be prone to fluid overload. Use of low sodium containing fluids (e.g., Lactated Ringer's or NaCl 0.45%) is usually preferred. The examples listed below should serve only as a guideline. Anesthetic protocol and dose ranges should be based on familiarity of the anesthetist and other veterinary staff with particular drugs, familiarity with the patient's temperament, physical exam and other findings, knowledge of the underlying disease, and the pharmacological effect the drug.

Patent Ductus Arteriosus (PDA)

Goals: It is important to identify if blood shunted through the PDA is moving from the left systemic circulation towards the pulmonary right circulation (L–R) versus right towards the left (R–L). Most patients with PDA have a L–R shunt, which means pulmonary circulation and oxygenation are usually good, but systemic cardiac output is reduced. Anesthesia goals are to avoid systemic hypotension and pulmonary hypertension as this can create a R–L shunt. A patient with R–L shunt can become extremely hypoxic and carries great anesthetic risk.

Anesthesia protocol: Induction with an opioid (e.g., fentanyl 1 mcg/kg IV) followed by diazepam (0.1 mg/kg) and etomidate (1 mg/kg). Maintenance with low dose isoflurane plus an infusion of opioids (fentanyl CRI 2–10 mcg/kg/h).

What to watch for: Aggressively treat hypotension with inotropes (e.g., dopamine 5–10 mcg/kg/min or dobutamine 5–10 mcg/kg/min). High tidal volume positive pressure ventilation (IPPV) should be avoided as it can increase intrapulmonary pressure. Monitoring should include basic monitoring plus an arterial line for invasive blood pressure measurement. Heart rate should be closely monitored and bradycardia aggressively treated with anticholinergics. Large bore IV catheters are critical for rapid fluid resuscitation in case of catastrophic hemorrhage during surgery. During compression of the PDA with surgical manipulation for placement of an aneroid constrictor, or during ligation of the PDA, watch for reflex bradycardia and have a dose of atropine or glycopyrrolate ready.

Mitral Regurgitation (MR)

Goals: Anesthetic goals are to reduce the regurgitation fraction, and to avoid increases in systemic vascular resistance and bradycardia. Arteriodilators are effective by reducing the ventriculo-atrial pressure gradient.

Anesthesia protocol: Induction can be achieved with most injectable anesthetics (etomidate, propofol, alfaxalone, or ketamine). Bradycardia will increase regurgitation fraction and worsen overall forward blood flow. Administer anticholinergics if bradycardia is present. Maintenance can be achieved with either propofol infusion or inhalant (isoflurane or sevoflurane) anesthetic. Adding constant rate infusions with drugs like lidocaine and opioids will reduce overall anesthesia requirement and reduce cardiac depression. Adding diazepam and/or an opioid will reduce induction drug doses and side effects. Isoflurane or sevoflurane are good choices for maintenance.

What to watch for: It is recommended to reduce total amount of fluid being administered and to avoid fluid boluses during the procedure. The use of fluid pumps and buretrols will ensure no fluid bolus is administered accidentally.

MR with Congestive Heart Failure (CHF)

Patients presenting with evidence of pulmonary edema and CHF are very poor anesthetic candidates. Anesthesia should be delayed if possible until the underlying heart failure has improved, or the patient be referred to a board-certified anesthesiologist. Aggressive diuretics, vasodilators, and oxygen supplementation will help to produce a more stable patient.

MR patients that have a history of CHF in the past are prone to decompensating during anesthesia. Be extremely conservative with fluid therapy (< 2–5 ml/kg/h) and consider low sodium fluids (0.45% NaCl with 2.5% dextrose).

Hypertrophic Cardiomyopathy (HCM)

Goals: Some patients with HCM have outflow tract obstruction due to systolic anterior motion of the mitral valve. This type of obstruction is dynamic and is accentuated by increases in contractility or heart rate. Patients with HCM are prone to sympathetic over-stimulation and are more sensitive to catecholamines. Maintaining a low stress environment is essential. Cats should be kept in a quiet room, away from dogs.

Anesthesia protocol: The plan should be aimed at mild myocardial depression with little or no increase in systemic vascular resistance. If the patient has confirmed dynamic outflow obstruction then a *low* dose of dexmedetomidine IM may be an acceptable sedative. Dexmedetomidine causes an increase in systemic vascular resistance, increase in afterload, decrease in heart rate, and decrease in myocardial contractility that may be useful to patients with forward dynamic outflow obstruction. Other sedation choices would be combinations of opioids (e.g., oxymorphone) and midazolam. Induction can be achieved with etomidate. Avoid using drugs that would increase heart rate, such as ketamine or the anticholinergics.

What to watch for: Monitor and treat arrhythmias. HCM patients are prone to development of ventricular tachyarrhythmias.

Q. What should I plan for with respect to post-operative care of these patients?
A. A Recent epidemiological study demonstrated that the majority of (peri)-anesthetic deaths happen during the immediate post-operative period [9]. Pain, hypothermia, and hypoventilation are some of the factors that cause decompensation in the recovery period. Patients should be

transferred to an intensive care unit or a surgical team member must be assigned to continue close monitoring until the patient is normothermic, breathing well after extubation, and with pulse oximeter readings > 95%.

References

1 Wagner C, Bick J, Johnson D, *et al.* Etomidate use and postoperative outcomes among cardiac surgery patients. *Anesthesiology* 2014; **120(3)**:579–589.
2 Komatsu R, You J, Mascha EJ *et al.* Anesthetic induction with etomidate, rather than propofol, is associated with increased 30-day mortality and cardiovascular morbidity after noncardiac surgery. *Anesthesia and Analgesia* 2013; **117(6)**:1329–1337.
3 Seravalli L Pralong F Revelly J *et al.* Adrenal function after induction of cardiac surgery patients with etomidate bolus: a retrospective study. *Annales Françaises d'Anesthésie et de Réanimation* 2009; **28(9)**:737–737.
4 Short CE, Bufalari A. Propofol anesthesia. *Veterinary Clinics of North America: Small Animal Practice* 1999; **29(3)**:747–778.
5 Glowaski M, Wetmore L. Propofol: application in veterinary sedation and anesthesia. *Clinical Techniques in Small Animal Practice* 1999; **14(1)**:1–9.
6 Muir W, Lerche P, Wiese A, *et al.* Cardiorespiratory and anesthetic effects of clinical and supraclinical doses of alfaxalone in dogs. *Veterinary Anesthesia and Analgesia* 2008; **35(6)**:451–462.
7 Ambros B, Duke-Novaloski T, Pasloske K. Comparison of the anesthetic efficacy and cardiopulmonary effects of continuous rate infusions of alfaxalone-2-hydroxypropyl-beta-cyclodextrin and propofol in dogs. *American Journal of Veterinary Research* 2008; **69(11)**:1391–1398.
8 Murrell JC, Hellebrekers LJ. Medetomidine and dexmedetomidine: a review of cardiovascular effects and antinociceptive properties in the dog. *Veterinary Anesthesia and Analgesia* 2005; **32(3)**:117–127.
9 Brodbelt D. Perioperative mortality in small animal anesthesia. *Veterinary Journal* 2009; **182(2)**:152–161.

33 Anesthetic Considerations for Gastrointestinal Disease

What did that dog eat?

Carrie Schroeder

Department of Surgical Science, School of Veterinary Medicine, University of Wisconsin, USA

KEY POINTS:

- Many commonly used anesthetic agents increase the incidence of vomiting and gastroesophageal reflux.

- Gastroesophageal reflux may be clinically silent and can lead to esophagitis, esophageal strictures, and aspiration pneumonitis.

- Obese patients present anesthetic challenges related to respiratory compromise; these patients may require peri-anesthetic oxygen supplementation to avoid desaturation and should be mechanically ventilated during anesthesia.

- Both laparoscopy and upper GI endoscopy may cause abdominal distension due to insufflation of the peritoneal cavity or stomach. This may lead to decreased venous return and respiratory compromise.

- Lower GI endoscopy can cause distension of the colon which can be associated with sudden increases in vagal tone.

- Vomiting and diarrhea may cause electrolyte abnormalities such as hypokalemia and hyponatremia and either metabolic acidosis or alkalosis. Measurement of electrolytes and evaluation of acid-base status should be performed prior to anesthesia and patients should be stabilized as necessary before anesthetic induction.

Q. What are the recommendations for fasting of patients prior to anesthesia?

A. The rationale for pre-operative fasting is to lower the incidence of peri-operative regurgitation and gastroesophageal reflux, thus decreasing the risk of post-anesthetic esophagitis and aspiration pneumonitis or pneumonia. It is generally recommended that food be withheld from adult dogs and cats for 8–12 h prior to surgery while free access to water may be allowed until the time of surgery. Some studies have shown, however, that

---

Questions and Answers in Small Animal Anesthesia, First Edition. Edited by Lesley J. Smith.
© 2016 John Wiley & Sons, Inc. Published 2016 by John Wiley & Sons, Inc.

prolonged fasting may actually increase gastric acidity and gastroesophageal reflux [1,2]. In dogs, the administration of a small meal of canned food 3 h prior to the induction of anesthesia did not significantly increase the volume of gastric contents and actually decreased gastric acidity [2]. This suggests that a very small meal of canned food 3 h prior to anesthetic induction may be of benefit to lower gastric acidity, potentially decreasing the risk of post-anesthetic esophagitis or pneumonitis.

Very young animals (< 12 weeks) should not have food withheld for more than 2 h due to decreased hepatic glycogen stores. Blood glucose should be checked immediately preceding anesthetic induction to verify normoglycemia.

Q. What are the consequences of gastroesophageal reflux (GER)?

A. GER reflux may lead to esophagitis, esophageal strictures, and, depending on the severity of reflux, aspiration pneumonitis or pneumonia. Considering that most anesthetic agents decrease the tone of the lower esophageal sphincter, it is not uncommon for patients to have passive or silent GER under anesthesia. Older patients and patients undergoing abdominal surgery have an increased risk of GER as compared to other surgeries, yet patient positioning, surprisingly, has no influence on the incidence of GER [3]. Unfortunately, GER is usually undetectable without the aid of an esophageal pH meter or esphagoscopy. Peri-anesthetic administration of anti-emetics, prokinetics, and antacids are variably effective in preventing GER. The anti-emetic maropitant and the prokinetic metoclopramide were ineffective at reducing GER, while the prokinetic cisapride and proton pump inhibitor omeprazole were both effective in reducing the incidence of peri-anesthetic GER [4–7].

Q. How do I avoid aspiration pneumonia?

A. Aspiration of gastric contents does not necessarily cause aspiration pneumonia. The aspiration of regurgitated or refluxed gastric content into the lungs may cause bronchospasm and pneumonitis, which can predispose a patient to bacterial colonization of the lungs and subsequent aspiration pneumonia. The lungs may be damaged by aspiration of greater than 0.3–0.4 ml/kg at a pH less than 2.5 [8]. As discussed previously, GER may be clinically silent and pre-emptive treatments may be ineffective. Prevention of aspiration of gastric contents should be geared towards airway management. It is important to rapidly intubate patients at high risk of GER with a cuffed endotracheal tube and inflate the cuff to properly seal the trachea. The cuff should be generously lubricated prior to insertion of the endotracheal tube to maximize the seal, as the lubricant fills in areas of less than perfect contact between the cuff and the inner wall of the trachea. Prior to extubation, the caudal oropharynx should be suctioned or swabbed if reflux or regurgitated matter are present and the tube should remain in place with the cuff inflated until the patient has regained proper airway reflexes. The nose should be positioned downward so as to allow drainage of regurgitated gastric contents rather than pooling in the caudal oropharynx.

Q. My patient is obese – how will this affect my anesthetic plan?

A. There are a number of problems associated with obesity in anesthetic patients. The primary peri-anesthetic concerns involve respiratory compromise, patient positioning, and dosing of anesthetic agents.

✓ Obesity may lead to rapid desaturation with hypoventilation, as detected by a drop in the measured S_pO_2.

- This can be managed by thorough pre-oxygenation prior to anesthetic induction: supply 100% oxygen by facemask at 5 l/min for 5 min.

- Following anesthesia, closely monitor SpO_2 and supplement oxygen via endotracheal tube or facemask as necessary in order to maintain S_pO_2 above 94%.

✓ The obese patient is also more prone to atelectasis and hypoventilation: the patient should be mechanically ventilated or receive assisted ventilation for the entire anesthetic period.

✓ When possible, dorsal recumbency and Trendelenburg positioning (head down position) should be avoided to prevent respiratory compromise. Dorsal recumbency in an obese patient will significantly reduce venous return because of compression of the vena cavae.

✓ In order to prevent overdosing of anesthetic agents, drug dosages should be based upon an estimated lean or ideal body weight. This includes sedatives, analgesics, induction agents, IV fluids, and local anesthetics.

Q. What are the anesthetic concerns in a patient undergoing upper GI endoscopy?

A. Most pre-anesthetic concerns are related to the patient's underlying disease and the reason upper GI endoscopy is necessary. Pre-anesthetic management and sedation should be geared towards the individual patient; there are no specific concerns related to the procedure. A study evaluating the effect of selected anesthetic agents on endoscopy found that commonly administered anesthetic agents such as hydromorphone and medetomidine did not adversely impact the time to pass an endoscope into the stomach and duodenum of cats, while a similar study in dogs found that the combination of morphine and atropine led to increased difficulty in passing an endoscope into the duodenum [9,10].

The major concern related to upper GI endoscopy is insufflation of the stomach. Massive distention of the stomach due to insufflation may lead to decreased venous return, respiratory compromise, and vasovagal stimulation. While endoscopy is performed, the anesthetist should periodically verify that the stomach is minimally distended. Should over-distention occur, air should be suctioned out immediately with the endoscope to prevent untoward effects.

Q. Is there anything different in the management of a lower GI endoscopy?

A. Lower GI endoscopy is considered a relatively safe procedure with a low incidence of adverse effects [11]. Similar to upper GI endoscopy, vasovagal stimulation may occur due to insufflation and distension of the colon. As with all anesthetic events, vigilant monitoring of cardiovascular parameters is warranted and clinically significant bradycardia may be treated with anticholinergic agents such as atropine or glycopyrolate.

Q. What are the anesthetic concerns in a patient undergoing laparoscopy?

A. Similar to endoscopy, there are minimal pre-anesthetic concerns specific to laparoscopic procedures. Anesthetic protocols should be geared towards any underlying conditions that may be present in the patient. Concerns specific to laparoscopy are related to insufflation of the abdomen with carbon dioxide. Much like endoscopy, dilatation of the peritoneal cavity may lead to decreased venous return and respiratory compromise. Mechanical ventilation is highly recommended as the distended abdomen may limit full excursion of the lungs and diaphragm. Furthermore, carbon dioxide that is used for insufflation may be absorbed across the peritoneum. It is important to closely monitor end-tidal carbon dioxide as hypercapnia may occur if ventilation parameters are not adjusted appropriately. At the completion of surgery, aspiration of carbon dioxide from the peritoneal cavity should be performed. Despite this, it is not uncommon for a small amount of gas to remain in the peritoneal cavity. Patients may be uncomfortable despite minimal incisions due to pneumo-peritoneum.

Q. What are the metabolic derangements commonly associated with vomiting and diarrhea?

A. Vomiting of gastric contents causes a loss of potassium, chloride, sodium, and bicarbonate. Patients may present with hypochloremia, hypokalemia, hyponatremia, dehydration, and metabolic acidosis. Pyloric outflow obstruction is an exception as vomiting of stomach acid may lead to metabolic alkalosis. Patients with prolonged or severe diarrhea may present with hypo- or hypernatremia, hypokalemia, and metabolic acidosis despite elevated bicarbonate.

Q. How can I deal with metabolic derangements seen with vomiting and diarrhea?

A. Patients with severe acute or chronic vomiting or diarrhea should have electrolytes and acid-base status checked prior to anesthesia. Anesthetic management should be geared towards each individual derangement and pre-anesthetic stabilization of severe electrolyte and acid-base abnormalities should be prioritized.

    ✓ Hypokalemia can be corrected at a rate not to exceed 0.5 mEq/kg/h. Anesthesia should be delayed, if possible, until the patient's potassium level can be stabilized above 2.5 mEq/l.

✓ Hyponatremia should not be corrected rapidly. Sodium supplementation to improve moderate to severe hyponatremia (< 120 mEq/l) should be spread over 24 h.

✓ Administration of bicarbonate is rarely indicated for metabolic derangements; peri-anesthetic administration of intravenous fluids and correction of the underlying problem are generally enough to manage acidemia.

✓ During anesthesia, it is important to maintain control of carbon dioxide either through manual ventilation or close monitoring of spontaneous ventilation to avoid additional respiratory acidosis caused by hypercapnia or respiratory alkalosis by hypocapnia.

Q. I need to provide analgesia to my vomiting patient, what can I give?

A. ✓ Opioids are powerful analgesics that may cause vomiting, especially when given subcutaneously or intramuscularly. Intravenous administration of opioids such as fentanyl, buprenorphine, hydromorphone, and oxymorphone generally do not cause vomiting and may be administered to vomiting patients.

✓ Nonsteroidal anti-inflammatory drugs (NSAIDs) are not recommended in patients with gastrointestinal compromise due to the potential for gastroduodenal ulceration [12]. NSAIDs should also be avoided in patients with severe vomiting or diarrhea as their use in volume-depleted patients may be associated with renal compromise [13].

✓ Maropitant, an anti-emetic, has demonstrated anesthetic drug-sparing effects in abdominal surgery that may suggest a potential role in managing visceral pain [14].

Q. What are the effects of common anesthetic drugs on the GI system?

A. See Table 33.1 for a list.

Table 33.1 Gastrointestinal side effects of some commonly used anesthetic drugs.

Drug	Effect	Notes
Acepromazine	Anti-emetic	Most effective if given 15 min prior to opioid administration [15]
Alpha-2 agonists	Emetic	Especially pronounced in cats at higher dosages
Anticholinergics	Decreased GI motility [16]	
Benzodiazepines	Anti-emetic	Effect seen in humans, not observed clinically in animals [17]
Opioids	Emetic	Variable effects on gastroesophageal reflux [18,19]
Volatile anesthetics	Increased gastroesophageal reflux	Not necessarily a direct drug effect [20]

References

1 Galatos AD, Raptopoulos D. Gastro-oesophageal reflux during anaesthesia in the dog: the effect of preoperative fasting and premedication. *Veterinary Record* 1995; **137(19)**:479–483.

2 Savvas I, Rallis T, Raptopoulos D. The effect of pre-anaesthetic fasting time and type of food on gastric content volume and acidity in dogs. *Veterinary Anesthesia and Analgesia* 2009; **36**:539–546.

3 Galatos AD and Raptopoulos D. Gastro-oesophageal reflux during anaesthesia in the dog: the effect of age, positioning, and type of surgical procedure. *Veterinary Record* 1995; **137(20)**:513–516.

4 Wilson DV, Evans AT, Mauer WA. Influence of metoclopramide on gastroesophageal reflux in anesthetized dogs. *American Journal of Veterinary Research* 2006; **67**:26–31.

5 Panti A, Bennett RC, Corletto F, *et al.* The effect of omeprazole on oesophageal pH in dogs. *Journal of Small Anima Practice* 2009; **50(10)**:540–544.

6 Zacuto AC, Marks SL, Osborn J, *et al.* The influence of esomeprazole and cisapride on gastroesophageal reflux during anesthesia in dogs. *Journal of Veterinary Internal Medicine* 2012; **26**:518–525.

7 Johnson RA. Maropitant prevented vomiting but not gastroesophageal reflux in anesthetized dogs premedicated with acepromazine-hydromorphone. *Veterinary Anesthesia and Analgesia* 2014; **41**:406–410.

8 Cameron JL, Caldini P, Toung JK, *et al.* Aspiration pneumonia: physiologic data following experimental aspiration. *Surgery* 1972; **72(2)**:238–245.

9 Smith AA, Posner LP, Goldstein RE, *et al.* 2004. Evaluation of the effects of premedication on gastroduodenoscopy in cats. *Journal of the American Veterinary Medical Association 2004;* **225(4)**:540–544.

10 Donaldson LL, Leib MS, Boyd C, *et al.* Effect of preanesthetic medication on ease of endoscopic intubation of the duodenum in anesthetized dogs. *American Journal of Veterinary Research* 1993; **54(9)**:1489–1495.

11 Leib MS, Baechtel MS, Monroe WE. Complications associated with 355 flexible colonoscopic procedures in dogs. *Journal of Veterinary Internal Medicine* 2004; **18(5)**: 642–646.

12 Forsyth SF, Guilford WG, Haslett SJ, *et al.* Endoscopy of the gastroduodenal mucosa after carprofen, meloxicam and ketoprofen administration in dogs. *Journal of Small Animal Practice* 1998; **39(9)**:421–444.

13 Surdyk KK, Sloan DL,Brown SA. Renal effects of carprofen and etodolac in euvolemic and volume-depleted dogs. *American Journal of Veterinary Research* 2012; **73(9)**:1485–1490.

14 Boscan P, Monnet E, Mama K, *et al.* Effect of maropitant, a neurokinin 1 antagonist, on anesthetic requirements during noxious visceral stimulation of the ovary in dogs. *American Journal of Veterinary Research* 2011; **72(12)**:1576–1579.

15 Valverde A, Cantwell S, Hernandez J. Effects of acepromazine on the incidence of vomiting associated with opioid administration in dogs. *Veterinary Anesthesia and Analgesia* 2004; **31**:40–45.

16 Burger DM, Wiestner T, Hubler M, *et al.* Effect of anticholinergics (atropine, glycopyrrolate) and prokinetics (metoclopramide, cisapride) on gastric motility in beagles and labrador retrievers. *Journal of Veterinary Medicine A: Physiology and Pathology in Clinical Medicine* 2006; **53(2)**:97–107.

17 Rodola F. Midazolam as an anti-emetic. *European Reviews in Medical Pharmacologic Science* 2006; **10(3)**:121–126.

18 Wilson DV, Evans AT, Miller R. 2005. Effects of preanesthetic administration of morphine on gastroesophageal reflux and regurgitation during anesthesia. *American Journal of Veterinary Research* 2005; **66**:386–390.

19 Wilson DV, Evans AT, Mauer WA. Pre-anesthetic meperidine: associated vomiting and gastroesophageal reflux during the subsequent anesthetic in dogs. *Veterinary Anesthesia and Analgesia* 2007; **34**:15–22.

20 Wilson DV, Boruta DT, Evans AT. Influence of halothane, isoflurane, and sevoflurane on gastroesophageal reflux during anesthesia in dogs. *American Journal of Veterinary Research* 2006; **67**:1821–1825.

34 Anesthetic Considerations for Hepatic Disease

An organ with some important jobs

Jane Quandt

College of Veterinary Medicine, University of Georgia, USA

KEY POINTS:

- The liver is important as it is involved in the production of glucose, albumin, and coagulation factors.

- The liver metabolizes anesthetic drugs and this can impact anesthetic recovery.

- Glucose is necessary for energy production and is vital for brain function.

- Albumin provides COP for fluid homeostasis.

- Coagulation factors are required to prevent hemorrhage.

- Anesthetic drugs that are used for patients with liver disease should be short-acting, reversible, or produce minimal cardiovascular and respiratory depression.

Q. What is the main blood supply to the liver?

A. Twenty percent of the cardiac output is delivered to the liver. Of that percentage, 30% of the blood flow and 90% of the oxygen is supplied by the hepatic artery and the remainder is provided by the portal vein [1].

Q. What are clinical signs of hepatic disease or insufficiency?

A. Clinical signs include ascites, depression, seizures, jaundice, hepatoencephalopathy, stunted growth, anorexia, and weight loss. Decreased blood values for albumin, urea nitrogen, glucose, and cholesterol can be seen with poor liver function. Coagulation times of prothrombin, partial thromboplastin can be prolonged and there can be increased fibrinogen values [1].

Blood ammonia concentration and bile acids are indicators of liver dysfunction. Bile acids are produced by the liver and excreted in the bile. An increase in postprandial bile acid concentration indicates a decrease in hepatic function or the presence of a portosystemic vascular shunt [1,2].

Questions and Answers in Small Animal Anesthesia, First Edition. Edited by Lesley J. Smith.
© 2016 John Wiley & Sons, Inc. Published 2016 by John Wiley & Sons, Inc.

Q. What are four primary functions of the liver that can affect anesthesia?

A. The liver has many functions, but the four primary functions that can impact anesthesia are:

✓ glucose homeostasis
✓ protein synthesis
✓ production of clotting factors
✓ drug metabolism and detoxification.

Glucose homeostasis (including formation, storage, and release) is an essential part of normal liver function. Blood glucose values should be closely monitored in the patient with liver dysfunction as hypoglycemia can be present. Hypoglycemia (less than 50 mg/dl) can result in neurological symptoms as glucose is the obligate energy source for the brain. Bradycardia and circulatory collapse may also occur. Hypoglycemia during anesthesia can result in a prolonged recovery [1,2]. If hypoglycemia is present, dextrose should be added to the crystalloid fluid therapy to maintain a blood glucose within the normal range [1,2,3]. The concentration of dextrose in the crystalloid fluid can be 2.5–5%. If the fluid rate delivery rate is high the concentration should be lower, that is 2.5%, to avoid hyperglycemia. A fluid delivery rate of less than 5 ml/kg/h may require a higher dextrose concentration to achieve normoglyemia. The patient's blood glucose value should be monitored every 35–40 min during the duration of anesthesia and recovery to avoid hypo- or hyperglycemia. There are specific dog or cat point-of-care glucometers that simplify this monitoring.

The liver is the only site for albumin synthesis. Low plasma albumin level will result in more free drug being available as there is less drug binding to protein. When administering anesthetic agents a lower dose may be needed to avoid an overdose.

Albumin accounts for 80% of the colloid oncotic pressure (COP) of plasma. When the albumin concentration is less than 1.5 g/dl the decrease in COP can result in redistribution of fluid to the extracellular spaces, leading to the development of edema. Fluid therapy may need to include a colloid such as hetastarch or plasma to improve the COP [1,4].

A low COP may contribute to ascites. A large amount of ascites may impinge on lung expansion and pulmonary function. Removal of ascites prior to anesthesia may be considered but should be done slowly as rapid removal of a large amount of fluid may cause a fluid shift from the vascular space to the abdominal cavity as ascites formation continues. This fluid shift can cause serious hypotension and cardiovascular compromise. This can also be seen intra-operatively if the ascites is removed rapidly via surgical suction. Intravenous fluids should be given during ascites removal to avoid cardiovascular collapse [1,2].

The liver also synthesizes all coagulation proteins except factor VIII. Antithrombin II, antiplasmin, and plasminogen are also produced by the liver. Coagulation can be affected by liver disease and a coagulation profile is recommended prior to surgery. There will be shortened half-lives of the coagulation factors with potential for disseminated intravascular coagulation and increased blood loss during surgery. A prolonged coagulation profile should be treated with fresh frozen plasma. Hypothermia can also slow coagulation times so the patient should be kept normothermic during surgery and into the recovery period [1,2,4].

Most anesthetic drugs and sedatives are metabolized by the liver. To improve liver metabolism, keep the patient normotensive to maintain hepatic blood flow and to keep metabolic rate normal. In addition consider use of drugs that have a short half-life or can be reversed to minimize recovery time [2,4].

Q. What effect does a portosystemic shunt have on anesthesia?

A. Portosystemic shunts are usually found in pediatric or juvenile patients, and because of their congenital hepatic disease these patients will have an increased risk for hypotension, hypoglycemia, and hypothermia. Intra- or extra-hepatic shunting will affect highly extracted drugs by increasing drug availability. Hepatic metabolism is the main elimination route for most lipophilic drugs. Hepatic clearance is determined by hepatic blood flow, protein binding, and intrinsic clearance via hepatic enzymes. The hepatic clearance of drugs with high extraction ratios depends largely on liver blood flow. A decrease in liver blood flow due to a shunt will affect the clearance of these drugs. Drugs that have poor hepatic extraction are influenced by changes in plasma protein binding and intrinsic metabolic clearance [5]. It is recommended to use agents with minimal cardiovascular depressant effects and those that can be antagonized or do not need hepatic function for metabolism and elimination from the body [6]. Benzodiazepines may be contraindicated in patients that exhibit hepato-encephalopathy. These patients may have increased central nervous system sensitivity to benzodiazepines due to the presence of endogenous benzodiazepine receptor ligands, which are increased in the blood of dogs with portosystemic shunts [2]. The reversal agent for benzodiazepines, flumazenil, can be used to reverse hepato-encephalopathy and coma to a certain degree. These patients may also have concurrent hypokalemia due to gastrointestinal loss via vomiting, diarrhea, or urinary loss. Hypokalemia should be corrected prior to anesthesia [1].

The chronic nature of portosystemic shunt may lead to increased GABA sensitivity and permeability of the blood–brain barrier. The effects of anesthetic drugs may be unpredictable, more profound, and longer in duration. Drugs that are highly dependent on hepatic metabolism for termination of action such as ketamine, tiletamine (telazol), acepromazine, alpha-2 agonists, and benzodiazepines should probably be avoided. Drugs that are highly protein bound, such as the barbiturates, are more active when hypo-albuminemia is present [1].

Q. What are some of the anesthetic considerations in patients with hepatic disease?

A. The patient with hepatic disease needs to be closely monitored intra-operatively and during recovery. Pre-operative blood work is necessary to assess blood glucose, coagulation times, protein levels, and electrolytes. When forming the anesthetic plan, consider use of those agents with short half-lives, minimal cardiovascular effects, and those that can be reversed. Mean arterial blood pressure should be maintained $\geq$ 70 mmHg to prevent further liver damage, hepatic ischemia, and to aid in drug metabolism [6]. Seizures due to hepato-encephalopathy may occur. Diazepam or phenobarbital used to treat seizures may have a prolonged duration of action as they are metabolized by the liver and hepatic disease may alter their pharmacokinetics. It is suggested that drugs that may induce seizure activity, such as ketamine and tiletamine, be avoided. There may be increased cerebral sensitivity to gamma aminobutyric acid (GABA) in some patients with hepatic disease. This increased sensitivity may enhance the depressant effects of the barbiturates and benzodiazepines [1,2]. There can be a prolonged recovery from anesthesia. The patient should be kept warm to avoid hypothermia, which can contribute to a long recovery and decrease drug metabolism.

Q. Why do patients with hepatic disease have an increased susceptibility to many anesthetic drugs?

A. ✓ The decrease in albumin will affect protein binding of anesthetic drugs, which are highly protein bound. Hypo-albuminemia will lead to more active drug being available with increased effects and duration.

  ✓ A decrease in drug metabolism may result in potentiated drug effect and toxicity and may also result in prolonged recovery times.

  ✓ There is an increased sensitivity of the CNS to anesthetic agents in patients with liver disease.

  ✓ Hepatic blood flow is altered with hypotension reducing portal blood flow so drugs that depend on high hepatic clearance may have a prolonged effect.

Q. How do inhalant anesthetics affect hepatic blood flow?

A. Total hepatic blood flow is maintained within a narrow limit. The inhalant anesthetic agents can decrease liver blood flow and therefore oxygen delivery. Hypotension will exacerbate this decrease in hepatic blood flow. The use of positive pressure ventilation will affect hepatic blood flow by decreasing venous return, especially in the patient that is hypovolemic [1].

Q. How would you monitor the patient with hepatic disease that is undergoing anesthesia?

A. All the standard monitoring should be employed: pulse oximetry, capnometry, ECG and heart rate, respiratory rate, body temperature, urine output, non-invasive or invasive blood pressure (if possible), PCV, TP, and blood glucose [1].

Q. What anesthetic drugs should be considered?

A. Premedication should be used to make the patient easier to handle, provide analgesia, and to decrease the amount of inhalant required. Opioids, that is pure μ agonists such as fentanyl, hydromorphone, methadone, oxymorphone, meperidine, and morphine, are commonly used as they provide good analgesia and can be reversed if necessary. Hydromorphone, oxymorphone, methadone, and fentanyl may be preferred if given IV over morphine or meperidine as the latter two agents may cause histamine release leading to hypotension. Fentanyl can be used as a CRI to allow for titration of analgesia that is individualized for the patient. Opioid induced bradycardia and respiratory depression can be side effects. The newest opioid, remifentanil, may be the opioid of choice for short procedures or for intra-operative analgesia as it does not require liver metabolism. Remifentanil has an extremely short duration of action and is highly lipid soluble, so its effects occur very quickly. Avoid rapid boluses of this drug and plan to administer it as a constant rate infusion in order to achieve consistent plasma levels [7,8].

Avoid acepromazine because of its hypotensive effects, its prolonged duration, and the lack of a reversal agent [1,2,4]. The alpha-2 agonists can lead to brady-arrythmias and increase blood glucose concentrations. The negative effect of these drugs on cardiac output and their vasoconstrictive effects can compromise organ blood flow and oxygen delivery. They may be considered if profound sedation is needed, and they can be reversed if necessary. The use of benzodiazepines in patients with liver disease is controversial due to their effect on GABA. Midazolam may be preferred as it is water soluble whereas diazepam can cause vessel irritation and hypotension when given IV due to the propylene glycol carrier.

Anesthetic induction can be achieved with propofol, etomidate, or alfaxalone following IV opioids [1,2,4]. Propofol may be the preferred induction agent for patients with hepatic disease as redistribution and metabolism is rapid. The total body clearance of propofol exceeds hepatic blood flow indicating other sites of elimination, such as the lung. The duration of action of propofol is not prolonged in patients with hepatic disease. Inhalant agents such as isoflurane and sevoflurane are used for maintenance of anesthesia.

Q. Can local anesthetics be used in patients with liver disease?

A. The local anesthetics of the amide class, lidocaine, mepivacaine, and bupivacaine, are directly metabolized by the liver. In patients with hepatic disease there may be a prolonged effect [2].

Q. How does biliary disease affect anesthesia?

A. Patients with gall bladder mucocoeles may have concurrent pancreatitis or bile peritonitis. They are usually older, sicker patients. Dogs with distention of the gall bladder or obstruction of the bile duct should not be given pure μ opioid receptor agonists for premedication, as there is concern they may cause constriction of the bile duct and possible gall bladder rupture.

Butorphanol and buprenorphine are less likely to cause this constriction and therefore may be preferred, but will also provide less analgesia. Propofol, alfaxalone, or etomidate may be preferred choices for induction agents. Inhalant anesthesia with isoflurane or sevoflurane is preferred. In patients that are extremely painful and may tend to become hypotensive with high levels of inhalants, a fentanyl CRI can be given. This will provide analgesia that can be titrated to effect and allow for a decrease in the amount of inhalant that is required. These patients will need cardiovascular support with fluids and possibly inotropes and vasopressors [6].

References

1 Green SA, Marks SL. Hepatic disease. In: Tranquilli WJ, Thurmon JC, Grimm KA (eds) *Lumb & Jones Veterinary Anesthesia and Analgesia*, 4th edn. Blackwell Publishing: Ames, IA, 2007:921–926.

2 Grubb TL. Anesthesia for patients with special concerns. In: Carroll GL (ed.) *Small Animal Anesthesia and Analgesia*. Blackwell Publishing: Ames, IA, 2008:193–238.

3 Koenig A. Hypoglycemia. In: Silverstein DC, Hopper K (eds) Small Animal Critical Care Medicine. *Saunders Elsevier: St.* Louis, MO 2009:295–299.

4 Weil AB. Anesthesia for patients with renal/hepatic disease. *Topics in Companion Animal Medicine* 2010; **25(2)**:87–91.

5 Bosilkovska M, Walder B, Bessen M, *et al.* Analgesics in patients with hepatic impairment. Pharmacology and clinical implications. *Drugs* 2012; **72**:1645–1669.

6 Clarke KW, Trim CM, Hall LW. Anesthesia of the dog. In: Clarke KW, Trim CM, Hall LW (eds) *Veterinary Anesthesia*, 11th edn. Saunders Elsevier: St. Louis, MO 2014:405–498.

7 7.Anagnostou TL, Kazakos GM, Savvas I, *et al.* Remifentanil/isoflurane anesthesia in five dogs with liver disease undergoing liver biopsy. *Journal of the American Animal Hospital Association* 2011; **47(6)**:e103–e109.

8 Pypendop BH, Brosnan RJ, Sial KT, *et al.* Pharmacokinetics of remifentanil in conscious cats and cats anesthetized with isoflurane. *American Journal of Veterinary Research* 2008; **69(4)**: 531–536.

35 Anesthetic Considerations for Renal Disease

Ins and outs of water and salts

Jane Quandt

College of Veterinary Medicine, University of Georgia, USA

KEY POINTS:

- Urine production is an important indication of renal perfusion.
- Urine output in the normal animal is 1 to 2 ml/kg/h.
- Maintaining a mean arterial blood pressure above 60 mmHg is needed to ensure adequate renal perfusion in a healthy animal.
- Animals with renal impairment may benefit from IV fluid therapy prior to anesthesia and into recovery. To avoid volume overload colloids can be part of the fluid therapy.
- NSAIDs are not recommended in animals with renal impairment.

Q. How is blood flow to the kidneys regulated?

A. Renal blood flow (RBF) is regulated by extrinsic nervous and hormonal control and by intrinsic autoregulation. Renal vasculature is highly innervated by the sympathetic nervous system that constricts blood flow in certain areas of the kidney under various physiologic conditions, including stress. Intrinsic autoregulation of RBF occurs when the mean blood pressure (MAP) is between 80 and 180 mmHg; in this pressure range the kidney can control blood flow by altering resistance in the glomerular afferent arterioles. At mean arterial blood pressures below 80 and above 180, autoregulation of RBF begins to fail. The kidneys receive 20–25% of the cardiac output. The kidneys have a high oxygen consumption, which makes them susceptible to ischemic insult if oxygen delivery is inadequate, either because of patient hypoxia or because of inadequate cardiac output and renal perfusion. This means that during anesthesia the respiratory and circulatory systems must be supported in order to adequately deliver oxygen to the kidneys [1].

Q. What is the recommended pre-operative preparation and blood work for the renal patient?

Questions and Answers in Small Animal Anesthesia, First Edition. Edited by Lesley J. Smith.
© 2016 John Wiley & Sons, Inc. Published 2016 by John Wiley & Sons, Inc.

A. A complete physical exam should be performed in all patients undergoing anesthesia. In the renal patient a serum chemistry analysis, urinalysis, and assessment of urine output is essential. A blood urea nitrogen (BUN), creatinine, and creatinine clearance are used to assess the glomerular filtration rate (GFR), although these may be rather insensitive tests to subclinical reductions in GFR. A reagent test strip (e.g., Azostix) reading is a very poor substitute for a measured BUN. Renal tubular function can be evaluated via urine specific gravity and urine osmolarity. Electrolytes (most importantly, potassium) need to be evaluated and acid-base determined, ideally with an arterial blood gas analysis. A patient with suspected chronic renal disease needs evaluation of the PVC and TP. The kidney produces erythropoietin and chronic renal disease can lead to decreased production and subsequent anemia [1,2]. TP can be low 2° to proteinuria, which can occur with chronic glomerulo-nephropathies.

Q. Why is azotemia harmful if my patient is going under anesthesia?

A. Azotemia causes CNS depression, which will be additive with the CNS depressant effects of sedative and anesthetic drugs. Other reasons to correct azotemia include improvement of acid-base status; patients with azotemia are commonly acidotic which will increase the fraction of unbound drugs in the plasma. This would require the use of lower doses of highly protein bound injectable agents to avoid a relative drug overdose. Hyperkalemia is often seen with acidosis and azotemia. Hyperkalemia should be corrected prior to anesthesia due to its deleterious effect on cardiac rhythm. An effort should be made to reduce any level of azotemia prior to anesthesia. Pre-renal azotemia 2° to dehydration should be corrected and peri-operative hypovolemia needs to be avoided [2,3].

Q. Are pre-anesthetic fluids recommended in patients with renal disease?

A. Cardiovascular depression under anesthesia can lead to impaired renal function. To help minimize this effect IV crystalloid fluids can be given prior to anesthesia, during anesthesia, and into recovery. Pre-operative IV fluids will help to put the animal is a mild state of diuresis with the goal of having the urine output between 0.5 and 2.0 ml/kg/h. Ideally, IV balanced isotonic crystalloids should be administered for a 12–24 h period prior to anesthesia, at rates of $\sim$ 2 ml/kg/h. The rate should be tailored to the individual patient and fluid deficits should be corrected in addition to the maintenance rate of $\sim$ 2 ml/kg/h. The patient should be closely monitored for volume overload [1]. Patients with oliguric or anuric renal failure will not tolerate even these rates of fluid administration and are at a high risk for volume overload.

Anemia causes decreased oxygen delivery. A chronic renal failure patient with a PCV < 20% should prompt consideration for a pre-operative blood transfusion. Because most of these patients suffer from chronic anemia, they are somewhat more tolerant of a low PCV because of chronic shifts in Hb affinity for oxygen; specifically an increased Hb affinity for oxygen (left-shifted Bohr curve). Regardless, patients with a PCV < 15% will most certainly benefit from a pre-operative blood transfusion to increase their oxygen carrying capacity.

Renal failure patients may also suffer from hypo-proteinemia, which can lead to more free anesthetic drug available and to a lower colloid oncotic pressure (COP), which puts the patient at higher risk for anesthetic induced hypotension and relative hypovolemia, as fluids do not remain in the intravascular space when COP is low. These patients may require additional fluid therapy with a colloid. When giving a colloid concurrently with a crystalloid the amount of crystalloid is usually decreased by 40–50% to avoid volume overload [1,3]. Commonly available colloids (e.g., hetastarch) can be given at rates no higher than 50 ml/kg/day (see Chapter 9 for more details).

Q. What electrolyte is of most concern with renal disease?

A. Potassium is commonly elevated in patient with renal disease.

Q. How is the level of hyperkalemia related to anesthetic risk, specifically cardiac effects?

A. Hyperkalemia can have detrimental effects on the heart because of unstable electrical activity. An ECG should be monitored when managing and treating hyperkalemia. The level of K^+ can be correlated to the changes in the ECG waveform. Mild hyperkalemia, 5.5–6.0 mEq/l, will result in T waves that become large and tented. Moderate hyperkalemia, 6.0–8.0 mEq/l, will result in a decreased R amplitude and a decreased P wave amplitude. The QRS and PR intervals will be prolonged and the ST segment will be depressed. The heart rate can begin to slow at K^+ levels of 6.5–7 mEq/l. At high K^+ levels, > 7.5 mEq/l, the heart rate becomes very slow and atrial standstill may occur, the T wave may or may not be large. Severe hyperkalemia, greater than 8 mEq/l, will lead to an absence of P waves and a wide QRS. At K^+ levels of 9.5 mEq/l or higher, ventricular flutter, ventricular fibrillation, and asystole are likely [1,2].

Q. What is the treatment for hyperkalemia?

A. A serum K^+ > 5.5 mEq/l should be lowered before the animal undergoes anesthesia. The goal of treatment is to drive the K^+ into cells to lower the intravascular levels. Calcium (calcium gluconate 50–150 ml/kg by slow IV bolus) can be given to help stabilize the cardiac cell membranes and prevent some of the deleterious cardiac effects of hyperkalemia. Acidosis will exacerbate hyperkalemia because H^+ is exchanged for K^+ by the cells in order to attempt to normalize pH, leading to higher extracellular K^+. Respiratory acidosis due to hypoventilation under anesthesia should be avoided. Many renal failure patients have chronic metabolic acidosis as well, so anesthetic-induced respiratory acidosis will lower the animal's pH to potentially dangerous levels. Purposeful assisted/mechanical hyperventilation will decrease serum K^+ by 0.5 mEq/l for every 10 mmHg reduction in P_aCO_2. P_aCO_2 should not be reduced below ~ 35 mmHg, however, due to deleterious effects on cerebral blood flow. Bottom line – avoid hypoventilation and respiratory acidosis in renal patients!

Judicious fluid therapy is the key to directly lowering serum potassium in renal failure patients. Mild hyperkalemia can be treated with fluid therapy consisting of 0.9% NaCl to dilute the K^+, increase GFR and increase urinary excretion of K^+. Lactated ringers solution could also be used due to its low K^+ content. Moderate to severe hyperkalemia can be treated with 0.9% NaCl infusion and 1.5 G/kg of 20–50% dextrose given IV to stimulate insulin release, which promotes the movement of K^+ into cells. Insulin can be given with the dextrose, 0.1 to 0.25 U/kg, to further promote movement of K^+ into cells. Effects on serum potassium start within one hour and last several hours. During treatment, serum K^+ should be monitored repeatedly [1,2].

Q. How does anesthesia affect the kidneys?

A. Kidney function, that is renal blood flow (RBF), glomerular filtration rate (GFR), urinary output and electrolyte excretion, are temporarily decreased during general anesthesia. All anesthetics can decrease the GFR by decreasing the RBF. Peri-anesthetic events such as stress, hypotension, acidosis, hypovolemia, and pain can result in reductions in perfusion pressure to the kidneys, release of catecholamines, and production of ADH, endothelin, nitric oxide, and prostaglandins, and activation of the aldosterone–renin–angiotensin system. The concern to the anesthetist is the development of acute kidney injury [2]. Even without clinical evidence of acute kidney injury, subclinical renal damage 2° to peri-anesthetic events as listed above may well shorten a patient's life long term due to the development of chronic renal failure in later years.

If the anesthetic episode is short with minimal complications, and the patient is monitored and cardiovascular and respiratory function are well-supported, then renal function and renal values should return to normal within hours. In patients with pre-existing renal compromise, prolonged anesthesia (> 1 h) and complicated procedures, pain, hypoxia, hemorrhage, hypotension, and stress can be detrimental to normal renal function and lead to acute renal injury [1].

Q. Are any anesthetic agents nephrotoxic?

A. Inhalant anesthetic agents are nephrotoxic in that they produce generalized reduction of renal function. Renal ischemia can occur due to anesthetic induced systemic hypotension and reduced cardiac output [2]. Sevoflurane, when used with "low flow" anesthesia, that is fresh gas flow rates < 10 ml/kg/min, and when administered in an anesthetic machine with dehydrated carbon dioxide absorbent, may produce Compound A, which has been shown to be nephrotoxic in rats. The clinical significance of this in dogs is debatable. Injectable agents also affect renal function, again because the reduction in systemic blood pressure will lead to a reduction in RBF and GFR. Pre-anesthetic hypovolemia will exacerbate the potential for renal hypotension.

Q. What anesthetic agents are recommended (or not) in patients with renal disease and what are their effects on renal function?

A. It important when planning anesthetic drug protocols for patients with renal disease to consider reducing the drug dosage. If the patient is hypoproteinemic, higher amounts of free active drug will be available leading to a more profound effect. Chronic renal failure patients are frequently cachectic and will have decreased muscle mass as well, resulting in less available depots for drug redistribution and a longer residence time in the plasma with greater and/or more prolonged CNS effects. Renal failure will also lead to impaired renal clearance, which causes a prolonged effect of drugs that are excreted in the renal system. A good example here is ketamine, which in cats is renally eliminated as the parent drug. Ketamine, in a cat with chronic renal failure, will have a longer residence time and prolonged duration of effect.

In patients with renal disease, anesthetic premedication is important in order to avoid stress and pain which can lead to sympathetic catecholamine release with resulting vasoconstriction and a decrease in renal blood flow. Premedication will decrease the amount of general anesthesia that is required and will better preserve cardiac output and blood flow. Sedatives may be used as part of premedication and can be combined with the opioids for a balanced approach. Acepromazine may create systemic hypotension due to vasodilation as result of its alpha adrenergic blockade effect. A low dose of acepromazine (0.01 to 0.02 mg/kg) may be used in the patient that has been adequately fluid loaded. The alpha blockade may protect the renal cortex from sympathetically mediated vasoconstriction. There can be prolonged sedation from acepromazine in azotemic patients.

Alpha-2 agonists are not recommended because of the reduction in cardiac output and decrease in organ blood flow that this class of drugs can cause. These drugs also inhibit ADH, leading to increased urine production, which should be avoided in the animal with urinary obstruction.

Benzodiazepines, midazolam or diazepam, are useful in that they have minimal cardiovascular effects and therefore less effect on RBF. Diazepam may have a prolonged effect in azotemic or oliguric patients due to the renal excretion of the active metabolite, oxazepam. The benzodiazepines can be reversed with flumazenil.

Opioids are preferred for anesthetic premedication. They have minimal effect on the cardiovascular system with only a small portion excreted via the kidneys. They provide analgesia which will help decrease pain related sympathetic catecholamine injury to the kidneys. An additional advantage to the use of opioids is that they can be reversed. So, bottom line for premedications? Your best choice is a combination of a pure μ agonist opioid and a benzodiazepine!

For anesthetic induction, the main goal is to reduce, as much as possible, the chance for hypotension. Low doses of propofol, alfaxalone, or etomidate have no direct negative renal effects. With opioid premedications, required doses of your induction drug can be low enough to minimize hypotension. Dissociatives, ketamine and telazol, may reduce RBF via increased sympathetic tone and vasoconstriction. Renal excretion of ketamine and the active metabolite, norketamine, may result in prolonged effects in azotemic or oliguric patients [1–3].

Q. What mean blood pressure is desirable to maintain renal perfusion?

A. A mean arterial pressure of 60 mmHg or higher is needed *in healthy normal patients* to achieve renal perfusion and urine production and provide blood flow to vital organs. In patients with renal failure, the mean arterial pressure should be maintained at 80 mmHg as this is the presumed lower limit of renal blood flow autoregulation and is especially important in those animals with pre-existing disease. Direct arterial blood pressure monitoring is ideal, but is not always possible. If indirect blood pressure monitoring is used, such as a Doppler, the systolic blood pressure should be maintained at 90 mmHg or better to ensure a mean arterial pressure greater than 60 mmHg [1–3].

Q. I've heard that dopamine can be used to improve RBF. Now I'm hearing about a new drug called fenoldapam – what is it?

A. Dopamine has historically been used to improve RBF in dogs as it stimulates DA-1 receptors. Stimulation of DA-1 receptors increases renal blood flow, induces diuresis, and decreases renal vascular resistance and variably increases glomerular filtration rate [1,4]. DA-1 receptors are present in low numbers in the feline kidney and low dose dopamine does *not* improve urine output, sodium excretion, glomerular filtration, or fractional sodium excretion in cats [4]. Clinical studies in both dogs and cats have been controversial with respect to any potential benefit of dopamine infusions on renal function. Fenoldopam is a selective DA-1 receptor agonist with no alpha or beta effects. The DA-1 receptors in the feline kidney have a greater affinity for the DA-1 agonist fenoldopam than for dopamine [4]. Fenoldopam infused in normal cats at 0.5 mcg/kg/min for 2 h increased urine production, sodium excretion, and GFR. There may be DA-1 mediated vasodilation which can cause a transient decrease in mean arterial blood pressure [4]. Fenoldopam has been used to treat oliguric renal failure in humans. Fenoldopam may be considered for treatment of cats with severe renal disease.

Q. Is it true that I should avoid NSAIDs in patients with renal failure?

A. YES. When the perfusion to the kidney decreases under anesthesia, the GFR decreases accordingly. Prostaglandins serve to vasodilate the afferent renal arteriole to maintain renal blood flow and GFR. Prostaglandins also stimulate the release of renin. This effect is mediated by the COX-1 and COX-2 enzymes. When NSAIDS are administered to a hypovolemic or hypotensive patient the prostaglandin-mediated effect of local vasodilation is diminished or even lost. This can lead to significant kidney damage and may lead to acute renal failure. COX-2 selective agents can increase the production of thromboxanes, which have a local vasoconstrictive effect and will worsen renal damage.

References

1 Grubb TL. Anesthesia for patients with special concerns. In: Carroll GL (ed.) *Small Animal Anesthesia and Analgesia*. Blackwell Publishing: Ames, IA, 2008:193–238.
2 Greene SA, Grauer GF. Renal Disease. In: Tranquilli WJ, Thurmon JC, Grimm KA (eds) *Lumb & Jones' Veterinary Anesthesia and Analgesia*, 4th edn. Blackwell Publishing: Ames, IA, 2007:915–919.
3 Weil AB. Anesthesia for patients with renal/hepatic disease. *Topics in Companion Animal Medicine* 2010; **25(2)**:87–91.
4 Simmons JP, Wohl JS, Schwartz DD, *et al.* Diuretic effects of fenoldopam in healthy cats. *Journal of Veterinary Emergency and Critical Care* 2006; **16(2)**:96–103.

36 Anesthetic Considerations for Post-Renal Urinary Tract Disease

Oh, for a steady stream!

Ann B. Weil

Department of Veterinary Clinical Sciences, College of Veterinary Medicine, Purdue University, USA

KEY POINTS:

- Patients with obstructive urinary tract disease may present with a wide variation in clinical status.
- Many will require fluid therapy to make up volume deficits prior to general anesthesia.
- Hyperkalemia is a life-threatening consequence of some urinary tract diseases.
- Hyperkalemia should be treated prior to general anesthesia.
- These patients require analgesia as part of an anesthetic or sedative plan.

Q. What are the most important considerations for anesthetizing a patient with a post-renal urinary tract problem?

A. Some examples of post-renal urinary tract disease requiring general anesthesia include:

✓ blocked cats

✓ dogs with urethral obstruction

✓ dogs and cats with ruptured bladders.

These patients will present with a wide range of morbidity and clinical problems associated with their disease process. The patient may be a healthy young cat with an acute urethral obstruction, or it may be nearly moribund from an untreated complete obstruction. One must take into consideration the overall health of the patient first, with the knowledge that post-renal urinary problems often present as emergency cases. These conditions can produce significant electrolyte changes, metabolic disturbances, and hypovolemia that must be addressed when making an anesthetic plan [1]. These

---

Questions and Answers in Small Animal Anesthesia, First Edition. Edited by Lesley J. Smith.
© 2016 John Wiley & Sons, Inc. Published 2016 by John Wiley & Sons, Inc.

patients are also very painful and their analgesic needs must be addressed. It may not be possible to completely normalize the patient prior to general anesthesia, presenting a challenge to the anesthetist.

Q. What abnormalities might be present?

A. Animals with a urethral obstruction or a ruptured bladder may be hypovolemic, azotemic, acidotic, hyperglycemic, and have a variety of electrolyte abnormalities. If a complete obstruction is present, they may be unable to pass any urine, making fluid therapy a challenge as you don't want to rupture the bladder. In order to relieve the obstruction, however, this patient will require sedation and/or general anesthesia with its attendant cardiovascular depression, so adequate circulating fluid volume is important. The patient should be stabilized with cautious intravenous fluid therapy so that it can undergo general anesthesia to relieve the obstruction as soon as possible. There are a variety of "recipes" available for expeditious fluid therapy, including mixtures of crystalloids and colloids. The emphasis should be on quick stabilization of the patient so the obstruction can be relieved. Azotemia will only resolve with IV fluid administration and resolution of the obstruction so that the intratubular pressure in the kidney is reduced and GFR can be improved [2]. Fluid administration should at least address the volume deficit of the patient and be continued during the procedure at a rate of 3–5 ml/kg/h with the obstruction relieved as quickly as possible to avoid bladder rupture.

Q. What electrolyte abnormalities should I anticipate?

A. These patients may suffer from hyperkalemia, hyperphosphatemia, hyponatremia, hypermagnesemia, and hypocalcemia [1]. Of these disturbances, hyperkalemia ($K^+ > 5.5$ mEq/l) is the most immediate life-threatening concern and should be corrected prior to general anesthesia if at all possible. Other electrolyte abnormalities should be corrected with ongoing fluid therapy throughout the peri- and post-operative period.

Q. How do you handle a hyperkalemic patient?

A. Treatment of hyperkalemia can depend on the level of the disturbance. Conditions such as ruptured bladders have a high likelihood of hyperkalemia. Patients suffering urethral obstruction may or may not be hyperkalemic, depending on the duration of the obstruction and whether it is partial or complete, but serum potassium concentration should be measured in every patient with urethral obstruction. Moderate to significant hyperkalemia ($K^+ > 6$ mEq/l) should be addressed prior to general anesthesia, due to the significant myocardial depression imposed by both general anesthetics and hyperkalemia. An ECG monitor should be used to evaluate for unstable electrical activity, but it is important to remember that the classic arrhythmias may not be seen due to the interactions of the other electrolyte abnormalities [3]. Control of CO_2 with the aid of mechanical ventilation (reducing acidosis) can also be helpful in managing hyperkalemic patients, in addition to medical therapy. This is because H^+ and K^+ are exchanged across cell membranes in order to normalize pH. If serum [H$^+$] is high, as in respiratory acidosis 2° to hypoventilation, the physiologic response is to move K$^+$ out of cells and into the vasculature in exchange for H$^+$. This will worsen the hyperkalemia.

Q. What steps can I take to treat the hyperkalemia?

A. Therapies to reduce serum potassium levels rely on dilution of serum potassium concentration by crystalloid fluid therapy and/or driving potassium back into cells. Calcium gluconate can be used for profound hyperkalemia to increase the myocardial cell's threshold membrane potential, thus reestablishing the cell's ability to depolarize despite the increased resting membrane potential [4]. Drug dosages for treating hyperkalemia are listed below [3,5]:

✓ saline (0.9% NaCl) diuresis
✓ dextrose bolus (0.5–1.5 g/kg) IV
✓ regular insulin (0.5 U/kg) with 2 g dextrose IV per 1 U insulin
✓ calcium gluconate (10%) bolus (0.5–1 ml/kg IV) slowly over 10 min
✓ sodium bicarbonate (1–2 mEq/kg IV slowly over 15 min).

Q. What anesthetic drugs can be used to unblock an obstructed cat?

A. It really depends on the systemic state of the cat. If the obstruction is relatively acute and the animal is in good shape, then there are many options, depending on drug availability and familiarity with the drug combination. A protocol that includes an analgesic, is short-acting, and provides excellent muscle relaxation is preferred by the author. If the cat has been obstructed for some time, then the animal's systemic condition will determine the optimal anesthetic protocol. Cats that are obtunded may be able to have a urinary catheter placed with only sedation. Hydration status should be addressed before general anesthesia begins. It is important to keep in mind that cats are easier to volume overload than dogs. See Table 36.1 for some suggested drugs and dosages.

Q. Are there any drugs that should be avoided?

Table 36.1 Drug doses for anesthetizing cats with urethral obstruction.

Premedication IV or IM		Induction agents	
Acepromazine	0.02 mg/kg	**Propofol (IV to effect)**	4–6 mg/kg
Midazolam	0.1–0.2 mg/kg	**Ketamine^a IV or IM**	1–5 mg/kg
Butorphanol	0.2–0.4 mg/kg		
Dexmedetomidine	0.005–0.010 mg/kg	**Alfaxalone IV or IM**	1–2 mg/kg
Buprenorphine	0.010–0.030 mg/kg		
Methadone	0.1–0.5 mg/kg		

^{a}Use lowest dose possible

A. The use of dexmedetomidine, medetomidine, or xylazine can be controversial in these cats. Alpha-2 agonists inhibit release of ADH, thus increasing urine volume in an animal that cannot void. They also cause a reduction in cardiac output that does not support optimal renal function. If an otherwise healthy cat is acutely obstructed and the practitioner is confident that a urinary catheter will pass, then dexmedetomidine can augment an anesthetic plan with excellent analgesia and muscle relaxation. It can be reversed after urinary catheter placement to enable a quick recovery. However, if the animal is azotemic and systemically ill, other drugs should be used to augment analgesia and muscle relaxation.

Ketamine is a dissociative anesthetic that has been commonly used for many years in the cat. It has been reported to be reliant on the kidney for elimination in this species, making it less desirable for use in the blocked cat that may have renal dysfunction. If it is the only injectable anesthetic available to the veterinarian, then a small IV dose is preferable to a larger dose administered intramuscularly.

Q. Are there any special considerations for anesthetizing a dog with urethral obstruction?

A. The basic principles are the same as when anesthetizing a cat with urethral obstruction. Dogs may be able to handle a higher fluid administration rate than the cat without volume overload. There are certainly some differences in dosing and expected drug effects between the two species. See Table 36.2 for some suggested drugs and dosages.

Q. How should these animals be monitored?

A. Complete anesthesia monitoring is recommended, as one should not assume a brief procedure is an innocuous process. Blood pressure, S_pO_2, CO_2, heart

Table 36.2 Drug doses for anesthetizing dogs with urinary tract disease.

Premedications		Induction agents	
Acepromazine IM, SC, IV	0.01–0.02 mg/kg	Propofol IV to effect	4–6 mg/kg
Midazolam IM, IV	0.1–0.2 mg/kg	Ketamine IV (combine with diazepam or midazolam)	5 mg/kg
Dexmedetomidine IM, IV	0.005–0.010 mg/kg	Alfaxalone IV to effect	2 mg/kg
Opioids IM, IV			
Hydromorphone	0.05–0.2 mg/kg		
Morphine IM	0.25 mg/kg		
Fentanyl IV	5 mcg/kg/hr		
Buprenorphine IM, IV	0.01–0.02 mg/kg		
Methadone IM, IV	0.1–0.5 mg/kg		

rate, respiratory rate, and eye signs should be monitored continuously during the procedure. ECG monitoring is particularly helpful in patients at risk for hyperkalemia. Mean arterial blood pressure should be maintained above 60 mmHg. Some practitioners may prefer to use a Doppler monitor to measure systolic blood pressure in the cat, which tends to be more likely to provide accurate readings in smaller patients. Systolic blood pressure should be >90 mmHg. Oxygen supplementation is almost always a good idea and can be provided via mask if the patient is sedated but is not intubated.

Q. How should I handle a patient with a ruptured bladder (or uroabdomen)?

A. Urine in the abdomen should be considered a medical emergency and needs to be removed. These patients are often azotemic and hyperkalemic due to absorption of potassium across peritoneal membranes. Potassium levels should be checked prior to anesthesia as well as throughout the procedure. Point of care cartridge-based monitors can be very helpful in these situations. If the patient is hyperkalemic, see previous question on hyperkalemia to address this. Hyperkalemia must be treated prior to anesthesia.

Q. How do I anesthetize a patient for cystotomy?

A. The patient's overall systemic health and analgesic needs will dictate the anesthesia protocol, as well as practitioner comfort with selected drugs. This surgical procedure warrants the use of a pure μ agonist opioid as part of a balanced anesthetic technique. Other premedication drugs could include acepromazine, dexmedetomidine, midazolam, or diazepam. Injectable choices for induction include propofol, ketamine, etomidate, or alfaxalone. Maintenance anesthesia with either isoflurane or sevoflurane is acceptable. Crystalloid fluids at 3–5 ml/kg/h should be administered.

Q. Are there any special considerations for anesthesia for cystoscopy?

A. Cystoscopy is a minimally invasive technique that still requires general anesthesia in animals. Butorphanol may be a good choice of opioid to include in the protocol if a quicker recovery from the procedure is desired. Cystoscopy can stimulate vagal tone, so the anesthesia provider should be prepared to administer an anticholinergic if necessary (atropine 0.02–0.04 mg/kg or glycopyrrolate 0.01 mg/kg). Crystalloid fluids at 3–5 ml/kg/h IV should be administered.

Q. What type of analgesia should be used for urinary tract procedures?

A. It is critical to remember that these patients are very uncomfortable if they have a urethral obstruction and an enlarged bladder. Opioids tend to be the most suitable analgesic agents for critical patients as they are not associated with depression of cardiac output. Alpha-2 agonists produce reliable analgesia, but they are associated with profound sedation and cardiac output reduction, as well as diuresis. The use of NSAIDs should be considered with caution and careful evaluation of the patient's renal function. If there are signs of renal function impairment, the NSAID should probably be avoided.

If there is no renal compromise, the use of a NSAID can be very useful in treating the inflammation and pain associated with urethral obstruction.

References

1 Lee JA, Drobatz KJ. Characterization of the clinical characteristics, electrolytes, acid-base, and renal parameters in male cats with urethral obstruction. *Journal of Veterinary Emergency and Critical Care* 2003; **13(4)**:227–233.

2 Bartges JW, Delmar RF, Polzin DJ, *et al.* Pathophysiology of urethral obstruction. *Veterinary Clinics of North America: Small Animal Practice* 1996; **26(2)**:255–264.

3 Thomovsky EJ. Managing the common comorbidities of feline urethral obstruction. *Veterinary Medicine* 2011; **106(7)**:352–359.

4 DiBartola SP, de Morais HA. Disorders of potassium: hypokalemia and hyperkalemia. In: DiBartola SP (ed.) *Fluid, Electrolyte, and Acid Base Disorders in Small Animal Medicine*, 3rd edn. St. Louis, Mo: Elsevier, 2006;91–121.

5 Grubb T. Anesthesia for patients with special concerns. In: Carroll GL (ed.) *Small Animal Anesthesia and Analgesia*. Blackwell Publishing: Oxford, 2008:193–238.

37 Anesthetic Considerations for Endocrine Disease

That gland is not bland

Berit L. Fischer

Department of Veterinary Clinical Medicine, University of Illinois at Urbana-Champaign, USA

KEY POINTS:

- In patients undergoing elective procedures, treatment or stabilization of endocrine disease prior to anesthesia is preferable.

- Knowledge of how individual endocrine diseases affect the body is imperative to anesthesia protocol development.

- Successful anesthesia of patients with endocrine disease is often a matter of identifying, preventing, and treating common complications (hypothermia, hypotension, hypoventilation, bradycardia, pain).

- Stable patients with *controlled* hypo- and hyper-thyroidism, hyperadrenocorticism, hypoadrenocorticism, and diabetes mellitus can be anesthetized safely with proper monitoring.

Q. What is endocrine disease?

A. Endocrine organs are responsible for secreting hormones that function on target organs throughout the body to regulate metabolism, growth, cellular function, and reproduction. Excessive secretion, impaired secretion, and/or neoplasia of endocrine organs can result in endocrine disease.

Q. What are common veterinary endocrine diseases?

A. Hyperadrenocorticism (Cushing's disease), hypoadrenocorticism (Addison's disease), diabetes mellitus, and hypothyroidism are common endocrine disease in dogs. Cats are more commonly afflicted with diabetes mellitus and hyperthyroidism. Other less common endocrine diseases that affect veterinary species include pheochromocytoma, insulinoma, acromegaly (cats), and hyperaldosteronism (cats).

Questions and Answers in Small Animal Anesthesia, First Edition. Edited by Lesley J. Smith.
© 2016 John Wiley & Sons, Inc. Published 2016 by John Wiley & Sons, Inc.

Diseases of the Thyroid Gland

Q. What role do thyroid hormones play in the body?

A. The thyroid hormones, triiodothyronine (T3) and thyroxine (T4), are synthesized in and released from the thyroid gland in response to thyroid releasing hormone (TRH) and thyroid stimulating hormone (TSH) from the hypothalamus and anterior pituitary respectively.

Once released, T3 and T4 act at the cellular level to regulate metabolic rate, influence protein synthesis, and assist in normal fetal development. These actions help to maintain rate and contractility of the heart, thermoregulation, and proper ventilatory responses to hypercapnia and hypoxemia.

Q. What is hypothyroidism and who does it affect?

A. Hypothyroidism is a deficiency in thyroid hormones caused by destruction of thyroid tissue through autoimmune disease, atrophy, or neoplasia. It is relatively common in older (>7 years) dogs and is over-represented in English Setters, Giant Schnauzers, Golden Retrievers, Dobermans, Boxers, Shetland Sheepdogs, and Cocker Spaniels [1]. It is rare in cats but, when present, occurs following radioiodine therapy or surgical thyroidectomy for hyperthyroidism.

Q. What are the effects of hypothyroidism on various body systems?

A. See Table 37.1.

Q. Prior to anesthesia, what tests should be performed?

A. Prior to anesthesia, a thorough physical exam should be performed with particular emphasis on the cardiovascular system. Standard biochemical tests

Table 37.1 Effects of hypothyroidism on various organ systems.

Body system	Effects	Clinical result
Cardiovascular system	Decreased number/affinity of beta receptors on heart	Decreased contractility and heart rate = decreased cardiac output (CO)
	Atherosclerosis from altered lipid metabolism	Bradyarrhythmias Hypotension Decreased end-organ perfusion
Respiratory system	Decreased sensitivity to increases in carbon dioxide and decreases in oxygen	Hypoventilation Hypoxemia Respiratory acidosis
Gastrointestinal tract	Delayed gastric emptying/ileus	Increased risk of regurgitation/aspiration
Metabolism	Decreased hepatic metabolism Obesity	Prolonged drug action Hypothermia Hypoventilation
Nervous system	Peripheral neuropathies	Motor/sensory deficits

may reveal mild anemia, and elevations in cholesterol and triglycerides; however these findings rarely impact anesthesia.

Q. What are appropriate premedications to use in patients with hypothyroidism?

A. Anesthetic drugs may have a more profound effect in the patient with hypothyroidism. Use of drugs that are reversible or titratable is advised. Opioids, such as morphine, hydromorphone, or methadone, in combination with a benzodiazepine, may provide sufficient premedication to allow catheter placement and pre-oxygenation prior to anesthetic induction. Doses should be tailored to represent lean body weight in obese patients.

Acepromazine is long-lasting and irreversible, can promote the development of hypothermia, and may exacerbate hypotension. When deciding to use acepromazine, the anesthetist should use low doses (0.01–0.02 mg/kg), ensure the patient is normovolemic and aggressively prevent and treat hypothermia. An alpha-2 agonist, such as dexmedetomidine, can exacerbate bradyarrhythmias. It can also promote hypothermia and hypotension. These drugs are reversible, however, and in stable hypothyroid patients, low doses (1–1.5 mcg/kg IV; 2–3 mcg/kg IM) may be used if sufficient sedation is not achieved with opioids and benzodiazepines alone.

Q. What are appropriate induction agents to use in patients with hypothyroidism?

A. In patients with mild hypothyroidism, most induction agents are acceptable. Because ketamine stimulates the sympathetic nervous system, it may cause a beneficial increase in heart rate, contractility, and cardiac output.

Q. Adjunct analgesia?

A. Additional analgesia should be considered in the hypothyroid patient. Dose-dependent vasodilation and hypotension from inhalant anesthetics can be minimized through the administration of additional opioids as a constant rate infusion (fentanyl 5–10 mcg/kg/h) or intermittent boluses.

Loco-regional techniques, such as nerve blocks and epidurals, are equally beneficial in reducing doses of other drugs. Be careful employing these techniques in patients who have evidence of a peripheral neuropathy since deficits could worsen post procedure. It is also worth noting that hair regrowth can be slow or absent in dogs with hypothyroidism. If an epidural is planned, forewarning owners that their pet may have a bald spot can prevent angst later.

Q. Are there specific concerns regarding anesthetic management in the hypothyroid patient?

A. Many of the concerns surrounding anesthesia in the hypothyroid patient can be addressed in proper pre-operative preparation. The anesthetist should confirm that the patient was fasted prior to anesthesia to minimize risk of regurgitation and aspiration. Likewise, ensuring patients are hydrated prior to anesthesia can help prevent hypotension and improve perfusion of vital organs. Finally, pre-oxygenation benefits hypothyroid patients since they are at risk of desaturation from impaired ventilatory responses.

Intra-operative support should include aggressive prevention and treatment of hypothermia. Hypotension is common and can be treated through good cardiovascular support as is covered in Chapter 17.

Q. Are there particular concerns in the recovery period in patients with hypothyroidism?

A. Recovery may be prolonged due to slowed hepatic metabolism of drugs. Patients should be kept warm and oxygenation in the post-anesthetic period should be monitored using pulse oximetry. If S_pO_2 readings are <94%, provide supplemental oxygen.

Q. What is hyperthyroidism and who does it affect?

A. Hyperthyroidism is excessive synthesis and secretion of T3 and T4 from the thyroid gland. It is the most common endocrine disease in cats older than 8 years of age [1]. It is uncommon in dogs, but when present, is often caused by thyroid carcinoma or excessive administration of levothyroxine for treatment of hypothyroidism.

Q. Is it safe to anesthetize patients with hyperthyroidism?

A. Unlike hypothyroidism, anesthesia of patients with hyperthyroidism carries significant risk. Every attempt to stabilize T4 levels prior to elective anesthesia should be made to minimize morbidity and mortality.

Q. What are the effects of hyperthyroidism of various body systems?

A. See Table 37.2.

Q. Prior to anesthesia, what tests should be performed?

Table 37.2   Effects of hyperthyroidism on various organ systems.

Body system	Effects	Clinical result
Cardiovascular system	Increased: O_2 demand, CO, myocardial work, sensitivity of heart to catecholamines, number/affinity of beta receptors on heart Vasodilation	Tachyarrhythmias, systemic hypertension, thyrotoxic cardiomyopathy, tissue hypoxia, cardiac failure Hypotension (anesthetized)
Respiratory system	Increased O_2 demand	Tissue hypoxia
Gastrointestinal system	Decreased transit time, impaired peristalsis	Vomiting/diarrhea with fluid losses
Metabolism	Increased basal metabolic rate	Cachexia Hyperthermia Increased/more frequent anesthetic drug dosing Hypothermia (anesthetized)

A. In addition to a thorough physical exam, blood pressure measurement should be performed. Patients may present with tachyarrhythmias, such as a gallop rhythm, bounding pulses, and a parasternal cardiac murmur. If discovered, a complete cardiac work-up with chest radiographs, echocardiography, and ECG is advised. Complete blood count (CBC) and biochemistry panels may show mild polycythemia, elevations in liver enzymes, and electrolyte changes, particularly hypokalemia. Because of the increase in cardiac output, BUN and creatinine levels can be falsely lowered. This can make diagnosis of concurrent renal disease difficult in affected patients and warrants further investigation if it is suspected.

Q. What are appropriate premedications to use in patients with hyperthyroidism?

A. Although it is ideal to postpone anesthesia until patients have undergone treatment for hyperthyroidism, there may be emergent scenarios where one cannot wait. In these situations, drugs causing stimulation of the sympathetic nervous system should be avoided. These include anticholinergics, such as atropine or glycopyrrolate, and ketamine.

Similar to hypothyroidism, titratable drugs that are short-acting are advised. Opioids and benzodiazepines make good premedications for patients with hyperthyroidism, but may not offer enough sedation, particularly in aggressive cats. Alpha-2 agonist use is controversial. It may be beneficial since it causes an overall reduction in sympathetic tone, but it may further increase blood pressure and cardiac work through initial vasoconstriction. Acepromazine should be used with caution since its long-lasting effects and vasodilation could lead to cardiovascular collapse.

Q. What are appropriate induction agents to use in patients with hyperthyroidism?

A. Ketamine increases myocardial oxygen demand and can promote tachyarrhythmias. It should be avoided in patients with hyperthyroidism. Propofol, alfaxolone, and etomidate are all suitable choices. Dose-dependent vasodilation from propofol administration can lead to an unexpected drop in blood pressure. This can be minimized by adding a co-induction agent, such as fentanyl (3–5 mcg/kg). Chamber or mask inductions should be avoided in patients with hyperthyroidism. Not only can they cause profound vasodilation and hypotension, but the stress the induction causes can lead to catecholamine release and sudden cardiac arrest.

Q. Adjunct analgesia?

A. Additional opioids in the form of intermittent boluses or constant rate infusion (CRI) can help to minimize inhalant concentrations and decrease release of catecholamines during surgery. Loco-regional techniques, such as ring blocks, should be utilized when possible to minimize stress response.

Q. How should anesthetic management of the hyperthyroid patient be handled?

A. Pre-operative preparation should include crystalloid administration with stabilization of all electrolytes. Stress should be minimized through good premedication and gentle handling. Pre-oxygenation is especially important in these patients because of high O_2 demands. If the patient is tolerant, monitoring equipment including ECG and blood pressure should be placed prior to induction. A difficult intubation should be anticipated in patients with signs associated with a thyroid-related cervical mass. Numerous sizes of endotracheal tubes, a stylet or soft guide-wire (a long polypropylene urinary catheter can work well for this), two laryngoscopes, and a tracheostomy kit should be available.

Many hyperthyroid patients have concurrent cardiac disease and extensive hemodynamic monitoring, including invasive blood pressure and central venous pressure (CVP) is ideal, if possible. It is advisable to keep mean arterial blood pressure (MAP) within $\sim 20\%$ of pre-operative blood pressure values to ensure adequate renal perfusion when systemic hypertension has been identified. Diligent monitoring of body temperature is essential since both hyperthermia and hypothermia can occur. Intermittent positive pressure ventilation, either by mechanical ventilator or via assisted hand ventilation, may be necessary to avoid hypoventilation, increased CO_2, and subsequent catecholamine release.

Q. What is thyroid storm?

A. Thyroid storm is a sudden release of thyroid hormones into the circulation from a precipitating event, such as anesthesia, trauma, or vigorous rubbing of the thyroid gland. It can cause life-threatening arrhythmias, hyperthermia, hypertension, and cardiac failure [2]. Treatment includes administration of beta blockers (esmolol 0.05–0.15 mg/kg followed by 50–200 mcg/kg/min CRI), antihypertensive agents (i.e., nitroprusside, magnesium sulfate), and supportive care, including active cooling, fluid administration, and mechanical ventilation.

Q. What concerns are there with recovery of hyperthyroid patients?

A. Since thyroid storms can occur in the post-operative period, hyperthyroid patients should continue to be monitored carefully. Minimization of stress, continued administration of antithyroid drugs, and excellent post-operative analgesia are imperative. In patients undergoing thyroidectomy, damage to the recurrent laryngeal nerve could cause laryngeal paralysis and post-operative hypoventilation. Because of high O_2 demand, a supplemental oxygen source is indicated.

Diseases of the Adrenal Glands

Q. What substances are produced by the adrenal glands?

A. The adrenal cortex produces cortisol, androgens, and aldosterone. Secretion is regulated via release of corticotrophin releasing hormone (CRH) from the hypothalamus and adrenocorticotropic hormone (ACTH) from the anterior pituitary. The adrenal medulla produces the catecholamines, norepinephrine, and epinephrine and acts as a sympathetic post-ganglionic neuron.

Q. What is hyperadrenocorticism and who does it affect?

A. Hyperadrenocorticism, also known as Cushing's disease, is caused by unregulated secretion of cortisol from the adrenal cortex either from a pituitary adenoma or a functional adrenal cortical tumor. Iatrogenic Cushing's disease can also occur in patients being treated with corticosteroids. Cushing's disease is the most common endocrine disease of middle-age to older dogs. It is over-represented in Terriers, Poodles, Beagles, and Dachshunds [1]. Primary Cushing's disease rare in cats.

Q. Is it safe to anesthetize a patient with Cushing's disease?

A. Similar to hypothyroidism, anesthesia of patients with Cushing's disease is common. Often, proper preparation and monitoring can help to minimize complications associated with this disease. If a patient has been recently diagnosed with Cushing's disease and is undergoing a loading phase of mitotane (Lysodren), postponing elective procedures should be considered. During this phase, patients are at risk of an Addisonian crisis (adrenal insufficiency) and may not tolerate stress from anesthesia.

Q. What are the effects of hyperadrenocorticism on various body systems?

A. See Table 37.3.

Q. Prior to anesthesia, what tests should be performed?

A. In addition to a thorough physical exam, blood pressure measurement should be performed prior to anesthesia. A CBC and biochemical panel can be helpful in identifying whether there are other underlying diseases present, such as renal failure. An arterial blood gas analysis may reveal hypoxemia which could signal the presence of a pulmonary thromboembolism.

Table 37.3   Effects of hyperadrenocorticism on various organ systems.

Body system	Effects	Clinical results
Cardiovascular system	Vasoconstriction	Systemic hypertension
	Atherosclerosis	Volume contraction/hypovolemia
	Increased effects of catecholamines	Decreased perfusion of end organs
Hematopoietic system	Increased erythropoiesis and production of clotting factors	Increased blood sludging-poor perfusion of organs
	Decreased antithrombin III	Increased risk of thromboembolism-PTE/stroke
Respiratory system	Muscle weakness	Hypoventilation
	Organomegaly	Respiratory acidosis
	Obesity	

Q. What are appropriate premedications to use in patients with Cushing's disease?

A. Patients with Cushing's disease who are also hypertensive are often volume-contracted due to the vasoconstrictive effects of cortisol. This may result in unexpected drops in blood pressure or more profound responses to anesthetic drugs than anticipated. Use of reversible drugs that can be titrated is recommended. A balanced anesthetic technique utilizing low doses of alpha-2 agonists (e.g., dexmedetomidine 2–4 mcg/kg IM), opioids, and/or benzodiazepines are all acceptable. Drugs should be dosed based on lean body weight to prevent overdose.

Q. What are appropriate induction agents to use in patients with Cushing's disease?

A. Most induction agents can be used in patients with mild to moderate Cushing's disease. To avoid excessive dose-dependent vasodilation, good premedication with or without the addition of a co-induction agent (lidocaine 1.0 mg/kg, midazolam 0.2 mg/kg, fentanyl 3–5 mcg/kg) is recommended.

Q. Adjunct analgesia?

A. Loco-regional techniques are highly desirable in patients with Cushing's disease. Their use can prevent prolonged recumbency and sedation associated with systemic analgesics. This may minimize the risk of pulmonary thromboembolism in the post-operative period.

The use of nonsteroidal anti-inflammatory drugs (NSAIDS) is controversial in patients with Cushing's disease. There is evidence that the concurrent use of corticosteroids and NSAIDS results in greater adverse gastrointestinal effects than either alone [3]. Since Cushing's patients have higher levels of circulating glucocorticoids, it can be inferred that this additive effect may also apply to them.

Q. What are the concerns regarding intra-operative anesthetic management in the Cushing's disease patient?

A. Muscle weakness, hepatomegaly, and obesity can all lead to hypoventilation and hypoxemia in the Cushing's patient. Pre-oxygenation and the use of mechanical or assisted ventilation along with monitoring capnography and pulse oximetry can help minimize this risk. In patients with systemic hypertension, keeping MAP within ~20% of pre-operative values, as recommended in humans, may help to ensure adequate renal perfusion.

Q. What concerns are there with recovery of patients with Cushing's disease?

A. Following extubation, many patients with Cushing's disease will hypoventilate leading to hypoxemia. Monitoring pulse oximetry can determine if supplemental oxygen via face mask, nasal prongs/catheter, or oxygen cage during the first few post-operative hours is needed.

Q. What is hypoadrenocorticism?

A. Hypoadrenocorticism, also known as Addison's disease, is caused by impaired secretion of mineralocorticoids (aldosterone) and/or glucocorticoids (cortisol) from the adrenal cortex. This depletion leads to an inability to handle stress and impairs fluid/electrolyte balance. In addition to primary hypoadrenocorticism, many patients may suffer from adrenal insufficiency because of sudden withdrawal of corticosteroid therapy or severe illness.

Q. What is an Addisonian Crisis?

A. An Addisonian Crisis is a severe manifestation of inadequate cortisol secretion with or without appropriate aldosterone secretion in response to stress, leading to cardiovascular collapse. Cortisol is required for maintaining vascular tone and vascular responses to catecholamines. Without it, patients can suffer from hypotension, low volume status, anemia from both impaired erythrocytosis and bleeding into the gastrointestinal tract, and impaired glucose regulation. Severe depletion of aldosterone leads to hypovolemia, metabolic acidosis, and life-threatening hyperkalemia.

Q. Is it safe to anesthetize a patient with hypoadrenocorticism?

A. Patients who have been diagnosed as having hypoadrenocorticism and are receiving appropriate glucocorticoid and mineralcorticoid replacement therapy can be safely anesthetized if proper measures are taken to ensure they are able to handle the stress involved with anesthesia, surgery, and hospitalization.

Q. How can hypoadrenocorticism affect anesthesia?

A. The additional stress from anesthesia, surgery, and hospitalization can put the Addisonian patient at risk. Hypotension and impaired tissue perfusion are probably the most common complications because of reduced vascular tone, sodium and chloride losses, and metabolic acidosis. Severe hyperkalemia can lead to arrhythmias and cardiac arrest, and anemia can compromise tissue oxygen delivery.

Q. Prior to anesthesia, what tests should be performed?

A. In patients previously diagnosed with hypoadrenocorticism who appear systemically healthy on physical exam, a minimum database evaluating hydration status and electrolyte and acid-base balance should be performed. Other biochemical tests should be undertaken as deemed necessary to evaluate organ function. Abnormalities identified on pre-operative biochemical tests should be corrected prior to anesthesia if possible.

Q. What are appropriate premedications to use in patients with hypoadrenocorticism?

A. Preparation for additional stress, as occurs with general anesthesia, is invaluable in patients with hypoadrenocorticism. This may require a 50–100% increase in glucocorticoid supplementation the day of anesthesia and during hospitalization followed by a slow taper. Minor elective procedures that are short in duration may not require any increase; however, those patients undergoing emergency anesthesia or prolonged, complicated procedures should receive additional supplementation.

In stable, hydrated Addisonian patients, most combinations of premedications (opioids, alpha-2 agonists, acepromazine, and benzodiazepines) are acceptable. Minimizing stress through premedication is beneficial for this population of patients. If volume status is unknown, use short-acting, reversible drugs.

Q. What are appropriate induction agents to use in patients with hypoadrenocorticism?

A. In well-regulated Addisonian patients, ketamine with a benzodiazepine, alfaxalone, or propofol are all appropriate choices for induction. In anemic patients, or those with electrolyte abnormalities, the indirect sympathetic actions of ketamine could increase oxygen demand or precipitate cardiac arrhythmias.

Although etomidate is an excellent induction agent in patients with cardiovascular instability, it also causes adrenocortical suppression via inhibition of 11-beta-hydroxylase. For this reason, its use in Addisonian patients is controversial.

Q. Are there specific concerns regarding anesthetic management in patients with hypoadrenocorticism?

A. Minimization of stress and perfusion of vital organs are of most concern in patients with hypoadrenocorticism. Ample fluid administration with crystalloids and/or colloids can help to optimize volume status. Monitor the ECG, particularly for changes due to hyperkalemia. Monitor blood pressure for hypotension and troubleshoot all normal causes. If other causes of hypotension have been excluded, adrenal insufficiency should be suspected. Supplementation with additional glucocorticoids, such as dexamethasone sodium phosphate at 0.05–0.2 mg/kg IV may be indicated.

Q. What concerns are there with recovery of patients with hypoadrenocorticism?

A. Reduce stress! Pain and hypothermia are both stressful, so pay attention to analgesic needs and maintain normothermia. If additional glucocorticoids were administered prior to or during anesthesia, patients should be continued on them during their hospital stay and then tapered off slowly.

Diabetes Mellitus

Q. What is diabetes mellitus (DM)?

A. Diabetes mellitus is an endocrine disease caused by impaired glucose homeostasis either due to a deficiency of insulin or an inability of the tissue to respond to it, otherwise known as "insulin resistance". It is most common in middle-age female dogs and male cats.

Table 37.4 Effects of diabetes mellitus on various organ systems.

Body system	Effects	Clinical results
Cardiovascular system	Increased vessel stiffness, atherosclerosis, vessel inflammation	Decreased organ perfusion (kidney/brain) Systemic hypertension Volume contraction/hypovolemia
Renal system	Glomerulosclerosis Osmotic diuresis Hypokalemia/ hyponatremia Metabolic acidosis	Renal failure Dehydration/hypovolemia Muscle weakness/Arrhythmias Decreased myocardial contractility/CO
Metabolism	Hyperglycemia Negative energy balance	Dehydration/hypovolemia Ketone formation Metabolic acidosis
Nervous system	Peripheral neuropathy Autonomic neuropathy	Pain, motor/sensory deficits Positional hypotension Tachycardia Delayed gastric emptying/ aspiration

Q. Is it safe to anesthetize a patient with diabetes mellitus?

A. Newly diagnosed diabetic patients are at higher risk of morbidity and mortality under anesthesia, therefore elective procedures should be postponed in this population until their disease is stabilized. Likewise, patients who present with diabetic ketoacidosis are also poor anesthetic candidates. Diabetics should be well-regulated and ketone-free to minimize risk associated with anesthesia.

Q. What are the effects of diabetes mellitus on various body systems?

A. See Table 37.4.

Q. What tests should be performed prior to anesthesia?

A. Important tests prior to anesthesia include evaluation of electrolytes, hydration status, prerenal or renal azotemia, urine or serum ketones, acid-base status, and blood glucose.

Q. What steps should be taken to prepare a diabetic patient for anesthesia?

A. There are numerous opinions and few studies on pre-anesthetic fasting and administration of insulin prior to anesthesia and surgery in veterinary patients. These include the administration of no insulin or food prior to checking blood glucose or the administration of anywhere between 25–100% of the usual dose of insulin with or without a small meatball of food [4]. How much insulin is required by an individual animal, however, may be more dependent on how well-regulated the patient is prior to anesthesia and the complexity of the scheduled surgical procedure. Regardless, in order to minimize waiting time and continued fluctuations in blood glucose, diabetic patients should be scheduled as the first anesthesia case of the day. Stress should be minimized to prevent release of counter regulatory hormones (cortisol) which increase blood glucose and insulin requirements. Patients that are dehydrated should receive IV fluids prior to anesthesia to improve circulating blood volume. Blood glucose should be preferably < 250 mg/dl (14 mmol/l) prior to induction. If glucose is higher than this, regular insulin at 0.1–0.3 U/kg can be administered subcutaneously or half intravenously and half subcutaneously. Blood glucose levels should be monitored carefully (i.e., every 30 min) following regular insulin administration.

Q. What are the goals when anesthetizing a diabetic patient?

A. ✓ Avoid hypoglycemia.
   ✓ Minimize hyperglycemia.
   ✓ Maintain electrolyte and acid-base balance.
   ✓ Minimize stress that could increase plasma glucose concentrations.
   ✓ Return to a normal eating and insulin schedule as quickly as possible.

Q. What are appropriate anesthetic premedications to use in patients with DM?

A. Prolonged sedation may affect the ability of patients to return to a normal eating schedule and should, therefore, be avoided by using short-acting and reversible drugs. Acepromazine, although long-lasting, may be an acceptable premedication at low doses (0.01–0.02 mg/kg) as long as patients are well-hydrated prior to anesthesia. Opioids are beneficial in many ways. The analgesia they provide minimizes sympathetic responses during surgery, and they are reversible if necessary. Benzodiazepines are also acceptable premedications. Alpha-2 agonists are controversial in diabetic patients since they directly inhibit insulin release from pancreatic beta cells. They also, however, decrease sympathetic tone and the benefits of this decrease may counteract any hyperglycemia caused by insulin inhibition.

Q. What are good induction agents to use in patients with DM?

A. Most induction agents are acceptable in well-regulated patients. The anesthetist should be aware that ketamine could increase blood glucose levels since it indirectly stimulates the sympathetic nervous system.

Q. Adjunct analgesia?

A. Excellent intra-operative analgesia can minimize sympathetic responses to surgical stimuli, thereby helping glucose homeostasis. Use of loco-regional blocks can be particularly effective in preventing a stress response; however, if patients have evidence of peripheral neuropathy as can occur with DM, local blocks may exacerbate neurologic signs post-operatively.

Q. What concerns are there regarding intra-operative anesthetic management in the diabetic patient?

A. Intra-operative monitoring should include serial blood glucose measurements every 30–60 min. Titration of either regular insulin (0.025–0.050 U/kg/h) or dextrose solutions (1.25–5%) should be used to maintain blood glucose between 150–250 mg/dl (8–14 mmol/l). Intra-operative hypoglycemia should be avoided since clinical signs are not apparent under anesthesia and may result in irreversible cerebral injury.

In addition to blood glucose, blood pressure monitoring is very important since significant hypotension is more prevalent in diabetic patients. Intra-venous fluids should be continued to support circulating blood volume and the dehydrating effects of hyperglycemia.

Q. What concerns are there with recovery of patients with diabetes mellitus?

A. Glucose homeostasis continues to be impaired in the post-operative period until the patient can resume normal eating and insulin schedules. Sedation should be minimized for this reason and blood glucose should be monitored hourly until the patient is eating. It is important to recognize that diabetic patients may require continued dextrose and/or insulin infusion during this time. Since pain itself could cause the release of counter-regulatory hormones, excellent post-operative analgesia is imperative.

Pheochromocytoma

Q. What is a pheochromocytoma?

A. A pheochromocytoma is a tumor of the chromaffin cells in the adrenal medulla. These cells are responsible for release of epinephrine and nore-pinephrine into the blood following stimulation of the sympathetic nervous system. When they become neoplastic, unregulated release of these neurotransmitters occurs resulting in severe hypertension and tachycardia.

Q. Is it safe to anesthetize a patient with a pheochromocytoma?

A. No! Patients with pheochromocytomas are at high risk of mortality when undergoing anesthesia, even with prior stabilization. In a patient with a known pheochromocytoma, extreme caution is advised. Often, patients with pheochromocytomas are anesthetized without knowledge that one is present since clinical signs can be vague or sporadic. Significant cardiovascular instability under anesthesia should prompt suspicion. If a patient is suspected of having a pheochromocytoma and requires anesthesia, referral to or consultation with a board-certified veterinary anesthesiologist is highly recommended.

Q. What are the effects of a pheochromocytoma on various body systems?

A. See Table 37.5.

Q. What events precipitate a pheochromocytoma crisis?

Table 37.5 Effects of pheochromocytoma on various organ systems.

Body system	Effects	Clinical results
Cardiovascular system	Activation of sympathetic nervous system	Systemic hypertension Increased myocardial O_2 demand/work Decreased tissue perfusion Volume contraction/hypovolemia Tachyarrhythmias/impaired filling Decreased cardiac output Cardiac failure Cardiac arrest
	Vessel occlusion (from tumor)	Edema Ascites Hypoventilation
Nervous system	Encephalopathy from hypertension/decreased perfusion Cerebral hemorrhage	Seizures Coma Stroke Death
Renal system	Decreased renal blood flow Decreased glomerular filtration rate	Renal failure

A. Multiple events can lead to sudden release of catecholamines from a pheochromocytoma. These include anesthesia induction, tumor manipulation during adrenalectomy, histamine release, increased intraabdominal pressure from either bladder expression or laparoscopy, and anything that increases sympathetic tone, such as elevations in CO_2, certain drugs, pain, and stress.

Q. What tests should be performed prior to anesthesia?

A. A complete blood count and biochemical profile should be evaluated in patients with suspected pheochromocytoma to determine the status of other organ systems. Other tests to evaluate the cardiovascular system specifically, including blood pressure measurements, an ECG, and thoracic radiographs are also warranted.

Q. What steps should be taken to prepare a patient with pheochromocytoma for anesthesia?

A. In preparation for anesthesia and surgery, it is recommended that patients with a suspected pheochromocytoma be placed on an alpha-1 antagonist for a minimum of 10–14 days and up to 4 weeks beforehand [5]. This does not prevent the rapid swings in heart rate and blood pressure, but allows the patient to vasodilate over time and normalize circulating blood volume. The most common drug used is phenoxybenzamine starting at 0.5 mg/kg orally twice daily. During treatment, blood pressure should be monitored every 3–5 days and the dose of phenoxybenzamine doubled until a maximum dose of 2 mg/kg orally twice daily is reached or signs of hypotension (weakness, lethargy, ataxia, collapse) are observed. Systolic blood pressure should be consistently < 160 mmHg and diastolic pressure should be <100 mmHg prior to undergoing anesthesia. If tachyarrhythmias are present, a beta blocker, such as atenolol (0.5–1.0 mg/kg orally once daily) or carvedilol (0.5 mg/kg orally twice daily), may also be added but *only* after alpha blockade has been established [6].

Q. What are appropriate anesthetic premedications to use in a patient with pheochromocytoma?

A. Decreasing stress is essential in patients with a pheochromocytoma. Also, appropriate pre-operative preparation with alpha- and beta-receptor blockade makes these patients much less risky under anesthesia. Generally, an opioid alone or in combination with a benzodiazepine is recommended. Morphine should be avoided because of its ability to induce histamine release.

Q. What are good induction agents to use in patients with pheochromocytoma?

A. Propofol, etomidate, and alfaxalone, in combination with good opioid/benzodiazepine premedications are all acceptable induction agents. Ketamine should be avoided due to its indirect stimulation of the sympathetic nervous system. Inhalant inductions are likewise not recommended since they cause undue stress in the patient.

Q. Adjunct analgesia?

A. The addition of other drugs to minimize sympathetic stimulation during anesthesia/surgery is recommended. Opioids, such as additional bolus doses of hydromorphone, oxymorphone, or methadone, or a constant rate infusion of fentanyl serve well in this purpose. Loco-regional techniques are often beneficial in reducing stress responses in patients with pheochromocytomas.

Q. What concerns are there regarding intra-operative anesthetic management in the patient with pheochromocytoma?

A. These cases are highly intensive and may be best referred to a facility with a board-certified veterinary anesthesiologist. Invasive monitoring is required in patients with pheochromocytoma. An arterial catheter to monitor direct blood pressure should be placed prior to anesthetic induction if possible. Central lines help to monitor trends in volume status and are beneficial in patients undergoing an adrenalectomy, where hypotension following excision is likely. Intermittent positive pressure ventilation should be instilled to avoid a sympathetic response from elevations in carbon dioxide. Hemodynamic drugs that are rapid-acting should be on hand as well as emergency drugs. During a pheochromocytoma crisis, beta blockers, such as esmolol can treat tachyarrhythmias, and nitroprusside, magnesium sulfate, or calcium channel blockers can help treat hypertension. The anesthetist should have experience using these drugs as unpredictable changes can occur.

Q. What concerns are there with recovery of patients with pheochromocytoma?

A. In patients undergoing an adrenalectomy, hypotension should be expected since the sympathetic receptors are downregulated. Treatment with fluids and vasopressors, such as vasopressin, may be required. Some patients may remain hypertensive, and monitoring of blood pressure and administration of an alpha-1 antagonist should continue in the post-operative period. Continue to monitor ECG, invasive blood pressure, and volume status. Oxygen supplementation is advised.

References

1 Feldman EC, Nelson RW. *Canine and Feline Endocrinology and Reproduction*, 3rd edn. Saunders: St. Louis, 2004.

2 Ward CR. Feline thyroid storm. *Veterinary Clinics of North America Small Animal Practice* 2007; **37**:745–754.

3 Boston SE, Moens NM, Kruth SA, *et al*. Endoscopic evaluation of the gastroduodenal mucosa to determine the safety of short-term concurrent administration of meloxicam and dexamethasone in healthy dogs. *American Journal of Veterinary Research* 2003; **64**:1369–1375.

4 Kronen PWM, Moon-Massat PF, Ludders JW, *et al*. Comparison of two insulin protocols for diabetic dogs undergoing cataract surgery. *Veterinary Anesthesia and Analgesia* 2001; **28**:146–155.

5 Herrera MA, Mehl ML, Kass PH *et al*. Predictive factors and the effect of phenoxybenzamine on outcome in dogs undergoing adrenalectomy for pheochromocytoma. *Journal of Veterinary Internal Medicine* 2008; **22**:1333–1339.

6 Domi R, Laho H. Management of pheochromocytoma: old ideas and new drugs. *Nigerian Journal of Clinical Practice* 2012; **15(3)**:253–257.

38 Anesthetic Considerations for Orthopedic Surgery

Give that dog a bone

Odette O

Ross University School of Veterinary Medicine, St. Kitts,

KEY POINTS:

- Patients requiring orthopedic surgery present commonly in veterinary practice.

- Orthopedic surgery can be used to correct either congenital or traumatic problems, and can be amongst the most painful procedures performed.

- An individualized anesthetic plan should be made for each patient depending on signalment, history, physical exam/laboratory findings, and orthopedic condition.

- A balanced anesthesia plan may include the use of loco-regional techniques and/or constant rate infusions.

- Pain management should be considered pre-, intra-, and post-operatively with frequent reassessment.

Q. What type of patient is most likely to need an orthopedic procedure?

A. Most patients present with either a congenital or traumatic orthopedic injury. A retrospective study from the UK found the frequency of cranial cruciate rupture in dogs to be 1.19%, with Rottweilers, West Highland White terriers, and Yorkshire terriers being over-represented. In addition, females, obesity, and dogs over 8 years of age were more likely to suffer cranial cruciate ligament rupture [1]. Another author looked at over 1 million dogs within a 40-year timeframe and found both hip dysplasia and cranial cruciate ligament rupture to be increasingly common over the study period. Also, they found that large and giant breed dogs were at greater risk for either or both of these orthopedic conditions [2]. Both studies also found a higher risk of these orthopedic problems in neutered animals.

Q. What are the most common orthopedic procedures performed in dogs and cats?

A. As previously stated, cranial cruciate ligament rupture and hip dysplasia are the most common orthopedic issues in dogs [3]. Fracture or luxation repair

---

Questions and Answers in Small Animal Anesthesia, First Edition. Edited by Lesley J. Smith.
© 2016 John Wiley & Sons, Inc. Published 2016 by John Wiley & Sons, Inc.

after a traumatic event is another leading cause of patient presentation to veterinary hospitals for orthopedic surgery. For cats, trauma is the most common reason for an orthopedic repair. However, radiographic evidence suggests that hip dysplasia, patellar luxations, and degenerative joint disease are becoming increasingly common in cats [4].

Q. How painful is an orthopedic problem and corrective surgery?

A. Severity of lameness has *not* been found to correlate with radiographic signs [5], so pre- and post-operative analgesic considerations should be based on clinical pain assessments and response to treatment. In human subjects, orthopedic pain is widely accepted as severe, with the incidence of moderate to severe pain in hospitalized patients being up to 76% [6].

Q. What type of pre-anesthetic workup is recommended for a patient before orthopedic surgery?

A. Depending on case presentation, a patient-specific pre-anesthetic workup should be planned (see Chapter 1). For young, healthy patients a minimum database of packed cell volume (PCV), total plasma solids, blood glucose, and blood urea nitrogen (BUN) will help determine overall patient status. Ideally, patients with a history of underlying disease or trauma should be stabilized as much as possible prior to an orthopedic procedure. A study of 100 dogs showed thoracic abnormalities in 57% of dogs presenting with traumatic orthopedic injury. Interestingly, 79% of these dogs had no evidence of thoracic lesions based upon physical examination findings [7]. A more detailed workup including complete blood count (CBC), biochemical profile, serum electrolytes, urinalysis, thoracic radiographs, electrocardiogram, and/or blood gas analysis should be considered along with appropriate supportive care for any patients presenting with a history of significant trauma.

Q. What are some general anesthetic considerations in patients presenting for orthopedic surgery?

A. General concerns may arise from specific history, physical examination findings, hydration status, and concurrent medications. In addition, the location of surgery will influence intravenous catheter placement location and positioning of the patient. Patient preparation is usually fairly standard (see Chapter 3). Patient comfort in these cases is of paramount importance. Multimodal analgesia is important for both treating acute and preventing the development of additional chronic pain.

Q. Should pre-anesthetic drugs be administered?

A. Yes! Pre-anesthetic medications are often given by the intramuscular route when the patient does not have an IV catheter in place. Use of premedications provides pre-emptive analgesia and muscle relaxation, facilitates minimal restraint and IV catheter placement, decreases patient anxiety, and decreases the amount of induction agent and inhalant required (Chapters 5, 6, and 8). Based on the potentially intense level of pain in patients presenting for an orthopedic procedure and the surgery itself, a pure μ agonist opioid such as morphine (0.3–1 mg/kg), hydromorphone (0.05–0.2 mg/kg), oxymorphone (0.05–0.2 mg/kg), methadone (0.5–1 mg/kg), or fentanyl (2–5 mcg/kg bolus followed by a constant rate infusion at 5–20 mcg/kg/h) and/or a loco-regional block is recommended. Sedative type and dosing will depend on the patient's signalment, history, and physical exam findings with most healthy, well hydrated, yet anxious patients benefiting from either acepromazine (0.01–0.05 mg/kg intramuscular) or dexmedetomidine (2–10 mcg/kg intramuscular). Benzodiazepines provide the least predictable sedation in many patients, and may best be reserved for calm patients or those cases where other sedatives are contraindicated.

Q. Which induction agents are the most suitable?

A. Depending on the patient's signalment, history, and presenting complaint a number of induction agents may be considered (see Chapter 10). Recall that the level of sedation provided by pre-anesthetic medication is inversely proportional to the amount of induction agent required, that is a patient with more profound sedation from premedication will require less induction agent. Patients who are healthy other than their orthopedic presenting complaints can most likely be induced with *any* of the currently available agents. Those who have suffered a traumatic injury presenting for orthopedic surgery after a period of stabilization/hospitalization may benefit from inclusion of an NMDA-antagonist such as ketamine in the induction protocol. The exception may be traumatic head injury, where the use of ketamine is still controversial. NMDA-antagonist use may help prevent central sensitization, a phenomenon resulting in chronic pain [8]. Although the pre-emptive effects of ketamine in chronic pain have recently come into question, it is still used in the treatment of this type of pain and its role in multimodal analgesia can also help to lower opioid dosing and related side effects as well as help prevent opioid-related hyperalgesia [9]. Ketamine in combination with a muscle relaxant such as a benzodiazepine or propofol can be used for induction and then serves as a loading dose if a constant rate infusion of ketamine is planned for surgical analgesia (see Chapter 22).

Q. Are there any specific inhalants that should be used for anesthetic maintenance?

A. Isoflurane and sevoflurane are the most commonly used inhalants in veterinary anesthesia today. The amount of inhalant required to maintain an ideal surgical plane of anesthesia can vary widely depending on other drugs used in the anesthetic plan (premedication, induction, constant rate infusions) and whether or not loco-regional anesthetics are used. More profound sedation, use of pure mu agonist opioid, and the addition of CRIs, or loco-regional anesthetic techniques will result in a greatly reduced inhalant requirement to maintain an ideal general anesthetic plane. For instance, use of analgesic constant rate infusions such as morphine, lidocaine, and ketamine can reduce isoflurane MAC by up to 48% [10]. A study that reported the amount of end-tidal isoflurane needed in dogs undergoing pelvic limb orthopedic surgery after receiving an epidural containing bupivacaine either alone, with morphine, or with dexmedetomidine showed an average isoflurane requirement of 0.73% [11].

Q. What are my options for providing good analgesia for these patients?

A. A number of intra-operative analgesic techniques are available to the practitioner. Systemic analgesic administration is often provided either by repeated IV bolus or constant rate infusion (see Chapter 22). A multimodal approach to creating a protocol allows us to decrease the amount of each drug used along with minimizing potential side effects. Pure mu agonist opioids (such as fentanyl 2–20 mcg/kg/h or morphine 0.1–0.2 mg/kg/h) are an appropriate choice based on potentially intense levels of pain +/– the addition of ketamine (2–10 mcg/kg/min) and lidocaine (25–50 mcg/kg/min). Epidural or spinal analgesia (see Chapter 23) is another reasonable option, but is appropriate only for pelvic limb procedures. Morphine with the addition of a local anesthetic such as lidocaine, ropivacaine, or bupivacaine is widely used for lumbosacral epidural administration, though bupivavaine alone has been found to provide similar and acceptable analgesia in a study comparing three protocols in 60 dogs [11]. Ultrasound guided or nerve stimulator guided regional anesthesia is another analgesic option for these patients, but these techniques require some advanced training and a fair amount of technical practice. A local anesthetic (ropivacaine or bupivacaine) with or without the addition dexmedetomidine is commonly used [12]. Regional techniques for the thoracic limb include the cervical paravertebral block (upper thoracic limb), brachial plexus block (elbow and distal structures), and RUMM block (distal thoracic limb). Regional techniques for the pelvic limb include a femoral and sciatic nerve block or a psoas compartment and sciatic nerve block. Recall, patients with these adjunctive techniques may demonstrate significant reductions in inhalant requirement and should be monitored closely for excessive anesthetic depth.

Q. What type and how much intravenous fluid should be administered?

A. Fluid therapy type, rate, and quantity should be determined based on patient status (see Chapter 9). Ideally, any patient requiring an orthopedic procedure should have their fluid status normalized if possible prior to surgical intervention. For most cases, a balanced electrolyte solution should be given at 5 ml/kg/h. Underlying cardiac or renal dysfunction may require more conservative fluid therapy, while hemorrhage or the use of large amounts of vasodilating agents (acepromazine, inhalant) may require more aggressive fluid therapy. It is important to continually monitor patient status throughout the procedure plus quantify and replace any significant surgical blood loss.

Q. Is a multi-parameter monitor necessary for these cases?

A. The old saying, "there is no such thing as safe anesthesia, just safe anesthetists" speaks truth! There is absolutely *no* replacement for diligence, constant patient monitoring, and being proactive in dealing with any abnormalities. There are recommended guidelines published by both the American College of Veterinary Anesthesia and Analgesia and American Animal Hospital Association regarding the monitoring of anesthetized patients [13,14]. Both advocate continuous monitoring and awareness of cardiovascular, respiratory, and CNS status with appropriate actions taken to address issues. To this end, use of pulse oximetry, capnography, non-invasive blood pressure monitoring, thermometer, and electrocardiogram are advocated whenever possible. For further reading about monitoring, Chapter 14 has more detailed information.

Q. What are some possible complications that may arise when dealing with a patient undergoing anesthesia for an orthopedic surgery?

A. General anesthesia is still the most common technique for patients undergoing orthopedic surgery. So, any concerns related to anesthetic and analgesic drug administration apply. The patient should constantly be monitored for hypotension, hypoventilation, hypoxemia, and hypothermia. From a management perspective, all patients scheduled for an orthopedic procedure should be considered to have some degree of risk for surgical bleeding. However, this varies depending on the type and location of surgery and also whether or not there is a history of trauma. Generally, spinal surgeries have the highest risk of significant blood loss and depending on their injuries, patients with traumatic fractures may also have significant risk. The popliteal artery can sometimes be incised during TPLO surgery, leading to acute hemorrhage.

Regurgitation and possible esophagitis leading to esophageal stricture or aspiration of gastric contents followed by pneumonia can be potentially fatal consequences of anesthesia. In a referral UK population, dogs undergoing orthopedic surgery were found to be 27 times more likely to regurgitate than those scheduled for diagnostic procedures [15]. This study also found that patients weighing > 40 kg were about 5 times more likely to regurgitate than those less than 20 kg.

Q. Is general anesthesia always required for orthopedic surgery?

A. Not necessarily. Although general anesthesia with the addition of systemic and/or local analgesia is still the most common technique in veterinary medicine, there is an increasing trend towards decreasing morbidity and mortality in human medicine through the use of sedation with local analgesia techniques for hip and knee surgeries [16]. In dogs, there is limited data on the use of procedural sedation with loco-regional anesthesia for pelvic limb orthopedic surgeries, but early case reports are promising. A report of 10 dogs undergoing pelvic limb surgery using femoral + sciatic nerve blocks (bupivacaine 0.5% with dexmedetomidine 0.5 mcg/ml at 0.1 ml/kg/nerve) after hydromorphone premedication (0.05 mg/kg IM), propofol (1 mg/kg) and dexmedetomidine (0.5 mcg/kg) IV induction and maintenance with propofol (0.07–0.15 mg/kg/min) and dexmedetomidine (1 mcg/kg/h) found satisfactory cardiovascular parameters and excellent anesthetic recoveries [17].

Q. What are important considerations after the orthopedic surgery?

A. It is very important to continue to monitor and provide supportive care to patients throughout the anesthetic recovery period. Chapter 24 covers basic recovery concerns.

Q. What post-operative pain management options are there?

A. Assessing and managing patient discomfort is integral to what we do. Pain assessments should be performed frequently (see Chapters 25 and 26). There are many options available to increase patient comfort (Chapter 27). Continuation of constant rate infusions for the immediate post-operative period is a good option (see Chapter 22). However, note that the infusion rates are often decreased during this period to prevent negative side effects such as nausea from lidocaine or dysphoria and significant respiratory depression from fentanyl in the awake patient. The patient should be assessed regularly and adjustments made accordingly.

Nonsteroidal Anti-Inflammatory Drugs (NSAIDs, see Chapter 6) are extremely effective in post-operative pain management after an orthopedic procedure. The anti-inflammatory effects and minimal to no sedation make them desirable in the post-operative period and beyond. For longer term use, it is important to use *as much as needed as little as possible*, monitor the patient regularly for adverse effects, and educate the client about signs to look for and report. Vomiting, diarrhea, renal/hepatic dysfunction, gastrointestinal ulceration, and hemostatic deficiencies make this class of drugs the largest group having adverse effects reported to US FDA Center for Veterinary Medicine [18]. The use of a client information sheet plus regular rechecks and communication are important tools to help increase patient safety.

Q. Are there adjunctive modalities that may help manage pain and facilitate recovery for orthopedic patients?

A. Yes! Rehabilitation therapy is aimed at promoting healing, re-establishing function, and increasing patient comfort. Orthopedic conditions are commonly treated by this modality both before and after an invasive procedure. Rehabilitation therapy is directed towards a patient and joint-specific plan. Some examples may include cryotherapy and/or supportive bandaging prior to the surgical event and range of motion, weight-bearing exercise, aquatic therapy, massage, transcutaneous or neuromuscular electrical stimulation, cold/hot packs, therapeutic ultrasound, and/or laser post-operatively [19].

Acupuncture is becoming increasingly popular in veterinary medicine as a tool to help manage both acute and chronic pain. This complex modality can relieve pain, promote tissue healing, and treat myofascial trigger points often associated with orthopedic abnormalities resulting from injury, muscle overuse, and/or abnormal posture [20].

Q. Will these patients be pain-free after surgery and the recovery period?

A. Unfortunately, even after a surgical procedure, most patients will likely develop osteoarthritis and possibly degenerative joint disease that will need life-long management. Weight management, nutraceuticals, and the use of NSAIDs are often employed for this purpose [21]. A retrospective owner questionnaire-based study looking at 226 dogs about 2.7 years after surgery to stabilize cranial cruciate ligament rupture found what was considered to be a good to excellent outcome in approximately 97% of pets. However, approximately 30% of these dogs still had significant scores on a validated chronic pain scale, while 12% of them received NSAIDs at some point for reasons related to stifle joint surgery [22]. This information emphasizes the importance of client education to help recognize pain not only in the post-operative and recovery period, but long afterwards as well!

References

1 Adams P, Bolus R, Middleton S *et al.* Incidence of signalment on developing cranial cruciate rupture in dogs in the UK. *Journal of Small Animal Practice* 2011; **52**:347–352.

2 Witsberger TH, Villamil JA, Schultz LG, *et al.* Prevalence of and risk factors for hip dysplasia and cranial cruciate ligament deficiency in dogs. *Journal of the American Veterinary Medical Association* 2008; **232**:1818–1824.

3 Johnson JJ, Austin C, Breur G. Incidence of canine appendicular musculoskeletal disorders in 16 veterinary teaching hospitals from 1980 through 1989. *Veterinary Comparative Orthopedics* 1994; **7**:56-69.

4 Sumner-Smith G. Musculoskeletal Diseases. In: Montavon PM, Voss K, Langley-Hobbs SJ (eds) *Feline Orthopedic Surgery and Musculoskeletal Disease*, 1st edn. Saunders Ltd., 2009: 39– 104.

5 Gordon WJ, Conzemius MG, Riedesel E, *et al.* The relationship between limb function and radiographic osteoarthrosis in dogs with stifle osteoarthrosis. *Veterinary Surgery* 2003; **32** 451–454.

6 Aubrun F, Valade N, Coriat P *et al.* Predictive factors of severe postoperative pain in the postanesthesia care unit. *Anesthesia and Analgesia* 2008; **106(5)**:1535–1541.

7 Selcer BA, Buttrick M, Barstad R, *et al.* The incidence of thoracic trauma in dogs with skeletal injury. *Journal of Small Animal Practice* 1987; **28(1)**:21–27.

8 Chaparro LE, Smith SA, Moore RA, *et al.* Pharmacotherapy for the prevention of chronic pain after surgery in adults. *Cochrane Database of Systematic Reviews* 2013, Issue **7**. Art. No.: CD008307. DOI: 10.1002/14651858.CD008307.pub2.

9 Niesters M, Martini C, Dahan A. Ketamine for chronic pain: risks and benefits. *British Journal of Clinical Pharmacology* 2013; **77(2)**:357–367.

10 Muir WW, Wiese AJ, March PA. Effects of morphine, lidocaine, ketamine, and morphine-lidocaine-ketamine drug combination on minimum alveolar concentration in dogs anesthetized with isoflurane. *American Journal of Veterinary Research* 2003; **64(9)**:1155–1160.

11 O O, Smith LJ. A comparison of epidural analgesia provided by bupivacaine alone, bupivacaine + morphine, or bupivacaine + dexmedetomidine for pelvic orthopedic surgery in dogs. *Veterinary Anesthesia and Analgesia* 2013; **40**:527–536.

12 Campoy L, Read MR. *Small Animal Regional Anesthesia and Analgesia*. Wiley-Blackwell, 2013.

13 American College of Veterinary Anesthesia and Analgesia: Small Animal Monitoring Guidelines. http://www.acvaa.org/ (accessed November 14, 2014).

14 American Animal Hospital Association: Veterinary Practice Guidelines: AAHA Anesthesia Guidelines for Dogs and Cats http://www.aahanet.org/publicdocuments/anesthesia_guidelines_for_dogs_and_cats.pdf (accessed November 14, 2014).

15 Lamata C, Loughton V, Jones M, *et al*. The risk of passive regurgitation during general anaesthesia in a population of referred dogs in the UK. *Veterinary Anesthesia and Analgesia* 2012; **39**:266–274.

16 Memtsoudis SG, Sun X, Chiu YL, *et al*. Comparative Effectiveness of Anesthetic Technique in Orthopedic Patients. *Anesthesiology* 2013; **118 (5)**:1046–1058.

17 Campoy L, Martin-Flores M, Ludders JW *et al*. Procedural sedation combined with locoregional anesthesia for orthopedic surgery of the pelvic limb in 10 dogs: case series. *Veterinary Anesthesia and Analgesia* 2012; **39**:436–440.

18 U.S. Food and Drug Administration/U.S. Department of Health and Human Services Veterinary Non-Steroidal Anti-Inflammatory Drugs (NSAIDs) Safety & Health. http://www.fda.gov/AnimalVeterinary/SafetyHealth/ProductSafetyInformation/ucm055434.htm (accessed November 14, 2014).

19 Davidson JR, Kerwin SC, Millis DL. Rehabilitation for the Orthopedic Patient. *Veterinary Clinics of North America: Small Animal Practice* 2005; **35**:1357–1388.

20 Fry LM, Neary S, Sharrock J, *et al*. Acupuncture for Analgesia in Veterinary Medicine Review Article. *Topics in Companion Animal Medicine*. 10.1053/j.tcam.2014.03.001 (accessed November 14, 2014).

21 Wilke VL, Robinson DA, Evans RB, *et al*. Estimate of the annual economic impact of treatment of cranial cruciate ligament injury in dogs in the United States. *Journal of the American Veterinary Medical Association* 2005; **227(10)**:1604–1607.

22 Mölsä SH, Hielm-Björkman AK, Laitinen-Vapaavuori OM. Use of an owner questionnaire to evaluate long-term surgical outcome and chronic pain after cranial cruciate ligament repair in dogs: 253 cases (2004–2006). *Journal of the American Veterinary Medical Association* 2013; **243(5)**:689–695.

39 Anesthetic Management of Common Emergencies in Small Animals

Or, who can think at 2 am?

Jane Quandt

College of Veterinary Medicine, University of Georgia, USA

KEY POINTS:

- Stabilize the patient prior to anesthesia. These efforts would include fluid therapy, possibly blood products, correction of acid-base and electrolyte abnormalities, and (for GDV) decompression of a distended stomach.

- Have all anesthesia equipment checked and in place to allow for a smooth and rapid induction with immediate and complete monitoring of the patient.

- The emergency patient may have a full stomach leading to potential regurgitation while under general anesthesia.

- Emergency patients may require more than one IV catheter in order to deliver fluids, blood products, and drugs,

- Be prepared to mechanically or hand ventilate the emergency patient.

Gastric Dilation-Volvulus

Q. What makes gastric dilation-volvulus (GDV) an emergency?

A. GDV leads to multiple systemic abnormalities with a high mortality rate. The distended stomach severely restricts ventilation by cranial displacement of the diaphragm and leads to hypoventilation. The hypoventilation can lead to hypercapnia and hypoxia, with decreased tissue oxygen availability and increased lactate, which can initiate cardiac arrhythmias. Pre-oxygenation prior to anesthesia, during the induction phase, is recommended. Acid-base abnormalities can vary. There can be metabolic alkalosis due to gastric sequestration of hydrogen ions, or metabolic acidosis can occur from decreased cardiac output and poor ventilation. Serum electrolytes, and acid-base status

---

Questions and Answers in Small Animal Anesthesia, First Edition. Edited by Lesley J. Smith.
© 2016 John Wiley & Sons, Inc. Published 2016 by John Wiley & Sons, Inc.

should be assessed prior to anesthesia and, if possible, corrected before anesthesia [1–3].

With GDV the abdominal distention can decrease cardiac output by up to 90% from normal. The severe gastric distention compresses the intra-abdominal veins, such as the caudal vena cava, portal vein, and the splanchnic vessels. This venous occlusion decreases the venous return which in turn decreases cardiac output and systemic blood pressure. There is also decreased hepatic and renal blood flow. Gastric decompression prior to surgery can improve ventilation and cardiac function [2]. Dogs with GDV commonly have cardiac arrhythmias that are mainly ventricular in origin. Arrhythmias are associated with increased mortality and can be present in up to 40% of patients with GDV [2] [3]. With gastric distension, the high intra-abdominal pressure significantly decreases blood flow to the GI tract which leads to intestinal ischemia and then to bacterial translocation, which can result in septic shock.

Q. Does measuring lactate levels provide any information?

A. The plasma lactate concentration at the time of hospital admission is a predictor of gastric necrosis and patient outcome [4]. Gastric necrosis appears to have a strong association with negative outcome and duration of hospital stay [4]. Plasma lactate concentration is normally 0.5–2.0 mmol/l. The plasma lactate concentration will increase with tissue hypoperfusion. A plasma lactate concentration of 7.4 mmol/l or higher is predictive of gastric necrosis and decreased chance of survival in dogs presenting with GDV [4].

Q. What fluids are used in resuscitation of the dog with GDV?

A. These dogs may present in both hypovolemic and septic shock. It is important to restore the circulating plasma volume using isotonic crystalloid fluids. After initial fluid volume resuscitation, a colloid such as hetastarch may be used to help in vascular fluid retention. The administration of large fluid volumes is best accomplished through the use of two large bore IV catheters in the cephalic or jugular veins [1,3]. Re-expansion of plasma volume will decrease the severity of cardiovascular depression prior to anesthetic induction. Crystalloids should be given at the rate of 20–40 ml/kg IV with a colloid such as hetastarch given at 10–20 ml/kg over 30 min [2].

Treatment with 7% hypertonic saline (4–5 ml/kg over 15 min) will help in the restoration of arterial blood pressure and perfusion. Hypertonic saline may provide additional benefits via modulation of systemic inflammation, increasing urine output, and intestinal motility [2,3]. It is *imperative*, however, that crystalloid fluids are given concurrently.

Q. Is it important to decompress the stomach in a GDV?

A. Gastric decompression should be done after fluid therapy has been initiated and the cardiovascular resuscitation has begun. Decompression will help to improve cardiovascular function but can result in hypotension due to the rapid release of endotoxins and ischemic by-products from reperfusion injury.

Decompression is done via passage of an orogastric tube. Intubation of the airway may be desirable to protect the airway and prevent possible aspiration. The dog can be sedated and general anesthesia induced to facilitate endotracheal intubation and passage of the orogastric tube. If passage of the orogastric tube is not possible, trocarization of the area of greatest tympany can be done to relieve the gastric distention, but this runs the risk of inducing septic peritonitis [3].

Q. What is the evidence for the use of lidocaine constant rate infusion (CRI) in the GDV patient?

A. Severe complications resulting from GDV occur from the ischemia-reperfusion injury and systemic inflammatory response syndrome seen following repositioning of the compromised stomach. Associated complications can include hypotension, acute kidney injury, disseminated intravascular coagulation, and cardiac arrhythmias. Lidocaine has been shown to decrease the severity of reperfusion injury and the systemic inflammatory response [5]. A recent study has shown that lidocaine at 2 mg/kg IV given at the time of presentation and then followed by a CRI of 50 mcg/kg/min IV for 24 h during and after surgery decreased the occurrence of cardiac arrhythmias, acute kidney injury, and hospitalization time in dogs that underwent surgery for GDV. Lidocaine also provides analgesia which will decrease opioid requirements [5].

Q. What anesthetic drugs are commonly used for GDV?

A. A combination of agents is commonly used for a multimodal analgesic and anesthetic plan. An IV opioid such as fentanyl, oxymorphone, or hydromorphone is used to provide analgesia, a benzodiazepine such as midazolam or diazepam gives muscle relaxation, lidocaine can be used to decrease reperfusion injury, and either propofol, ketamine, alfaxalone, or etomidate are given to facilitate intubation. These drugs are given IV and should be titrated to effect to achieve the lowest dose possible. The opioids should not be given IM because of the risk of vomiting, which can lead to aspiration pneumonia or potentially a stomach rupture due to increased intra-abdominal pressure. The decision of which induction agent to use may be influenced by the dog's heart rate. If the dog is tachycardic then propofol, alfaxalone, or etomidate with benzodiazepine may be preferred as ketamine increases the heart rate. Following intubation, a CRI of lidocaine can be started to continue its anti-inflammatory effects; in addition, fentanyl or ketamine (one or both) can be used as CRIs to enhance analgesia (see Chapter 22 for more details on CRIs). Maintenance can be with either isoflurane or sevoflurance. Nitrous oxide should be avoided with GI distention as it will equilibrate with the gas in the stomach and increase the intragastric volume and pressure [1]. Anesthetic monitoring should include ECG, pulse oximetry, capnometry, invasive (if possible) or non-invasive blood pressure, heart rate, respiratory rate, and temperature.

Gastric or Intestinal Foreign Bodies

Q. What makes a foreign body in the GI tract an emergency?

A. Dogs and cats commonly ingest objects that can become lodged in the pylorus or small intestine. Partial obstruction will allow limited passage of gas and fluid while a complete obstruction does not. A complete obstruction results in more severe distention of the intestine with gas and fluid. As the fluid and gas accumulate there is venous congestion and increased intraluminal pressure; this leads to mucosal ischemia and eventually necrosis with bacterial migration of toxins into the systemic circulation and peritoneal cavity. This will cause sepsis and shock. Proximal obstructions can cause persistent vomiting leading to electrolyte imbalances, dehydration, and hypovolemia [6].

Q. How is a linear foreign body different and is it also an emergency?

A. Part of the linear foreign body lodges either at the base of the tongue or at the pylorus and the remainder advances into the intestinal tract. Peristalsis can lead to obstruction or, as the linear foreign body becomes taut, it can cut into the mucosa, causing multiple perforations and peritonitis. This is associated with a high mortality rate. Cats seem more prone to ingestion of linear foreign bodies than dogs [6].

Q. What pre-operative therapy should be initiated?

A. Fluid resuscitation is vital to maintaining tissue perfusion. Crystalloids should be given IV at 10–20 ml/kg/h to treat any dehydration or volume loss. The goal is to maintain the mean arterial pressure at 60 mmHg or better to provide tissue perfusion. If the total protein is less than 4 g/dl or the albumin less than 1.5 g/dl, a colloid such as hetastarch IV at 5–10 ml/kg/hr should be added in order to maintain good oncotic pressure [6].

Q. If the animal develops septic shock, what additional therapy is used to maintain tissue perfusion?

A. Inotropes and or vasopressors may be needed to maintain blood pressure and perfusion. These should be given in addition to crystalloids and colloids. Commonly used inotropes are dopamine and dobutamine (2–10 mcg/kg/min IV). These agents have a short half-life necessitating the use of a CRI, but this does make it easy to titrate to effect. Vasopressors, which cause vasoconstriction, consist of norepinephrine, phenylephrine, and vasopressin (ADH). They should be used carefully as intense vasoconstriction can occur, which will increase blood pressure but will decrease blood flow to vital organs [7].

Q. What anesthetic agents are commonly used for GI surgery?

A. An opioid premedication will provide analgesia and decrease the amount of inhalant agent required. It is best to avoid IM opioids, if possible, to prevent vomiting. The animal should be receiving IV fluid therapy, in which case anesthetic premedication can be given IV. Induction can be achieved with a benzodiazepine and ketamine, alfaxalone, or etomidate. Propofol can be used, but with caution if the patient is hypotensive as propofol can exacerbate hypotension [7]. In the dog lidocaine can be incorporated into the induction technique and then given as a CRI. Anesthesia can be maintained with any of the modern inhalants other than nitrous oxide, because of the risk of GI distension. Monitoring should be complete and include ECG, pulse oximetry, capnometry, invasive or non-invasive blood pressure, heart rate, respiratory rate, and temperature.

Q. Is a lidocaine CRI used in cats undergoing GI surgery?

A. Lidocaine CRIs are not recommended in cats. The dose of lidocaine needed to improve analgesia in anesthetized cats creates greater cardiovascular depression then seen with isoflurane alone. This depression can be very severe in healthy cats, therefore it would be expected to be unacceptable in the critically ill cat [8,9].

Intervertebral Disk Disease

Q. What are the special concerns with intervertebral disk disease (IVDD)?

A. Dogs commonly present for emergency imaging and surgery for neurological deficits. Imaging now commonly consists of an MRI or a CT scan to diagnosis the disk herniation, although myelography may still be employed. These dogs are typically not fasted and require immediate anesthesia for diagnostics and surgery to relieve a compressive disk in the spinal canal.

Q. What are the major concerns with myelography?

A. Myelography involves injection of contrast material into the spinal subarachnoid space while the animal is under general anesthesia. Potential complications from this procedure include neurologic signs ranging from muscle fasciculation to generalized seizures and worsening of the patient's neurologic condition [10]. The incidence of seizures depends on the lesion location, severity of the neurologic deficit, what contrast medium was used, and what volume was injected and whether it was injected at the lumbosacral space or at the cisternal space.

Q. How can the seizure risk be minimized?

A. Careful and slow injection of contrast media may help lower the incidence of seizures. After the contrast has been given, elevation of the patient's head will reduce the risk of contrast flowing cranially [10]. IV fluids should be given to maintain diuresis and help the patient clear the contrast agent renally.

Q. What is an anesthetic protocol for imaging?

A. These patients are generally healthy other than their IVDD, so most anesthetic protocols can be considered. Premedications with opioids and sedatives such as benzodiazapines or low doses of acepromazine are standard. These patients don't usually require an alpha-2 agonist for sedation, but one could be used if necessary. Induction and maintenance, as well as monitoring, can be standard. If the patient requires surgery to relieve the disc herniation, then CRIs of fentanyl, lidocaine, and ketamine alone or in combination can be used to enhance analgesia and decrease the amount of inhalant that is required. The CRI can be carried into recovery at a reduced dose to provide post-operative analgesia.

Q. What are the concerns with CT or MRI and contrast agents?

A. Intravenous iodinated contrast media is often given during a CT scan. These contrast media consist of meglumine and/or sodium salts of iothalomate or diatrizoate. They are ionic and hyperosmolar which can lead to hypotension, tachycardia, ST segment depression, and prolonged QT intervals. These adverse reactions are usually seen within the first 5–10 min following administration of the contrast media and are potentiated by dehydration. Fluid therapy is important to correct dehydration and to treat mild hypotension and tachycardia. Fluid therapy will also promote contrast clearance [11]. Anaphylactic reactions have been reported in dogs receiving these contrast media. The contrast media used in MRI is the paramagnetic element gadolinium. An increased IV fluid rate is used to treat hypotension and tachycardia associated with its administration [11].

Q. What post-operative complications may there be following surgery for IVDD?

A. Dogs that have undergone anesthesia for diagnosis and treatment of IVDD have an increased incidence of post-operative pneumonia. The relevant risk factors for development of pneumonia in these patients include multiple anesthetics (one for diagnostic imaging and one for surgery), a long duration of anesthesia, having a cervical lesion, having tetraparesis prior to undergoing anesthesia, and vomiting or regurgitation after anesthesia [12].

Q. Are there any additional analgesic techniques that can be used?

A. Extradural morphine provides long-lasting analgesia. In one report, preservative free morphine at a dose of 0.1 mg/kg diluted with saline to a minimum volume of 0.4 ml was placed on the spinal cord and then covered with a collagen patch prior to surgical closure. Meticulous hemostasis is crucial to decrease the chance of dilution and systemic absorption. The analgesia provided may have a duration of 12–24 h [13].

Hemoabdomen

Q. Why is a hemoabdomen a surgical emergency?

A. These patients are typically bleeding from their liver or spleen and blood rapidly fills the peritoneal cavity, causing distension and relative hypovolemia. The PCV of blood in the abdominal cavity may be equal to or even greater than the peripheral PCV of the patient. Hypovolemia, anemia, and respiratory compromise due to the abdominal distension are all reasons to control the abdominal bleeding relatively quickly.

Q. How should I stabilize a dog with a hemoabdomen?

A. IV crystalloid fluids, colloids, and/or blood products should be administered as needed based on measured non-invasive blood pressure, heart rate, and PCV/TP. A goal would be to administer resuscitative fluids to reach, minimally, a mean arterial pressure of 60 mmHg and a PCV of 20% prior to anesthesia.

Q. How should I manage anesthesia for these patients?

A. Because of significant volume depletion, drugs that reduce cardiac output or blood pressure should be avoided. Generally, IV μ agonist opioids and benzodiazepines are used for premedication, followed by very low doses of either propofol, alfaxalone, etomidate, or ketamine. If the animal is tachycardic, ketamine will worsen the tachycardia and should be avoided. Maintenance can be with inhalants but the goal of anesthetic maintenance should be to use as little inhalant as possible, so plan for supplementing with CRIs of fentanyl, lidocaine, and ketamine. Invasive and complete monitoring should be performed.

Often blood loss will continue into and during surgery, or the patient may ooze significantly due to consumptive coagulopathy. Additional blood products, including packed red blood cells and fresh frozen plasma (to replace clotting factors and albumin) should be on hand. Blood pressure support with inotropes, such as dobutamine or dopamine, or vasopressors such as vasopressin may be necessary.

Q. How would you stabilize the patient with a diaphragmatic hernia?

A. Stabilize the patient by placing an IV catheter and administering an isotonic crystalloid fluid to treat for possible shock. Assess the level of trauma and degree of respiratory embarrassment. Do a CBC and chemistry. Oxygen therapy may be indicated as these patients are often in respiratory distress. Assess the animal for other injuries as a diaphragmatic hernia is often the result of trauma. Obtain thoracic radiographs to determine the severity of the diaphragmatic rupture, how much viscera is within the thoracic cavity and the presence of other thoracic trauma such as rib fractures. The abdomen also should be radiographed and ultrasound performed to identify any traumatic injury.

Q. What abdominal organs are commonly herniated?

A. The liver, stomach, small intestines, omentum, and spleen are commonly herniated.

Q. What are the indications for surgery?

A. Indications for surgery include a herniated stomach, strangulated bowel or organ, inability to oxygenate properly, and ruptured viscera. Early surgical intervention, within 24 h of admission, comes with an excellent prognosis for the acute case.

Q. Why is it important to know which side the hernia is on?

A. When preparing the patient for surgery, the side with the hernia should be placed in the dependent position. One should not place the non-herniated side down as the dependent lung will become atelectic and this will cause profound hypoxemia as the herniated side is poorly oxygenated as well. The animal should have the surgery site clipped while awake, if possible, and while standing them on their rear legs to allow for improved oxygenation.

Q. What kind premedication is recommended?

A. A rapid sequence induction is preferable to gain control of the airway. The animal should be pre-oxygenated prior to induction. Agents to consider will depend on the condition of the animal and any underlying disease. Monitor the heart rate and rhythm as myocardial damage can predispose to arrhythmias. ECG and pulse monitoring should continue into recovery as arrhythmias can take up to 36 h to develop. Anesthetic agents can be given IV if the catheter is in place for fluid therapy. Drugs that cause vomiting should be avoided. Opioids are indicated for analgesia but should be given IV if possible to prevent vomiting.

Q. What agents should be used for induction?

A. Most induction drugs can be used, titrated to effect to minimize the risk of overdose. Ketamine and a benzodiazepine, propofol, or alfaxalone are all appropriate. Etomidate should probably be avoided because of its tendency to cause retching. Additional analgesia can be provided with a fentanyl CRI of 3 to 10 mcg/kg/h for both the dog and cat. A loading dose of 3–5 mcg/kg IV is given prior to beginning the CRI; this loading dose can be incorporated into the induction technique. In the dog, lidocaine can be added for analgesia and oxygen free radical scavenging. A loading dose of 1 to 2 mg/kg IV is given (this too can be used as part of the induction) and then a CRI of 25–50 mcg/kg/min is recommended.

Q. What agent should be used for maintenance?

A. The inhalants can be used for maintenance. To minimize the hypotension commonly seen with inhalants, the use of a fentanyl CRI in the cat, and a fentanyl or lidocaine CRI or a combination of both can used in the dog to decrease the amount of inhalant required.

Q. When should ventilation begin?

A. Intermittent positive pressure ventilation should begin as soon as the animal is intubated to maintain and improve oxygenation. As soon as the abdominal incision is made the animal is dependent on the ventilator as the diaphragm is incompetent and negative intrathoracic pressure is impossible for spontaneous ventilation. The inspiratory pressure should be kept below 20 cm of H_2O to avoid barotrauma. The respiratory rate will be 10–20 breaths per minute with a tidal volume of 10–15 ml/kg. The pulse oximeter and capnograph should be used to monitor for oxygenation and appropriate ventilation.

Q. What is a common complication during surgery?

A. Be prepared to treat hypotension as this can occur as soon as the animal is placed in dorsal recumbency due to organ compression on the heart and vessels. When the viscera are removed from the thoracic cavity, blood pressure may drop further due to vasodilation of the abdominal organs, sequestration of blood, and potential reperfusion injury. Do not treat the hypotension with an excessive bolus of crystalloid fluids as this may lead to pulmonary edema upon the return of vascular tone. Hypotension can be treated with an infusion of dopamine or dobutamine at 1–10 mcg/kg/min IV.

Q. How do you re-inflate the lung?

A. Re-expansion should occur slowly. Maintain the set tidal volume, inspiratory pressure, and respiratory rate. Do not give artificially high tidal volumes or inspiratory pressure in an attempt to re-expand the lungs. Doing so can cause barotrauma and life-threatening pulmonary edema.

Q. What is re-expansion pulmonary edema?

A. This is a complication that results from the release of endotoxins and oxygen free radicals, decreased surfactant concentrations, negative interstitial pressures, or chronic hypoxia causing increased vascular permeability and protein-rich pulmonary edema [14]. This is seen upon release of the trapped organs and subsequent return of blood flow to the organs and the lungs. There is an increased incidence of re-expansion pulmonary edema if the lung has been collapsed for longer than 72 h. Keep the peak airway pressure below 20 cm of H_2O during ventilation. Pleural air should be evacuated slowly post-operatively.

Q. How should the patient be recovered?

A. These patients benefit from being recovered in an oxygen cage or with oxygen supplemented by placing nasal cannulas. Analgesia can be provided by giving an opioid intermittently or by maintaining a fentanyl CRI at a lower dose rate. The pulse oximeter should be used to monitor oxygenation status following extubation. ECG monitoring should continue for the next 48 h to identify any potential arrhythmias.

References

1 Greene SA, Marks SL. Gastrointestinal disease. In: Tranquilli WJ, Thurmon JC, Grimm KA (eds) *Lumb & Jones' Veterinary Anesthesia and Analgesia*, 4th edn. Blackwell Publishing: Ames, IA, 2007:927–932.

2 Clarke KW, Trim CM, Hall LW. Anesthesia of the dog. In: Clarke KW, Trim CM, Hall LW(eds) *Veterinary Anesthesia*, 11th edn. Elsevier Saunders: St. Louis, MO 2014:405–498.

3 Volk SW. Gastric dilatation-volvulus and bloat. In: Silverstein DC, Hopper K (eds) *Small Animal Critical Care Medicine*. Elsevier Saunders: St. Louis, MO 2009:584–588.

4 Beer KA, Syring RS, Drobatz KJ. Evaluation of plasma lactate concentration and base excess at the time of hospital admission as predictors of gastric necrosis and outcome and correlation between those variables in dogs with gastric dilatation-volvulus: 78 cases (2004-2009). *Journal of the American Veterinary Medical Association* 2013; **242(1)**:54–58.

5 Bruchim Y, Itay S, Shira BH, *et al.* Evaluation of lidocaine treatment on frequency of cardiac arrhythmias, acute kidney injury, and hospitalization time in dogs with gastric dilatation volvulus. *Journal of Veterinary Emergency and Critical Care* 2012; **22(4)**:419–427.

6 Fossum TW, Dewey CW, Horn CV, *et al.* Surgery of the digestive system. In: Fossum TW, Dewey CW, Horn CV (eds) *Small Animal Surgery* 4th edn. Elsevier Saunders: St. Louis, MO 2013:386–583.

7 Fossum TW, Dewey CW, Horn CV, *et al.* Surgery of the abdominal cavity. In: Fossum TW, Dewey CW, Horn CV (eds) *Small Animal Surgery* 4th edn. Elsevier Saunders: St. Louis, MO 2013:356–385.

8 Pypendop BH, Ilkiw JE. Assessment of the hemodynamic effects of lidocaine administered IV in isoflurane anesthetized cats. *American Journal of Veterinary Research* 2005; **66(4)**:661–668.

9 Pypendop BH, Ilkiw JE, Robertson SA. Effects of intravenous administration of lidocaine on the the the thermal threshold in cats. *American Journal of Veterinary Research* 2006; **67(1)**:16–20.

10 Lexmaulova L, Zatloukal J, Proks P, *et al.* Incidence of seizures associated with iopamidol or iomeprol myelography in dogs with intervertebral disk disease: 161 cases (2000-2002). *Journal of Veterinary Emergency and Critical Care* 2009; **19(6)**:611–616.

11 Cornick-Seahorn JL, Grimm J, Marks SL. Selected Diagnostic Procedures. In: Tranquilli WJ, Thurmon JC, Grimm KA (eds) *Lumb & Jones' Veterinary Anesthesia and Analgesia*, 4th edn. Blackwell Publishing: Ames, IA, 2007:1027–1032.

12 Java MA, Drobatz KJ, Gilley RS, *et al.* Incidence of and risk factors for postoperative pneumonia in dogs anesthetized for diagnosis of treatment of intervertebral disk disease. *Journal of the American Veterinary Medical Association* 2009; **235(3)**:281–287.

13 Aprea F, Cherubini GB, Palus V, *et al.* Effect of extradurally administered morphine on postoperative analgesia in dogs undergoing surgery for thoracolumbar intervertebral disk extrusion. *Journal of the American Veterinary Medical Association* 2012; **241(6)**:754–759.

14 Clarke KW, Trim CM, Hall LW. Anesthesia for intrathoracic procedures. In: Clarke KW, Trim CM, Hall LW (eds) *Veterinary Anesthesia*, 11th edn. Elsevier Saunders: St. Louis, MO 2014:599–609.

40 Anesthetic Management of Brachycephalic Breeds

These deserve a chapter all their own!

Lesley J. Smith

Department of Surgical Sciences, School of Veterinary Medicine, University of Wisconsin, USA

KEY POINTS:

- Try to avoid heavy sedation prior to anesthesia.
- Pre-oxygenate for induction.
- Be prepared with a good laryngoscope and many different tube sizes.
- Watch for bradycardia during anesthesia due to increased vagal tone.
- Monitor closely at recovery and extubate only when they "spit out the tube."

Q. What are common brachycephalic breeds of dog?

A. Common breeds include the English Bulldog, French Bulldog, Boston Terrier, Shih tzu, Pekinese, Pug, and Brussels Griffon [1]. Among these breeds, a given individual dog may be more or less affected by the brachycephalic syndrome, so "true" brachycephalics (e.g., the English Bulldog) should be considered on a spectrum with other breeds that share some of the same anatomic features. For example, the Boxer and the American Bulldog are not considered true brachycephalic breeds but do commonly have a relatively long soft palate and other anatomic features that resemble brachycephalic syndrome. Other breeds, for example the Shar Pei or Bull Mastiff, may share some brachycephalic features.

Q. What makes brachycephalic breeds more challenging to anesthetize?

A. These breeds typically have four anatomic abnormalities involving their upper airway that makes them more difficult to intubate and more at risk for airway obstruction and hypoxemia during periods of sedation or during anesthetic recovery [2]. The four abnormalities are: (i) stenotic nares, (ii) elongated soft palate, (iii) everted laryngeal saccules, and (iv) hypoplastic trachea. All of these abnormalities increase the resistance to airflow. The elongated soft palate and everted laryngeal saccules can make visualizing the larynx more difficult during intubation, and the hypoplastic trachea

---

Questions and Answers in Small Animal Anesthesia, First Edition. Edited by Lesley J. Smith.
© 2016 John Wiley & Sons, Inc. Published 2016 by John Wiley & Sons, Inc.

means that you may be unprepared with your tube sizes for just how small an endotracheal tube will fit!

After pre-anesthetic sedation and especially at recovery, the stenotic nares and relaxation of the elongated soft palate make the dog much more prone to airflow obstruction or just reduced airflow. These dogs have an increased work of breathing due to the increased resistance of the upper airway, and when they are not fully awake they may not be able to mount as much respiratory effort as they need to stay well oxygenated.

Q. How do I prepare for intubation in these patients?

A. It is important to try to avoid "heavy" sedation in these breeds. Typically, their temperaments are fairly cooperative, so try to use premedication that results in light sedation (e.g., midazolam 0.1 mg/kg and hydromorphone IM 0.05–0.2 mg/kg) and/or is reversible (e.g., dexmedetomidine IM 2–5 mcg/kg). Aggressive restraint should be avoided in these patients because many of them have a shallow orbit and can proptose an eye if they are violently struggling against restraint. If the patient will easily allow it, IV premedication is another option, but reduce your doses by 25–50% if going IV.

Prior to induction, if the patient will accept it, pre-oxygenation will help to increase the P_aO_2, which buys you a "window of time" during intubation before hypoxemia occurs. This is just a safety measure in case you run into trouble intubating. In order to effectively pre-oxygenate, you must run the O_2 flow on your anesthetic machine at, minimally, 2–3 l/min and use a canine mask preferably with the diaphragm fitted over the dog's muzzle. If the dog will not tolerate the diaphragm (many feel suffocated), then just use the mask but increase the O_2 flow to 4–5 l/min. Pre-oxygenate for at least 5 min prior to induction. Leave the mask on while you administer induction drugs and remove it only when you are ready to intubate.

Q. How do I intubate these patients?

A. Have a lot of different tube sizes ready! Choose several that seem appropriate for a "normal" dog of that size, then 2–3 that are several sizes down from that. It is not unheard of for a 30 kg Bulldog to take a 5 mm ID endotracheal tube! Many of these breeds err on the side of overweight, so base your endotracheal tube size on ideal body weight. Pre-oxygenate! Have a long laryngoscope blade with a good light.

After you've given your induction drug of choice to effect (many clinicians prefer propofol because of the excellent muscle relaxation it affords), make sure your assistant holds the mouth open as wide as possible. Use the blade of your laryngoscope or a tongue depressor to push the soft palate dorsally out of the way (you may see a wall of pink tissue on your first glance – that is the soft palate hanging down in the oropharynx). Once the soft palate is pushed out of the way, the larynx should be visible behind it. Use the beveled tip of the endotracheal tube to push between the laryngeal saccules. If it feels like you are forcing the tube, then go down a size until you find one that fits well. Secure the tube, inflate the cuff, and proceed as with any other patient at this point. It helps to tie around the tube and then behind the ears rather than over the muzzle, as the muzzle is so short in these dogs that you may not achieve a very secure tie.

Q. What about recovery?

A. These patients need close supervision in recovery. Monitoring pulse oximetry is important, at least until the patient is awake enough that they won't tolerate the pulse oximeter probe. Watch their color. Extubation should not occur until the dog is able to hold its head up and literally spit the tube out. Never extubate too early, as this is when the risk for airway obstruction and hypoxemia is high! These dogs commonly will remain intubated for much longer than "normal" dogs, so patience is key. It is also important, if possible, to keep them sternal during recovery with their head propped up on a towel or other support. A "head down" position will increase swelling in the nasal passages, which only adds to their airway resistance after they are extubated.

Q. What else should I know about brachycephalic dogs and anesthesia?

A. Many of these dogs have increased vagal tone. They can be relatively bradycardic under anesthesia. One option is to pre-treat with an anticholinergic before anesthesia. Another approach is to monitor heart rate during anesthesia and administer your anticholinergic only if the heart rate becomes unacceptably low. In this situation, an IV dose of glycopyrrolate (0.005–0.01 mg/kg) is a good choice.

References

1 American College of Veterinary Surgeons. Brachycephalic Syndrome. http://www.acvs.org/small-animal/brachycephalicsyndrome/ (accessed January 10, 2015).

2 Lodato DL, Hedlund CS. Brachycephalic Airway Syndrome: Management. *Compendium Continuing Education Veterinary* 2012; **34(8)**:E4.

41 Anesthetic Considerations for Other Canine Breeds

(considerations or myths....?)

Lesley J. Smith

Department of Surgical Sciences, School of Veterinary Medicine, University of Wisconsin, USA

KEY POINTS:

- There are few *true* breed sensitivities to anesthetics.

- Breed idiosyncrasies to various anesthetic, sedative, and analgesic drugs should be considered when formulating an anesthetic plan.

- Some herding breeds (e.g., Collies, Australian shepherds) have an MDR-1 receptor polymorphism that renders them potentially more sensitive to certain sedative drugs.

- Dachshunds are more prone to bradycardia 2° to increased vagal tone than other small breeds of dogs.

- Northern breeds of dogs (e.g., Malamutes) may become dysphoric in response to opioids more commonly than other breeds of dogs.

Q. Aren't some dog breeds more sensitive to anesthesia or anesthetic drugs?

A. Although many dog breed publications will report anesthetic sensitivity to certain drugs (e.g., ketamine, acepromazine), or to anesthesia in general, there are very few scientifically documented breed sensitivities to anesthesia. When owners or dog breeders present their animal and express concern about perceived anesthetic risk based on the animal's breed, it is important for the veterinarian to educate them on the general risks of anesthesia in all breeds/species and to reassure the client that the particular breed of the animal will be considered but that it is unlikely that there is a heightened risk based on the breed.

The one known and scientifically documented anesthetic drug sensitivity based on breed is that of greyhounds having delayed recoveries after thiobarbiturates (thiopental). This delayed recovery is due in part to the typically lean body type of these dogs such that there is little adipose tissue to which the drug can redistribute; however, the primary reason for the delayed recovery is that this breed has delayed cytochrome P450 hydroxylation of the drug compared to mixed breed dogs [1]. The same is also true of propofol with

Questions and Answers in Small Animal Anesthesia, First Edition. Edited by Lesley J. Smith.
© 2016 John Wiley & Sons, Inc. Published 2016 by John Wiley & Sons, Inc.

regard to greyhounds; however under clinical conditions propofol does not cause a delayed recovery in this breed likely because of its rapid redistribution characteristics and some extra-hepatic metabolic pathways [2]. Most anesthesiologists empirically extend this breed sensitivity to other sight hound breeds as well (Whippets, Italian Greyhounds, Borzois, Afgan Hounds) even though these breeds have not been specifically studied. Thiopental is no longer commercially available in the USA; however, it is still used clinically in other countries and may return to the US market in the future.

Q. Don't some dog breeds respond differently to sedatives and analgesics?

A. Some herding breeds of dogs, notably Collies, Shetland Sheepdogs, Old English Sheepdogs, and Australian Shepherds may be homozygous recessive or heterozygous for the "multidrug resistance" gene, or MDR1 [3]. In a survey from the Northwest US, 35% of Collies were homozygous recessive and 42% were heterozygous for this genetic polymorphism [4]. Genetic mutations in the MDR1 gene render the animal potentially more sensitive to certain drugs that are P glycoprotein substrates, the most infamous being ivermectin. Among anesthetic drugs, none have been scientifically proven to have altered pharmacokinetics in MDR1-mutant dogs. That said, the lab that has done the most work on this genetic mutation publishes a list of "suspect" drugs, and among these are acepromazine and butorphanol [5]. Anecdotal reports suggest prolonged and profound sedation from these two drugs in MDR1 mutant dogs. Currently, these drugs are recommended to be avoided or to be administered at a 25–50% reduced dose.

Q. I've heard that you shouldn't give acepromazine to Boxers. Is this true?

A. Anecdotal reports suggest that boxer dogs *may* be more sensitive to the hypotensive effects of acepromazine. In these individuals, acepromazine appears to produce profound sedation with bradycardia and dramatic decreases in blood pressure. While this "sensitivity" has not be scientifically documented, it may be prudent to use acepromazine cautiously or at low doses, and monitor blood pressure throughout the procedure, in this breed of dog.

Q. Aren't giant breeds more sensitive to sedative drugs and anesthetics?

A. Some general guidelines should be considered when making sedative/analgesic drug choices and calculating dosages in dogs. As a rule, giant breeds of dogs have a lower body surface area to volume ratio, and, as such, require much lower doses of sedative/analgesic drugs on a mg/kg basis. When choosing drug doses for a giant breed dog, err on the side of the lowest recommended dose of the range provided. Give induction drugs to effect.

Q. Can you give opioids to Northern breeds like Huskies and Malamutes? Don't these drugs make them dysphoric?

A. Some dog breeds do not sedate well with opioids, the Northern Breeds of dogs being the best example [6]. These dogs tend to get very dysphoric and vocal with opioids. In humans, genetic variations in the μ opioid receptor have been identified, with some of these variations being associated with variable responses to opioids (reduced clinical response and/or increased side effects). One study, with a small number of dogs represented, suggested that dogs that were dysphoric after opioid administration had a higher prevalence of a mutation in the μ opioid receptor than dogs that did not display dysphoria [7]. In Northern breeds, concurrent sedation with alpha-2 agonists may be necessary when using μ agonist opioids. Regional analgesic techniques, when they are an option, are a great alternative for pain management in these dogs.

Q. Why are Dachshunds often bradycardic under anesthesia?

A. It has been reported that, compared to other small breeds of dogs, Dachshunds have an increased incidence of bradycardia under anesthesia, despite similar body temperatures and anesthetic protocols [8]. The reason for this breed predilection is unknown but a good working hypothesis is that Dachshunds have higher resting vagal tone and/or respond with more dramatic increases in parasympathetic tone after administration of drugs like opioids and alpha-2 agonists.

References

1 Robinson EP, Sams RA, Muir WW. 1986. Barbiturate anesthesia in greyhound and mixed-breed dogs: comparative cardiopulmonary effects, anesthetic effects, and recovery rates. *American Journal of Veterinary Research 1986*; **47(10)**:2105–2112.

2 Court MH, Hay-Kraus BL, Hill DW, *et al.* Propofol hydroxylation by dog liver microsomes: assay development and dog breed differences. *Drug Metabolism and Disposition* 1999; **7(11)**:1293–1299.

3 Mealey KL, Meurs KM. Breed distribution of the ABCB1-1Delta (multidrug sensitivity) polymorphism among dogs undergoing ABCB1 genotyping. *Journal of the American Veterinary Medical Association* 2008; **233(6)**:921–924.

4 Mealey KL, Bentjen SA, Waiting DK. Frequency of the mutant MDR1 allele associated with ivermectin sensitivity in a sample population of collies from the northwestern United States. *American Journal of Veterinary Research* 2002; **63(4)**:479–481.

5 Washington State University, College of Veterinary Medicine, Veterinary Clinical Pharmacology. Multidrug Sensitivity in Dogs: Problem Drugs. http://vcpl.vetmed.wsu.edu/problem-drugs/ (accessed January 12, 2015)

6 Hofmeister EH, Herrington JL, Massaferro EM. Opioid dysphoria in three dogs. *Journal of Veterinary Emergency and Critical Care* 2006; **16**:44–49.

7 Hawley AT, Wetmore LA, Identification of single nucleotide polymorphisms within Exon 1 of the canine mu-opioid receptor gene. *Veterinary Anesthesia and Analgesia*. 2009; **37(1)**:79–82.

8 Harrison RL, Clark L, Corletto F. Comparison of mean heart rate in anaesthetized dachshunds and other breeds of dog undergoing spinal magnetic resonance imaging. *Veterinary Anesthesia and Analgesia* 2012; **39(3)**:230–235.

42 Anesthetic Considerations for Cats

An everyday challenge

Paulo Steagall and Javier Benito

Département de Sciences Cliniques, Faculté de Médecine Vétérinaire, Université de Montréal, Canada

---

KEY POINTS:

- Particular anesthetic considerations in cats include laryngospasm and the use of mouth-gags.
- Route of administration impacts analgesia.
- Loco-regional anesthetic techniques are crucial in pain management.
- Anesthesia for spay-neuter programs presents certain challenges including pediatric cats and large volume surgical clinics.
- Aggressive cats can be challenging to safely anesthetize.

Q. Is anesthetic risk higher in cats than in dogs?

A. The risk of anesthetic-related death in cats varies between 0.1 and 0.3%. A recent study in the UK reported a mortality rate of 0.24% in cats, which was higher than the 0.17% reported in dogs [1]. Poor health status (ASA status), age, extremes of body weight, endotracheal intubation, and the lack of anesthetic monitoring or fluid therapy are among risk factors that have been associated with peri-operative mortality in this species. Monitoring of anesthesia is associated with reduced anesthetic risk. Cats should have intravenous access and fluid therapy should be administered.

Q. What are the key points about anesthetic premedication in cats?

A. Sedation will decrease stress and anxiety to facilitate handling while possibly providing analgesia and reducing the requirements for general anesthetics. Sedation should not be considered safer than general anesthesia since some sedatives can cause significant cardiorespiratory depression. All of the beneficial aspects of anesthetic premedication (see Chapters 5, 6, and 8) apply to cats. Generally, a sedative drug is combined with an opioid for analgesia. The desired degree and choice of sedation should be evaluated on a case-by-case

---

Questions and Answers in Small Animal Anesthesia, First Edition. Edited by Lesley J. Smith.
© 2016 John Wiley & Sons, Inc. Published 2016 by John Wiley & Sons, Inc.

Table 42.1 Sedative and premedication drugs in cats.

Drug	Dosage regimens	Comments
Acepromazine	0.03–0.05 mg/kg IM, IV, SC	Mild sedation in cats.
Diazepam	0.1–0.5 mg/kg IV	Poor absorption after IM administration. Commonly used in combination with ketamine or propofol for anesthetic induction.
Midazolam	0.1–0.5 mg/kg IM or IV	Commonly used in combination with ketamine or propofol for anesthetic induction.
Xylazine	0.2–1 mg/kg IM, IV	Sedation when (dex) medetomidine is not available.
Dexmedetomidine	3–20 µg/kg IM, IV	Lower doses are used for neuroleptanalgesia while high doses are administered for anesthesia in combination with ketamine and opioid ("kitty magic").
Medetomidine	6–40 µg/kg IM, IV	Same for dexmedetomidine.
Ketamine	3–10 mg/kg IM or PO	Ketamine may be used for sedation in cats when combined with midazolam and an opioid.

basis. Table 42.1 shows doses and routes of administration of sedative agents in cats. Table 42.2 shows doses and routes of administration for opioids in cats. Other drugs: ketamine (3–5 mg/kg) or alfaxalone (2–3 mg/kg) have been administered by the intramuscular route for premedication in the "difficult" cat. Ketamine (5 mg/kg) is combined with an opioid (e.g., buprenorphine 0.02 mg/kg) and midazolam (0.25 mg/kg), or acepromazine (0.05 mg/kg) to facilitate handling.

Q. Does the route of administration impact analgesic efficacy of opioids in cats?

A. Yes. The route of administration influences pharmacokinetics and analgesic effects of opioids. This has been clearly demonstrated with buprenorphine and hydromorphone. Subcutaneous administration of buprenorphine at the current dosage regimens (0.02 mg/kg) and concentrations available (0.3 mg/ml) may induce euphoric behavior and mydriasis but without effective analgesia. A clinical study showed that buprenorphine may produce better post-operative analgesia and lower requirement for rescue analgesia when administered by the intravenous or intramuscular route in cats when compared with the subcutaneous or the oral transmucosal routes [2]. However, this concept should not be applied with the new formulation of buprenorphine (Simbadol® 1.8 mg/ml) that is currently approved for subcutaneous administration in cats in the USA. An open-access review has published guidelines on the clinical use of buprenorphine in cats [3]. Similar findings have been reported with hydromorphone. The subcutaneous route

Table 42.2 Dosage regimens and routes of administration of opioid analgesics in cats.

Opioid analgesic	Dosage regimens	Comments
Butorphanol	0.2–0.4 mg/kg IM, IV	Synergistic sedation when given with the sedative drugs listed in Table 42.1. Poor and short-acting analgesic effects.
Buprenorphine	0.02–0.04 mg/kg IM, IV, PO 0.24 mg/kg SC (Simbadol® every 24h for up to 3 days)	Good analgesia for moderate pain when combined with NSAIDs. Euphoric behavior.
Hydromorphone	0.025–0.1 mg/kg IV, IM	Reliable pain relief. Possible vomiting.
Oxymorphone	0.025 – 0.1 mg/kg IV, IM	Same for hydromorphone. Expensive.
Meperidine	3–5 mg/kg IM	Do not administer IV. Short duration of action.
Morphine	0.1–0.3 mg/kg IM	Vomiting and salivation.
Methadone	0.1–0.4 mg/kg IM, IV, PO	Rarely causes vomiting.
Fentanyl (CRI)	2–3 µg/kg loading dose followed by 3–20 µg/kg/h IV	Dose-dependent analgesia. Possible post-operative dysphoria. See text. Transdermal patches are also available at 12.5 and 25 µg/h.
Naloxone	0.01–0.04 mg/kg IV, IM	Opioid antagonist. It can be diluted in 5 ml of saline 0.9% and given to effect to reverse agitation and respiratory depression.

of administration produced a higher prevalence of adverse effects such as vomiting, and shorter duration of analgesia when compared with the intramuscular or intravenous routes. Meperidine and morphine may cause histamine release and hypotension when given intravenously.

The oral transmucosal route has been used for opioid administration in cats. Buprenorphine is commonly given for post-operative pain by this route. However, recent studies showed a lower bioavailability and potentially more limited application than previously reported. Nevertheless, the authors still find it an adequate option for post-operative analgesia in cases of moderate pain, and when combined with an NSAID. Methadone may be an alternative option for transmucosal administration and post-operative analgesia with similar physicochemical properties to buprenorphine. However, further studies are required in order to provide clinical recommendations. Most importantly, dosages and intervals of administration should be individualized since opioid "non-responders" have been reported. A multimodal analgesic approach is recommended.

Q. How about transdermal analgesia in cats?

A. Transdermal patches of fentanyl have been reported to produce variable plasma concentrations and inconsistent analgesia in the clinical setting, however some patients respond well and this technique may be an option for "hands-off" analgesia in some cases. A new transdermal formulation of fentanyl (Recuvyra™) that can be administered topically in dogs *is not approved nor recommended* for use in cats. The transdermal patch of buprenorphine did not produce adequate analgesia in one study in cats and further clinical investigations are required before any recommendation [4].

Q. There is a general fear of NSAID toxicity in cats. Is this a true concern or are NSAIDs actually an important tool in pain management in this species?

A. Yes, clinicians should be aware of potential toxicity with NSAIDs in any species. However, if dosage regimens, intervals of administration, and contraindications are respected, NSAIDs may be administered safely to cats. *These drugs play an essential role in pain management due to their anti-inflammatory, analgesic, and anti-pyretic effects.* Some strategies may help avoid adverse effects after NSAID administration in the peri-operative period: a thorough physical examination, hematocrit, total protein, and BUN may be a good start to identify potential contraindications to NSAID therapy. Contraindications include vomiting, anorexia, gastrointestinal disease, hypovolemia, hypotension, coagulopathy, hypoproteinemia, hepatopathy, and concomitant administration of corticosteroids. Peri-operative fluid therapy should be administered for kidney protection; hypotension should be avoided with blood pressure monitoring since COX inhibition is detrimental to renal perfusion. These drugs should not be administered to kittens. NSAIDs may be administered at the end of surgery or at recovery if the veterinarian is concerned about anesthetic-related hypotension.

Q. Cats can have degenerative joint disease. What is the current knowledge with NSAID therapy for these patients?

A. For chronic pain, NSAIDs have been shown to be potent analgesics while improving quality of life in cats [5]. Meloxicam (0.05 mg/kg PO daily) has been approved for daily administration in cats in the European Union. However, cats should be screened for other diseases since degenerative joint disease (DJD) and chronic kidney disease (CKD) commonly co-exist in these patients. A recent retrospective study has shown that long-term treatment with meloxicam (0.02–0.03 mg/kg PO every 24 h) did not result in adverse effects in cats with pre-existing CKD (even those at stages II and III) [6]. However, concurrent periodontal disease should be addressed and CKD must be stable. Frequent monitoring and good client communication is advised. The concept of minimum effective dose is important. Some cats with DJD have been successfully treated with two or three low doses of NSAIDs per week. Robenacoxib has shown a great safety and efficacy profile in cats. However, more prospective, randomized, clinical studies are required in patients with naturally occurring disease before recommendations are given.

Q. Laryngospasm is a possible life-threatening anesthetic complication in cats. How is laryngospasm is best avoided and/or treated?

A. Feline airways are small and more sensitive and reactive to laryngeal trauma, spasm, and edema than other species. The larynx may "close" during attempts to intubate; rapid respiratory depression, cyanosis, hypoxia followed by death can occur. In fact, endotracheal intubation has been identified as one of the risk factors of anesthesia in cats. A study in the UK reported that a 63% of cats that died after surgery had endotracheal intubation compared to 48% of non-intubated cats [1]. However, this information can be misleading because high-risk cases (ASA III-V) will most likely be intubated and these data may only represent cats that were already at risk before intubation.

Prevention: Topical desensitization of a cat's laryngeal mucosa via lidocaine administration is the primary means of avoiding laryngospasm. Local anesthetic sprays at concentrations of 10% must be avoided due to the risk of toxicity, edema, and cell damage which seems related to the drug carrier, and not the local anesthetic *per se*. Instead, the anesthetist may "splash" the larynx with 0.05–0.1 ml of lidocaine 2% using a 1-ml syringe via direct visualization using the laryngoscope. Gentle manipulation of the adjacent structures is mandatory. The arytenoids should not be touched at any time. If the anesthetic procedure is short (10–15 min), the larynx may be still desensitized in the recovery period. Endotracheal intubation in cats is commonly facilitated with good sedation and muscle relaxation. Anesthetic depth at induction should be sufficient to prevent gagging or coughing. A plastic stylet may be used within the endotracheal tube to guide intubation. Extubation is commonly performed when palpebral reflexes are strong and before the cat swallows. If extubation is delayed until there is active swallowing, the larynx may spasm upon removal of the tube.

Treatment: The cat should be re-induced with an induction agent and re-intubated. Provide 100% oxygen and then extubate when the cat begins to show signs of palpebral reflexes but is not yet swallowing.

Q. I've heard that mouth gags used in veterinary dentistry or endoscopy may cause blindness in cats. Is this a real concern, and what should one do to prevent this issue?

A. Yes. Mouth gags have been reported as a risk factor following anesthesia in cats [7]. Case reports describing temporary and permanent post-anesthetic blindness following dentistry or endoscopy procedures have now been published in cats. Mouth gags apply a continuous force against the teeth of the maxilla and mandible which can compress the maxillary artery. The latter is the main source of blood flow to the retina and brain in cats, whereas dogs have ancillary arterial supply to the brain and retina via the basilar artery. Opening the mouth will narrow the distance between the medial aspect of the angular process of the mandible and the rostrolateral border of the tympanic bulla; the maxillary artery courses between these two osseous structures [8].

In particular, spring-loaded mouth gags may reduce maxillary artery blood flow and compromise vascular supply to the brain and retina. Therefore, the use of mouth gags should be minimized or used intermittently, or not used at all. If absolutely needed, small mouth gags (20 mm needle caps) can be used and are placed between any teeth of the upper and lower jaws without interference with imaging.

Q. Why do some cats get subcutaneous emphysema?

A. This complication is related to tracheal tears that may occur during intubation or during movement of the intubated cat during a procedure. The tracheal wall of cats is much less resistant to pressure or torque than that of the dog. The endotracheal tube cuff should be inflated only to the point that there is no leak in the circuit (i.e., to effect), rather than arbitrarily inflated by 1–2 ml. During movement of the cat, as might occur when changing sides during a dental cleaning, the cat and the endotracheal tube should be disconnected from the anesthetic circuit so that there is no "drag" on the tube while the cat is being moved. Subcutaneous emphysema usually resolves with time, but is disconcerting and difficult to explain to the owner. Severe cases may progress to pneumothorax, requiring evacuation via chest tube. In the worst case scenario, death can result.

Q. I understand that anesthetic monitoring is essential to avoid morbidity and mortality. Is there anything particular about monitoring in cats that is different than in dogs?

A. Yes. Non-invasive blood pressure (NIBP) measurement relies on the placement of an occluding cuff either via oscillometric or Doppler ultrasonography method. Optimal width for cuff placement is approximately 40% of the limb circumference. The accuracy of the oscillometric technique in cats appears to be highly dependent on the device. The accuracy of the Doppler technique for indirect systolic blood pressure measurement usually correlates better with invasive technique measurements. However, in general the Doppler will underestimate systolic blood pressure in cats. In the clinical setting, blood pressure values of > 70 mmHg via Doppler are considered to be acceptable in cats. Most importantly, continuous monitoring will give an idea of blood pressure trends and should be part of the "big picture" (mucous membrane color, pulse monitoring and pulse oximetry, respiratory rate, etc). On the other hand, measurement of end-tidal carbon dioxide partial pressure ($ETCO_2$) via capnography will often display lower values than P_aCO_2. This is particularly true in side-stream capnography devices using non-rebreathing systems. The mixing of inspired and expired gases using relative high fresh gas flows, associated with the small tidal volume of cats, is the reason for this artifact. Some pulse oximetry devices may not work properly in cats due to their bulky size. Body temperature should be closely monitored to avoid hypothermia. Cats have been reported to also become hyperthermic after the administration of various opioids (see Chapter 20).

Q. Why should one perform loco-regional anesthetic techniques in cats?

A. Loco-regional anesthesia may provide peri-operative analgesia while providing inhalant anesthetic-sparing effects in a cost-effective manner. However, local anesthetic toxicity may occur when dosage regimens and intervals of administration are not properly calculated. In cats, it is well accepted that doses higher than 10 mg/kg of lidocaine (2%) and 2 mg/kg of bupivacaine might induce clinical signs of toxicity such as seizures, cardiorespiratory depression, coma, and death [9]. Bupivacaine must not be administered intravenously. *Clinicians should always check for negative aspiration of blood and resistance to injection to avoid intravenous administration, hematoma, or nerve damage.* The administration of lidocaine spray for endotracheal intubation should be taken in consideration for dose calculations. Overall, loco-regional anesthesia is crucial in the management of peri-operative pain and part of a multimodal analgesic approach. The use of these techniques becomes mandatory when other analgesic options are not available, or are contraindicated (for example NSAIDs).

Q. What are the most common and practical loco-regional anesthetic techniques in cats?

A. Various techniques are described in Chapters 23 and 28, but the most common ones used in cats are:
- ✓ epidural/spinal
- ✓ declaw
- ✓ dental blocks
- ✓ incisional blocks
- ✓ intra-testicular block.

Q. Can you provide what a "typical" anesthetic plan would be if you were managing a healthy and relatively friendly cat scheduled for a dental cleaning with extractions?

A. A combination of a pure μ agonist opioid (methadone, hydromorphone, oxymorphone, or morphine) with a sedative (acepromazine or dexmedetomidine) is commonly administered for pre-medication. Anesthetic induction is performed with either ketamine-diazepam, propofol, or alfaxalone. These drugs are usually given "to effect." Cats are intubated with a cuffed endotracheal tube after the anesthetist has "splashed" the larynx with 0.05–0.1 ml of lidocaine 2% using a 1 ml syringe via direct visualization using the laryngoscope. It is important to perform the "leak" test properly after intubation because debris, liquid, and other content could enter the airways during the procedure. Maintenance of anesthesia is performed with isoflurane or sevoflurane in 100% oxygen. A constant rate infusion of fentanyl can be administered during the procedure if several dental extractions and pain are expected. "Dental blocks" (mandibular, infra-orbital, maxillary, and mental block) are also extremely effective in managing pain during extractions. Bupivacaine (0.2–0.3 ml/site) is used due to its prolonged duration of action in comparison with lidocaine. This local anesthetic is cardiotoxic and total dose should not exceed 2 mg/kg. Negative aspiration of blood is required before injection. Fluid therapy is recommended with an isotonic crystalloid solution at maintenance rates (2–5 ml/kg/h). If there are no contraindications for NSAID administration, these drugs should be given according to the drug label. Monitoring should be "standard" using "hands-on" techniques (pulse palpation, respiratory rate, mucous membranes colors, etc.) in addition to devices such as a Doppler for blood pressure, pulse oximetry, and capnograph. Blood pressure should be monitored to ensure adequate renal perfusion especially when NSAIDs are administered. Post-operative analgesics should be administered until pain is managed. Full mouth extractions may require hospitalization for pain control.

Q. Spay-neuter programs are becoming crucial in our society for the control of overpopulation of cats. What are the general considerations for anesthesia in these programs?

A. The Association of Shelter Veterinarians veterinary medical care guidelines for spay-neuter programs has provided useful insight on how these programs are best implemented and performed [10]. The anesthetic protocol should include drugs that will produce analgesia, muscle relaxation, immobility, and loss of consciousness. Low-volume (literally!) protocols with a wide margin of safety and possible reversibility (especially for alpha-2 agonists) are key parts of the anesthetic regimen. The recovery from anesthesia should be rapid and smooth. The specific anesthetic protocol depends on the number and type of cats (i.e., feral), the skill and efficacy of technical assistance, timing and surgical competence, financial constraints of the program, drug availability, equipment and facilities. It is important to remember that cats have limited glucuronidation and ketamine is actively excreted by the kidneys in this species. Slow and prolonged recoveries can be a problem.

Q. Provide an overall view of the anesthetic management and specific drug protocols in spay-neuter programs.

A. ✓ *Fasting* should be performed according to the age of the cat; pediatrics (6–12 weeks) are usually fasted for only 2 h to avoid hypoglycemia while adult cats are fasted for at least 6 h.

✓ *Hypothermia* may be minimized by avoiding conductive heat loss, limiting body cavity exposure, avoiding excessive hair removal and the use of excessive antiseptic solutions, and by using low-oxygen flows.

✓ *Endotracheal intubation* may not be practical in a feline spay-neuter programs but may be required for treatment of hypoventilation and hypoxemia, and respiratory arrest.

✓ *Intravenous access* is recommended for female cats and may be important for administration of "top-ups" during anesthesia or emergency drugs.

✓ *Local anesthetic techniques* such as incisional, intraperitoneal, and intra-testicular blocks should be administered as part of the multimodal protocol for post-operative analgesia.

✓ *NSAIDs* should be given according to the veterinarian's discretion, the patient's health status, and the exclusion of contraindications to therapy. NSAIDs play a major role in pain relief post-operatively.

✓ *Anticholinergics* are sometimes administered for pediatric cats where cardiac output is more dependent on heart rate, but this is rather the exception than the rule.

✓ *"Hands-on"* monitoring is commonly used for assessment of anesthetic depth (pulse palpation, heart rate, respiratory rate, mucous membrane colors, and neurological reflexes), however some sort of equipment monitoring such as pulse oximetry and capnography may be important to identify and aid treatment of early hypoxemia and hypercapnia.

✓ A protocol for *anesthetic emergencies* should be in place with standard kits and equipment readily available (i.e., source of oxygen, airway and ven-tilation, drugs and reversal agents, charts with volumes, body weights, etc).

✓ *Anesthetic protocols* should be improved *"on the go"* with adjustments of dosage regimens and techniques. Table 42.3 suggests some anesthetic protocols for spay-neuter programs. A successful program includes necropsy and tentative diagnosis of any accidental deaths, and review of anesthetic records.

Q. Can you provide an overall view of anesthesia for the aggressive cat?

A. Aggressive cats may present a particular challenge to veterinarians. Every clinic should be trained, equipped, and have a general protocol in place for the aggressive cat. The aggressive cat is handled in a safe and calm envi-ronment with doors and windows closed. Equipment may include leather gloves, squeeze cages, and anesthetic induction chambers. Historical anes-thetic records should be reviewed and adjustments should be made to the protocol accordingly. The set-up for catheter placement, anesthetic induc-tion, equipment and monitoring should be ready including antagonist drugs. The cat should be handled minimally to avoid stress and injuries to personnel and the patient.

If an intramuscular injection *cannot* be given, transmucosal administration of ketamine (10 mg/kg) with or without dexmedetomidine (15–20 µg/kg) can be an option. The drug(s) are "sprayed" while the cat is hissing at the veterinarian. Ketamine produces profuse salivation, however sedation may be enough for physical restraint and intravenous catheter placement. Intra-venous anesthetics can be used safely for induction and given to effect.

If an intramuscular injection can be given, a combination of tiletamine and zolazepam (telazol) with xylazine have been suggested (see protocols for spay-neuter programs). The alpha-2 agonist (xylazine or dexmedetomidine)

Table 42.3 Anesthetic protocols for spay-neuter programs[a].

Premedication and induction	Comments
Buprenorphine Dexmedetomidine Ketamine	In one syringe of 2 ml, add 1 ml buprenorphine (0.3 mg/ml), 1 ml dexmedetomidine (0.5 mg/ml) and 1 ml ketamine (100 mg/ml). The dose is 0.1–0.15 ml/kg of the mixture IM.
"TKX" Tiletamine/Zolazepam Ketamine Xylazine[b]	In one bottle of tiletamine/zolazepam, add 4 ml of ketamine (100 mg/ml) and 1 ml (100 mg/ml) of xylazine. Each ml contains 80 mg of ketamine, 20 mg of xylazine, 50 mg tiletamine and 50 mg zolazepam. The dose is 0.25 ml for a 3 kg cat IM [11]. The addition of an opioid such as buprenorphine (0.02 mg/kg) IM is recommended. Supplemental doses of 0.05–0.1 ml IV or IM (total) may be required.
"TTDex" Tiletamine/Zolazepam Butorphanol Dexmedetomidine	In one bottle of tiletamine/diazepam, add 2.5 ml of dexmedetomidine and 2.5 ml of butorphanol. Each ml contains 50 mg tiletamine, 50 mg zolazepam, 0.25 mg dexmedetomidine and 5 mg butorphanol. The dose is 0.03–0.04 ml/kg IM for surgical anesthesia [12].

[a]Monitoring and oxygen therapy are always recommended. If needed and possible, maintenance of anesthesia in female cats can be performed with proper intubation and low concentrations of isoflurane (0.5%). Atipamezole (0.2 mg/kg, IM) or yohimbine (0.4 mg/kg) can be given to hasten anesthetic recovery when dexmedetomidine or xylazine has been used, respectively. NSAID administration is recommended if there are no contraindications.
Intraperitoneal and intra-testicular blocks will provide additional analgesia.
[b]When dexmedetomidine is not available or cost-prohibitive.

can be reversed after induction of anesthesia. These cats are extubated before full recovery of consciousness once palpebral reflexes are present. The intravenous catheter is removed before moving the cat into its kennel where the patient is closely watched.

References

1 Brodbelt DC, Pfeiffer DU, Young LE *et al*. Risk factors for anaesthetic-related death in cats: results from the confidential enquiry into perioperative small animal fatalities (CEPSAF). *British Journal of Anesthesia* 2007; **99** 617–623.

2 Giordano T, Steagall PV, Ferreira TH, *et al*. Postoperative analgesic effects of intravenous, intramuscular, subcutaneous or oral transmucosal buprenorphine administered to cats undergoing ovariohysterectomy. *Veterinary Anesthesia and Analgesia* 2010; **37**:357–366.

3 Steagall PV, Monteiro-Steagall BP, Taylor PM. A review of the studies using buprenorphine in cats. *Journal of Veterinary Internal Medicine* 2014; **28**:762–770.

4 Murrell JC, Robertson SA, Taylor PM *et al*. Use of a transdermal matrix patch of buprenorphine in cats: preliminary pharmacokinetic and pharmacodynamic data. *Veterinary Record* 2007; **28**:578–583.

5 Lascelles BD, Court MH, Hardie EM *et al.* Nonsteroidal anti-inflammatory drugs in cats: a review. *Veterinary Anesthesia and Analgesia* 2007; **34**:228–250.

6 Gowan RA, Baral RM, Lingard AE *et al.* A retrospective analysis of the effects of meloxicam on the longevity of aged cats with and without overt chronic kidney disease. *Journal of Feline Medicine and Surgery* 2012; **14**:876–881.

7 Stiles J, Weil AB, Packer RA *et al.* Post-anesthetic cortical blindness in cats: Twenty cases. *The Veterinary Journal* 2012; **193**:367–373.

8 Barton-Lamb AL, Martin-Flores M, Scrivani PV *et al.* Evaluation of maxillary arterial blood flow in anesthetized cats with the mouth closed and open. *The Veterinary Journal* 2013; **196**: 325–331.

9 Pypendop BH, Ilkiw JE. Assessment of the hemodynamic effects of lidocaine administered IV in isoflurane-anesthetized cats. *American Journal of Veterinary Research* 2005; **66**:661–668.

10 Looney AL, Bohling MW, Bushby PA *et al.* The Association of Shelter Veterinarians veterinary medical care guidelines for spay-neuter programs. *Journal of the American Veterinary Medical Association* 2008; **223**:74–86.

11 Williams LS, Levy JK, Robertson SA *et al.* Use of the anesthetic combination of tiletamine, zolazepam, ketamine, and xylazine for neutering feral cats. *Journal of the American Veterinary Medical Association* 2002; **220**:1491–1495.

12 Ko J, Berman A. Anesthesia in shelter medicine. *Topics in Companion Animal Medicine* 2010; **25**:92-97.

43 Anesthetic Management of Rabbits and Ferrets

Darn those little critters!

Katrina Lafferty

University of Wisconsin-Madison, University of Wisconsin Veterinary Care, USA

KEY POINTS:

- Rabbits are a high stress species, which makes working with them stressful for the anesthetist as well. Good premedications can make for a smoother anesthetic event.

- Most of the anesthetic information relevant to ferrets (intubation, catheter placement, monitoring equipment used, local blocks, etc.) is very similar to techniques used in cats.

- Rabbits can be challenging to intubate. However, there are several intubation techniques described in the text and with practice, one can master rabbit intubation.

- Rabbits and ferrets under anesthesia benefit from the same monitoring equipment as canine and feline patients.

- Rabbits and ferrets should be fasted before anesthesia, however, the time requirements are much less than adult canine and feline patients. The fasting times for rabbits and ferrets are more closely in line with neonatal and pediatric patients.

- Rabbits and ferrets are at increased risk for hypothermia; warming devices should be on hand for any case. Judicious monitoring of temperature is advised as overzealous warming can quickly lead to hyperthermia.

Q. What are common reasons to anesthetize a rabbit or ferret?

A. Rabbits commonly present for anesthesia to address dental issues, ocular trauma, urinary calculi, and for castration or ovariohysterectomy. Rabbits are high-stress creatures; with agitated patients it may be safer and less stressful to anesthetize them, rather than physically restrain, for minor procedures like radiographs or large volume venipuncture. Ferrets are rarely sold intact, so anesthesia for spays and neuters is uncommon. Ferrets regularly present for anesthesia to address adrenal or pancreatic tumors. Both species often require anesthesia for bite wounds, orthopedic repair, spinal trauma, and abdominal exploratory.

Questions and Answers in Small Animal Anesthesia, First Edition. Edited by Lesley J. Smith.
© 2016 John Wiley & Sons, Inc. Published 2016 by John Wiley & Sons, Inc.

Q. Are there any concerns when restraining rabbits or ferrets?

A. *Rabbits*: Rabbits require extra care with restraint for several reasons. Lagomorphs have highly developed lumbar and pelvic-limb muscles which allow for rapid bursts of speed when escaping predators. Relative to their size, these muscles are larger and more powerful than those of a horse. When a rabbit is lifted or restrained without securing the hindlegs, it is possible for them to fracture or dislocate lumbar vertebrae, causing spinal damage and potential paralysis [1,2]. Rabbits are at increased risk of hyperthermia during physical restraint. They have thick, dense fur and are not able to effectively control temperature through panting or perspiration. Rabbits have large, highly vascular ears that account for up to 12% of total body surface area. The ears are involved in thermoregulation and if covered during restraint hyperthermia can develop [1–3].

    Ferrets: Ferrets may be nippy, but are fairly easy to restrain using the "scruff and stretch" method. The patient is held with one hand grasping the loose skin over the shoulders and the other hand circling the hips firmly. A gentle stretch is used to restrain the patient, without pulling on the hindlimbs. Ferrets will yawn frequently whenever they are held by the scruff [4].

Q. What should be included in a pre-anesthetic exam?

A. The pre-anesthetic examination requirements for rabbits and ferrets are the same as for any other mammal. General information should include accurate weight, body condition score, hydration status, abdominal palpation, and auscultation of the heart and lungs. If possible blood should be collected for laboratory work; packed cell volume, total protein, and blood glucose are the bare minimum needed before anesthesia. If necessary, venipuncture can be done using sedation [2–4]. Table 43.1 includes a list of normal physical and hematologic parameters for rabbits and ferrets.

Q. For how long should rabbits or ferrets be fasted before anesthesia?

A. *Rabbits*: As a general rule, rabbits are fasted for 0–4 h, depending on nutritional status of the patient. Rabbits are often called a "non-vomiting" species. This group has a highly developed cardiac sphincter which prevents vomiting or regurgitation of food material. Rabbits utilize hind-gut fermentation and may suffer gastrointestinal stasis if held off-feed for extended periods. Some

Table 43.1 Normal values for rabbits and ferrets.

Parameter	Rabbit	Ferret
Temperature (°F)	101.3–104	100–104
Heart rate (beats/min)	135–325	200–400
Respiration rate (breaths/min)	30–60	33–36
Hematocrit (%)	33–50	36–48
Total protein (g/dl)	5.4–8.3	4.5–6.2
Glucose (mg/dl)	75–155	80–117

sources recommend withholding food to decrease stomach and intestinal volume, which may affect ventilation under anesthesia, but such fasting does not seem to produce any clinically appreciable results. If the patient will tolerate it, carefully rinsing or swabbing the mouth before anesthesia can remove large food particles. Water should be made available until surgery [5].

Ferrets: Ferrets have a rapid gastrointestinal transit time, only 3–4 h, and are at higher risk for hypoglygemia. Generally ferrets are held off-feed for 4–6 h; fasting time should be less than 2 h if there is a known insulinoma. Water should be made available until surgery [6,7].

Q. Should I include anesthetic premedication for rabbit or ferret patients?

A. Most patients (regardless of species) should receive premedication before general anesthesia. Premedication will reduce fear, stress, and anxiety. This is of crucial importance in these small mammalian species due to their normally high stress levels, which only increase during hospitalization.

Q. What anesthetic premedications can be used for rabbits and ferrets?

A. When creating an anesthetic plan for any patient, consider the procedure and choose an appropriate combination of sedative and analgesic. For non-painful procedures (radiographs, venipuncture, etc.) it is acceptable to use sedatives alone. For situations where pain is anticipated, a balanced anesthetic approach involving sedatives and analgesics should be provided. There is much research demonstrating pain to be detrimental to the healing process. Many veterinary professionals are concerned about side effects associated with premedication in exotic species, primarily sedation, respiratory depression, and ileus. However, the benefits of providing appropriate analgesia (faster wound healing, reduction of pain-induced ileus, humane patient care) greatly outweigh the risks. With careful and conscientious monitoring many of these concerns can be assuaged [8]. Table 43.2 includes dosages and routes for sedative and analgesic drugs.

Q. What are the preferred sites for intramuscular or subcutaneous injections?

A. Injection sites in rabbits and ferrets are very similar to those in cats and dogs. For subcutaneous injections, the loose skin over the shoulders and back can be used. For intramuscular injections, the lumbar muscles are preferred. Injections in the caudal aspect of the pelvic limbs may irritate the sciatic nerve and cause self-mutilation, particularly in rabbits [2].

Q. Where are the preferred sites for intravenous catheters?

A. *Rabbits*: IV catheters can be placed in the cephalic, lateral saphenous, marginal ear, and jugular veins. Female rabbits often have a large fold of skin under the chin called a dewlap that may make jugular catheter placement challenging [8,9]. Size 22–26 g intravenous catheters are typically used. Figure 43.1 shows catheter placement in the marginal ear vein of a rabbit. This is the preferred site for long-term catheters.

Ferrets: IV catheters can be placed in the cephalic, lateral saphenous, and jugular veins. Size 20–24 g intravenous catheters are typically used. Ferrets

Table 43.2 Sedative and analgesic drug doses.

Drug	Rabbit Dose in mg/kg	Ferret Dose in mg/kg	Comments
Sedatives:			
Acepromazine	0.25–1 (IM,SC)	0.1–0.25 (IM,SC)	May cause hypotension
Dexmedetomidine	0.05–0.1 (IM)	0.04–0.1 (IM)	May cause bradycardia
	0.0005–0.001 (IV)	0.0005–0.001 (IV)	
*Atipamezole	Equal VOLUME to dexmedetomidine (IM,SC,IV)	Equal VOLUME to dexmedetomidine (IM,SC,IV)	Reverses dexmedetomidine
Midazolam	0.25–2 (IM,SC,IV)	0.25–0.5 (IM,SC,IV)	Reverses midazolam
*Flumazenil	0.05–0.1 (IM,SC,IV)	0.05–0.1 (IM,SC,IV)	
Ketamine	5–50 (IM,SC)	5–50 (IM,SC)	Should not be used as a single agent
Analgesics:			
Buprenorphine	0.01–0.05(IM,SC,IV)	0.01–0.03(IM,SC,IV)	Q6–12 h
Butorphanol	0.2–2.0(IM,SC,IV)	0.05–0.4(IM,SC,IV)	Q2–4 h
Oxymorphone	0.05–0.2(IM,SC,IV)	0.05–0.2(IM,SC,IV)	Q6–8 h
Hydromorphone	0.05–0.2(IM,SC,IV)	0.1–0.2(IM,SC,IV)	Q6–8 h
*Naloxone	0.01–0.1(IM,SC,IV)	0.01–0.1(IM,SC,IV)	Opioids reversal (reverses ALL analgesia)
Morphine	0.1 (epidurally)	0.1 (epidurally)	Use preservative-free formulation
Bupivacaine	1.0 (epidurally)	1.0 (epidurally)	Use preservative-free formulation

IM=intramuscular; IV=intravenous; SC=subcutaneous

have tough skin and it may be necessary to make a small nick in the skin using a hypodermic needle at the catheter insertion site. This will prevent the catheter from snagging at placement. The jugular catheter may be difficult to maintain as the tube-like structure of the ferret body can make it hard to secure. Ferrets also resent having bandage material around the neck and may become depressed and anorexic as a result [4,10].

Q. When would you use an intraosseous (IO) catheter? What is the technique?

A. IO catheters are necessary in any patient where the intravenous approach is unattainable. For very small animals, or critical patients suffering from severe dehydration, shock, or circulatory collapse, IO access is often the only choice. The technique for placing an IO catheter in rabbits and ferrets is the same as for canine or feline patients. Preferred sites of IO placement in rabbits are the proximal femur, humerus, or tibia. For additional descriptions on how to place an IO catheter in exotic mammals, the listed reference has excellent information [11]. In ferrets the preferred sites are proximal tibia or proximal femur. IO catheter size will vary based on patient size but range from 18 to 23 g hypodermic needles or 18 to 22 g spinal needles. When using a hypodermic needle it may be necessary to place surgical wire in the lumen, acting as a stylet, to prevent plugging of the needle [2,4].

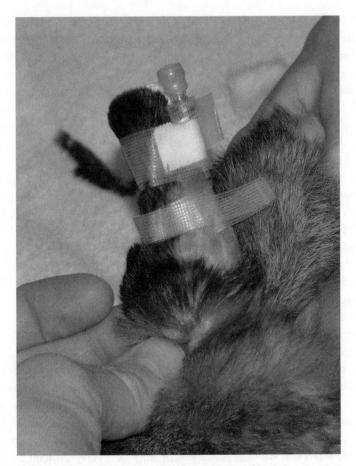

Figure 43.1 Catheter placement in the marginal ear vein of a rabbit.

Q. How should I induce anesthesia in rabbits and ferrets?

A. These patients are usually induced via delivery of inhalant and oxygen by face mask. Rabbits and ferrets should be premedicated before mask induction. Unlike cats and dogs, exotic patients are usually not sedate enough from premedication to place an intravenous catheter. In rabbits, intubation can be challenging and it is therefore not advisable to use induction drugs that are likely to cause apnea. Premedication serves to smooth the mask induction process and decrease the amount of inhalant required. An experienced handler should restrain the rabbit or ferret, taking care not to over-wrap the patient and restrict ventilation or cause hyperthermia. Take care to avoid corneal damage or ocular pressure with the edge of the mask, particularly in rabbits. Pre-oxygenate the patient if possible before starting the inhalant anesthetic. The generally accepted method to induce rabbits or ferrets is for the anesthetist to start with a high level of inhalant until the patient is anesthetized, then decrease to maintenance level. The author tends to start with 3–4% isoflurane, or 4–5% sevoflurane for induction, maintaining that inhalant level only until the patient becomes more relaxed. This is a quicker method of induction, but increases the risk of inhalant overdose. While every case is different and requires an individualized plan, with appropriate pre-medication and analgesia it is reasonable to expect to run patients at 1–2% on isoflurane or 1–3% on sevoflurane. Careful monitoring of the patient is nec-essary throughout the process. Once the patient is sufficiently anesthetized, they should be intubated and have an IV or IO catheter placed [5,12].

Q. What kind of breathing circuits are recommended for rabbits and ferrets?

A. Most rabbits and ferrets will weigh under 5 kg and should be placed on a non-rebreathing circuit. Any standard system – Mapleson, Magill, Bain, Ayre's T-piece – are acceptable types. These systems are lightweight and allow for rapid changes in inspired anesthetic levels. In the absence of carbon diox-ide absorbents, a higher oxygen flow rate is required. 150–200 ml/kg/min will provide adequate patient oxygen levels and effectively remove carbon dioxide from the system. If respiratory rates are higher than 40 breaths/min, the oxygen flow rate should be increased to 300 ml/kg/min [5].

Q. How do you intubate a ferret or rabbit?

A. Generally speaking, endotracheal tubes should be of a size to allow for easy placement and ability to form a good seal within the lumen of the trachea. Most patients should be intubated; intubation facilitates adequate delivery of anesthetic gases to the patient without exposing personnel to waste gases. Intubation also provides a patent airway to provide positive pressure ventila-tion as needed. There are some cases in which intubation may not be feasible. Rarely is this the case with ferrets, which are much like cats in terms of intu-bation. However, in some situations it may be overly difficult to intubate rabbit patients. Extensive oral trauma or dental disease in rabbits may render them physically impossible to intubate. Rabbits are, admittedly, challenging to intubate. In the author's opinion intubation should always be attempted, however, after two or three unsuccessful attempts the animal should be main-tained on a mask. Repeated intubation attempts can lead to a vagal response in many rabbits, particularly those that are not adequately premedicated.

Rabbits: Rabbits have a small oral opening, large, fleshy, firmly attached tongue, and a narrow trachea. For most rabbits endotracheal tubes range from size 1 mm to 3.5 mm [13]. There are four standard techniques for rabbit intubation, three techniques involve orotracheal intubation, the last involves nasotracheal intubation. With all types of intubation, placement can be confirmed through visualization of condensation within the tube, end-tidal carbon dioxide readings on a capnometer, or auscultating bilateral breath sounds during positive pressure ventilation. Intubation of rabbits requires patience and practice. Of the four described methods, the author has found the blind intubation technique to be both the easiest to learn and to teach to others.

✓ "Blind" intubation: As with direct visualization, the rabbit is placed in sternal recumbency with the head and neck in hyperextension. The goal with this restraint technique is to place the trachea in a straight line from mouth to thoracic inlet. The endotracheal tube is placed to one side of the incisors and advanced until condensation appears in the lumen of the endotracheal tube. Condensation in the tube signals exhalation, clearing of the tube signals inspiration. The tube should be advanced gently on inspiration, when the endotracheal tube clears. Very delicate rotation of the tube can displace the epiglottis and allow passage. Figure 43.2 shows blind oral intubation in a rabbit, using an end-tidal carbon dioxide monitor to aid in correct placement.

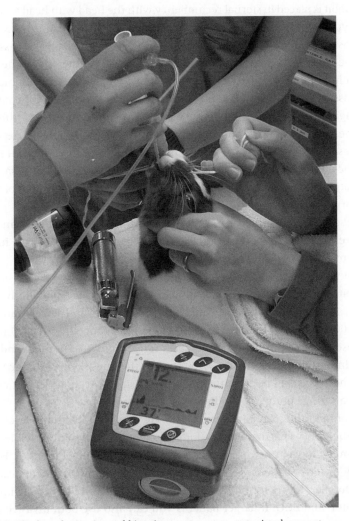

Figure 43.2 Blind intubation in a rabbit using a capnometer to assist placement.

✓ Direct visualization of the glottis: The rabbit is placed in sternal recumbency with the head and neck in hyperextension; gauze or IV tubing can be used behind upper and lower incisors to hold the mouth open. Using a small laryngoscope with a good light source, the blade is used to push the tongue down and visualize the glottis. It is advisable to place a small amount of lidocaine on the glottis to prevent laryngeal spasms. The tube is advanced with or without the use of a stylet.

✓ Indirect visualization of the glottis: This technique is accomplished using an endoscope. The endotracheal tube is passed either next to or over the endoscope. This technique can take much time to master and does require specialized equipment.

✓ Nasotracheal intubation: As with both indirect and direct visualization, the rabbit is placed in sternal recumbency with the head with head and neck in hyperextension. A small endotracheal tube – usually size 1.0–2.5 mm – is passed through the nasal opening, aiming ventro-medial, and passing into the trachea. It is advisable to use lidocaine gel on the end of the tube to help facilitate passage. There will be a certain amount of resistance when passing the endotracheal tube through the tight confines of the nasal passage. At no point should there be any feeling of "crunching" – this means the tube is off track and in the nasal turbinates. As rabbits are obligate nasal breathers, only one side of the nose should be attempted for nasotracheal intubation. If both sides are used and suffer trauma or nasal edema, patients may wake with varying degrees of respiratory distress or respiratory obstruction.

Ferrets: Intubation in ferrets is very straightforward. The glottis can be easily seen using a laryngoscope and positioning similar to that used for feline patients. Size 2.0–3.0 mm endotracheal tubes are required [14].

Q. What fluid rate should I use for anesthetic maintenance?

A. Rabbits and ferrets have higher fluid requirements than many other mammals. Standard maintenance fluid rates for rabbits and ferrets range from 40–100 ml/kg/day. Under anesthesia, fluid rates range from 10–20 ml/kg/h. In cases of shock or hemorrhage, rates range from 30–80 ml/kg and should be administered over 20 min. Even though the rates seem high, the volumes may be very small because the patients are small. Accuracy is best achieved with a syringe pump, IV fluid pump, or buretrol [4].

Q. What monitoring equipment is commonly used for rabbits and ferrets?

A. The short answer is to use everything you would on a canine or feline patient. The much longer answer is broken down by each type of monitor. For most rabbit or ferret patients you can reasonably use a pulse oximeter, capnometer, Doppler flow detector (for pulse and heart rate monitoring), temperature monitor, and ECG. In larger patients you can also use both invasive (in rabbits) or non-invasive blood pressure (both rabbits and ferrets) monitoring.

Regardless of the equipment used, nothing replaces a dedicated person to monitor, hands-on monitoring, and a good stethoscope.

Q. Where would you place a pulse oximeter probe?

A. Options include the tongue, toes, tail, and (in rabbits) scrotum, vulva, and ears. Caution should be used with clip-style probes as these can have a tourniquet effect on small tongues or appendages. Flat reflectance probes can be placed in the mouth, esophagus, or rectum. As with any other species, saturation readings should be at 95% or above. The challenge in obtaining accurate readings often lies in the limitations of the machine. Many monitors have difficulty maintaining accuracy in the face of heart rates over 300. A pulse oximeter is a useful monitoring tool, but cannot be relied upon as a sole indicator of patient stability [3,5].

Q. Can you use end-tidal carbon dioxide monitoring?

A. Yes! $ETCO_2$ monitoring works well in intubated patients. Capnometry is useful as an early alert system for airway occlusion, monitoring respiratory rate, assessing cardiac output, and evaluating ventilation. That said, mainstream capnometers are cumbersome and may add too much weight to the end of the endotracheal tube. Side-stream monitors require a sampling draw of up to 200 ml/min, which may lead to inaccurate and very low readings because of dilution of the sampled gas. There are side-stream capnometers available that require a sampling draw of less than 50 ml/min, providing more accurate numbers in these small patients [5].

Q. Is noninvasive blood pressure monitoring useful?

A. A Doppler ultrasonic flow detector is an invaluable piece of equipment. A probe alone can be placed over any artery to obtain heart rate and rhythm. When an ultrasonic flow probe is placed on a distal limb (carpal is preferred in rabbits; either carpal or tarsal is acceptable in ferrets) in conjunction with a blood pressure cuff, a systolic blood pressure measurement can be obtained. As with most other species, correct blood pressure cuff size is approximately 40% the circumference of the limb. Under anesthesia, systolic blood pressure should be maintained ≥ 90 mmHg [15]. In some larger patients with lower heart rates, oscillometric blood pressure monitors may be able to provide readings. The accuracy of these numbers is difficult to validate, but can be useful in monitoring trends over the duration of the anesthetic episode.

Q. Do I need to worry about thermal support?

A. Small patients are at increased risk of hypothermia due to their increased surface area to volume ratio. Patient temperatures can drop several degrees within minutes. Hypothermia can result in prolonged elimination of anesthetic drugs, bradycardia, respiratory depression, and increased morbidity and mortality. Monitor temperature using either a flexible rectal thermometer or an esophageal temperature probe. Body temperature should be maintained using warming devices such as circulating water blankets, covered warming pads, or warm air convection devices. Take care that patients are not overheated with external warming devices, because while these small patients cool down quickly, they also heat up quickly with iatrogenic heating [4,5].

Q. What do you define as bradycardia in rabbits and ferrets and how do you treat it?

A. In rabbits and ferrets, a heart rate below 200 beats per minute requires intervention. Atropine can be readily administered to ferrets. Many rabbits have high circulating levels of atropine-ase, an enzyme that will rapidly hydrolyze atropine, and thus rabbits require a much higher dose of atropine, or glycopyrrolate may be a better choice. Anticholinergics can have the added benefit of decreasing mucus production, which may in turn reduce the risk of mucus plugs in the endotracheal tube. However, while production is decreased, glycopyrrolate and atropine can increase the viscosity of the mucus, making it harder to remove plugs that do form. Use of anticholinergics for reduction of mucus production is a controversial subject [13]. See Table 43.3 for a list of common emergency drugs and doses.

Q. Are any loco-regional techniques used in rabbits and ferrets?

A. Epidural analgesia is an integral part of pain management in canine and feline patients and has definite applications for rabbits and ferrets. Epidurals can be used for any procedure where abdominal or hindlimb pain is anticipated. Epidurals can also be useful for surgeries involving the anus or external urinary tract. The technique for epidural placement in rabbits and ferrets is essentially the same as for other species, as described in Chapter 23. Preservative-free morphine can be used for both species. Analgesia lasts from 12–24 h in most cases. Preservative-free bupivacaine can be added to the epidural for more comprehensive pain management.

Table 43.3 Emergency drug doses.

Drug	Rabbit Dose in mg/kg	Ferret Dose in mg/kg	Comments
Atropine	0.1 (IM,SC,IV, IO, IT)	0.04 (IM,SC,IV, IO, IT)	
Glycopyrrolate	0.01–0.05 (IM,IV)	0.01–0.05 (IM,IV)	Longer onset and longer duration than atropine
Epinephrine (1:1000)	0.01–0.1 (IM,IV,IO,IT)	0.01–0.1 (IM,IV,IO,IT)	Dilute for IV use
Lidocaine	1–2 (IV)	1–2 (IV)	
Atipamezole	Equal VOLUME to dexmedetomidine (IM,SC,IV)	Equal VOLUME to dexmedetomidine (IM,SC,IV)	Reverses dexmedetomidine
Flumazenil	0.05–0.1 (IM,SC,IV)	0.05–0.1 (IM,SC,IV)	Reverses midazolam
Naloxone	0.01–0.1(IM,SC,IV)	0.01–0.1(IM,SC,IV)	Reverses opioids (reverses ALL analgesia)

IM=intramuscular; IV=intravenous; SC=subcutaneous; IT=intratracheal; IO=intraosseous

Many other loco-regional analgesic techniques are relevant in rabbit and ferret patients. Line blocks, ring blocks, brachial plexus blocks, and intra-testicular blocks are all useful analgesic techniques. Generally speaking the techniques for the listed blocks are the same as in canine or feline patients. A dose of 2 mg/kg of lidocaine or 1 mg/kg of bupivacaine can be used. The amount and volumes of the drugs used can be very small, so make certain to double (or triple) check mathematic calculations [5,12].

Q. What emergency drugs should be available?

A. Treat a respiratory or cardiac arrest as you would for any species. Obtain an airway and venous access. Begin chest compressions immediately in the case of cardiac arrest. The same drugs should be available as for any emergency situation: atropine, epinephrine, lidocaine, and appropriate reversal agents [5]. For resuscitation drug doses, see Table 43.3.

Q. What are the considerations for recovery?

A. Patients should be held, wrapped in a towel and without restricting the chest, until all righting reflexes have returned. The patient should be able to stand unsupported and with good balance. Rabbits that are let go too soon may kick or flail and cause vertebral dislocation or other trauma. Keep patients in a warm, quiet area where they can be monitored closely, but without distressing the animal. Heart rate, respiratory rate, and temperature should be monitored regularly for at least 3 h post-anesthesia. Watch the IV catheter carefully as most rabbits or ferrets will try to chew it out once fully awake [5,13].

Q. Do you ever reverse the any anesthetic drugs?

A. If the patient still seems "sleepy" or is taking a long time to recover, the sedative can be reversed. Rabbits, in particular, seem to have a lengthy recovery when given midazolam. This is not a reason to avoid using it as an anesthetic premedication. See Table 43.2 for doses of reversal agents.

Q. Can nonsteroidal anti-inflammatory drugs (NSAIDs) be used in rabbits and ferrets?

A. NSAIDS can and should be used as part of a multimodal analgesic plan for appropriate cases. The usage of NSAIDs in rabbits and ferrets carries the same concerns as with canine and feline patients. NSAIDs should not be given to dehydrated patients or those suffering gastrointestinal, hepatic, or renal dysfunction. Any rabbits or ferrets receiving long-term NSAID treatment should have blood chemistry values checked regularly [5,13]. See Table 43.4 for NSAID drugs and dosage information.

Q. How soon after anesthesia should rabbits or ferrets be offered food?

A. Rabbits are hindgut-fermenters and require food to be continually moving through the gastrointestinal tract in order to prevent ileus or GI stasis [2]. Ferrets have an extremely short gastrointestinal transit time and may be at increased risk of hypoglycemia if they have an insulinoma present [4]. For these reasons, food should be offered to rabbit and ferret patients as soon as they are awake, aware, and able to stand reasonably well.

Table 43.4   NSAID drug doses.

Drug	Rabbit Dose in mg/kg	Ferret Dose in mg/kg	Comments
Carprofen	1.5–5.0 (PO,SC)	2–5 (PO, SC)	Q12–24 h
Ketoprofen	1–3 (IM)	1–3 (SC, IM)	Q12–24 h
Meloxicam	0.1–0.3 (PO, SC)	0.1–0.3 (PO, SC)	Q24 h

PO=by mouth; SC=subcutaneous

References

1 Vella D, Donnelly T. Basic anatomy, physiology, and husbandry (rabbits). In: Quesenberry KE, Carpenter JW (eds) *Ferrets, Rabbits, and Rodents: Clinical Medicine and Surgery*, 3rd edn. Elsevier Saunders: St. Louis, 2012:157–173.

2 Graham J, Mader DR. Basic approach to veterinary care (rabbits). In: Quesenberry KE, Carpenter JW (eds) *Ferrets, Rabbits, and Rodents: Clinical Medicine and Surgery*, 3rd edn. Elsevier Saunders: St. Louis, 2012:174–182.

3 Heard DJ. Lagomorphs (Rabbits, hares, and pikas). In: West G, Heard D, Caulkett N (eds) *Zoo Animal and Wildlife Immobilization and Anesthesia*, 1st edn. Blackwell Publishing: Ames, 2007:647–653.

4 Quesenberry KE, Orcutt C. Basic approach to veterinary care (ferrets). In: Quesenberry KE, Carpenter JW (eds) *Ferrets, Rabbits, and Rodents: Clinical Medicine and Surgery*, 3rd edn. Elsevier Saunders: St. Louis, 2012:13–26.

5 Hawkins MG, Pascoe PJ. Anesthesia, analgesia, and sedation of small mammals. In: Quesenberry KE, Carpenter JW (eds) *Ferrets, Rabbits, and Rodents: Clinical Medicine and Surgery*, 3rd edn. Elsevier Saunders: St. Louis, 2012:429–451.

6 Muir WW, Hubbel JAE, Bednarski RM, *et al.* Anesthetic procedures in exotic animals. In: *Handbook of Veterinary Anesthesia*, 4th edn. Mosby Elsevier: St. Louis, 2007:438–484.

7 Evans T, Springsteen KK. Anesthesia of ferrets. *Seminars in Avian and Exotic Pet Medicine* 1998; **7(1)**:48–52.

8 Johnston MS. Clinical Approaches to analgesia in ferrets and rabbits. *Seminars in Avian and Exotic Pet Medicine* 2005; **14(4)**:229–235.

9 Lichtenberger M. Transfusion medicine in exotic pets. *Clinical Techniques in Small Animal Practice* 2004; **19(2)**:88–95.

10 Castanheira de Matos RE, Morrisey JK. Common procedures in the pet ferret. *Veterinary Clinics of North America: Exotic Animal Practice* 2006; **9(2)**:347–365.

11 Lennox AM. Intraosseous catheterization of exotic animals. *Journal of Exotic Pet Medicine* 2008; **17(4)**:300–306.

12 Wenger S. Anesthesia and analgesia in rabbits and rodents. *Journal of Exotic Pet Medicine* 2012; **21**:7–16.

13 Lichtenberger M, Ko J. Anesthesia and analgesia for small mammals and birds. *Veterinary Clinics of North America: Exotic Animal Practice* 2007; **10**:293–15.

14 Lennox AM, Capello V. Tracheal intubation in exotic companion mammals. *Journal of Exotic Pet Medicine* 2008; **17(3)**:221–227.

15 Bailey JE, Pablo LS. Anesthetic monitoring and monitoring equipment: application in a small exotic pet practice. *Seminars in Avian and Exotic Pet Medicine* 1998; **7(1)**:53–60.

44 Anesthetic Management of Birds

A fine feathered friend!

Katrina Lafferty

University of Wisconsin-Madison, University of Wisconsin Veterinary Care, USA

KEY POINTS:

- Birds should always be sedated/premedicated before handling and anesthesia. Most birds seen in a clinical setting are prey species and thus are easily stressed by handling. Premedications can reduce stress levels allowing for more thorough physical examination and smoother anesthesia.

- Avians have many unique anatomic differences that impact handling and anesthesia. Extra care should be used when handling birds not to restrict the chest. Birds do not have a diaphragm and must use thoracic muscles to breathe.

- Compared to many other species, avian patients are easy to intubate. Most birds lack a glottis and visualization of the trachea is straightforward.

- Anesthetized birds should always be intubated. Avian patients do not ventilate well under anesthesia. Their complex and highly efficient respiratory system cannot handle any periods of apnea.

- Most monitors used in traditional canine and feline patients can be used on avian patients. There is a need from some modifications in placement locations, but standard monitors (pulse oximetry, capnometry, Doppler flow detector, etc.) can and should be used to monitor anesthetized patients.

- Most birds should be fasted before anesthesia. Healthy birds should be fasted for about 1 h per 100 g of body weight. Compromised patients may not tolerate any degree of fasting.

Q. What are common reasons that birds require anesthesia?

A. There are numerous cases where an avian patient may require anesthesia. Leg, wing, and beak fractures are common presentations. Birds often suffer reproductive issues requiring surgical intervention. Examples include repairing a prolapsed cloaca or removing a retained egg. Endoscopically-guided crop, liver, and gastrointestinal biopsies are routinely required for a diagnosis and will require general anesthesia. In some cases it may be safer, easier,

---

Questions and Answers in Small Animal Anesthesia, First Edition. Edited by Lesley J. Smith.
© 2016 John Wiley & Sons, Inc. Published 2016 by John Wiley & Sons, Inc.

and less stressful to anesthetize a bird, rather than physically restrain it, for minor procedures such as beak trims, implant placements, radiographs, or larger volume venipuncture [1].

Q. Are there any concerns when restraining avian patients?

A. Birds have a unique respiratory system that is easily compromised by overzealous restraint. Birds have no diaphragm and utilize thoracic muscula-ture for both inhalation and exhalation [2]. Restriction of the thoracic cavity will inhibit adequate breathing/tidal volume. Birds have complete tracheal rings, but these can be collapsed during aggressive manual restraint [1].

Q. What should be evaluated in a pre-anesthetic exam?

A. The pre-anesthesia examination requirements in birds are essentially the same as for canines and felines. Basic information should include weight, body condition, hydration status, and auscultation of the heart, dorsal lungs, and ventral air sacs [1,3]. If possible, blood should be collected for laboratory work; packed cell volume (range 35–55%), total protein (range 3.5–5.5 g/dl), and blood glucose (~200 mg/dl) are the bare minimum needed before anesthesia. The benefits of pre-anesthetic blood work should be weighed against the risks of restraint [1]. Venipuncture can also be done after sedation.

Q. For how long should avian patients be fasted before anesthesia?

A. Having an empty crop and stomach reduces the potential for regurgitation and aspiration of gastric contents. For patients in dorsal recumbency, fast-ing can decrease pressure on the lungs from the weight of the stomach and intestines. The suggested duration of fasting is generally 1 h per 100 g of body weight. For example, a parrot weighing 600 g should be fasted for about 6 h. For birds less than 100 g, fasting is not recommended. In critical cases fasting may not be an option before anesthesia. In these situations intubation is a must. Keeping the head elevated during anesthesia and recovery may reduce the risk of regurgitation and aspiration [4].

Q. Should avian patients receive premedication before anesthesia?

A. All avian patients (regardless of species) should receive premedication before general anesthesia. Premedication reduces fear, stress, and anxiety in patients. Handling of unsedated birds can cause a physiologic stress response that may result in decompensation, collapse, or death. Sedation of avian patients reduces stress and can facilitate minor procedures such as examination, venipuncture, and radiographs [5]. Premedication makes for a smoother induction to general anesthesia and reduces the amount of inhalant anesthetics required for induction and maintenance [3].

Q. What sedatives are safe to use in birds as premedications?

A. Benzodiazepines are considered safest for avian sedation. They cause little respiratory or cardiovascular depression and are reversible. Unlike mammalian species, birds become quite sedate after benzodiazepines are administered. Midazolam is the preferred choice; it is water-soluble and

Table 44.1 Sedation and analgesia drug doses [1,6–8].

Drug	Dose	Comments
Midazolam	0.2–2.0 mg/kg (IM,IV,IN)	Generally lower doses needed IV High doses result in more profound sedation
Flumazenil	0.02–0.1 mg/kg (IM,IV,IN)	Reverses benzodiazepines
Butorphanol	0.5–4 mg/kg (IM,IV)	
Butorphanol CRI	0.075 mcg/kg/min (IV)	May require loading dose
Naloxone	0.01–0.04 mg/kg (IM,IV)	Reverses opioids (reverses ALL analgesia)

IM=intramuscular; IV=intravenous; IN=intranasal

safely administered by various routes. Higher doses result in more profound sedation; this may or may not be desired depending on procedure and patient temperament. Midazolam is reversed with flumazenil [1,6]. See Table 44.1 for drugs and doses.

Q. What opioids are safe to use in birds?

A. For non-painful procedures (radiographs, venipuncture, etc.) it is acceptable to use sedatives alone. For any situation where pain can be expected, however, a balanced anesthetic approach involving sedatives and analgesics should be provided. Much conflicting information exists on which analgesics work best for birds. Current research suggests that, unlike mammals, most avian species receive adequate levels of analgesia from butorphanol [1,6–8]. In psittacines, butorphanol can be given as a constant rate infusion to maintain analgesia [6]. See Table 44.1 for suggested doses.

Q. What are the preferred sites for injections?

A. Small volumes of isotonic fluid are commonly given to birds subcutaneously. Taking care not to over expand the area, 5–10 ml per site can be instilled over the inguinal, axillary, or scapular regions [1]. Birds possess a complex renal-portal system with specialized valves that control the flow of venous blood through the body. Epinephrine release (sympathetic stimulation) causes relaxation of the valve and blood from the hindlimbs enters into the body's central circulation. However, acetylcholine release (parasympathetic stimulation) causes contraction of the valve and blood from the legs is shunted directly through the kidneys. The impact of the renal portal system is complicated and not completely understood, but there is concern regarding intramuscular injections of nephrotoxic drugs (e.g., antibiotics) in the hindlimbs. As a general rule it is safe to give any IM injections in the pectoral muscles. IM injections in the legs should only be use for drugs that do not have a negative impact on the kidneys [9].

Q. Is the intranasal route of injection an option?

A. Midazolam, and its reversal agent flumazenil, both work well administered intranasally (IN). One study showed that 2 mg/kg midazolam IN resulted in adequate sedation for restraint and examination within a few minutes. Flumazenil given IN at 0.05 mg/kg reversed sedation within 10 min [5]. This is an ideal route for birds that may be too compromised for handling and IM injections.

Q. After sedation, how do I induce anesthesia in a bird?

A. In birds, induction is almost always performed by delivery of oxygen and inhalant by mask. An experienced handler should restrain the bird, taking care not to restrict ventilation. The beak and nares are completely covered by a face mask. There are many avian species and attendant facial shapes, so it may be necessary to fashion an induction mask to fit the patient. These can be created used various sizes of soda bottles or syringe cases. For small birds, the entire head can fit inside the mask. Avoid ocular damage with the edge of the mask. There are two ways to induce a bird with inhalant anesthetics. The first is "low to high" where the anesthetic is set at a low level and incrementally increased. This method may take slightly longer and causes more of an excitement phase, but it decreases exposure of patient and staff to excessive levels of inhalant. The second method is "high to low" whereby the anesthetist starts with a high level of inhalant until the patient is anesthetized, then decreases to maintenance level. This is a quicker method of induction, but increases the risk of inhalant overdose [3].

Q. How do you intubate a bird?

A. Birds over 80 g should always be intubated [3]. It may not be possible to intubate birds less than 80 g due to lack of available equipment. As discussed further on, birds have a very efficient respiratory system but cannot tolerate apnea. Intubation allows for control of ventilation, improved monitoring capabilities, and a secure airway in case of emergency [1]. Technically speaking, most species of birds are relatively easy to intubate. Endotracheal tube size varies based on species but can range from an 18 gauge intravenous catheter (e.g., Cockatiels, Parrots, Lovebirds) to a 7 mm endotracheal tube (e.g., Pelicans, Eagles, large Turkeys, large Geese, Cranes). Most pet birds will fall into the 2.5–5 mm range (Cockatoos, Macaws, African Greys, large Conures). Birds lack an epiglottis making visualization of the airway very simple. The glottis is typically located at the base of the tongue. Birds have complete tracheal rings and un-cuffed endotracheal tubes should be used for intubation. If a cuffed tube is used, the cuff should not be inflated in order to prevent ischemic damage to the trachea. Use extreme care not to move the endotracheal tube once placed; the friction from movement may cause tracheal tears, ruptures, or strictures [9]. The tube should be secured with tape

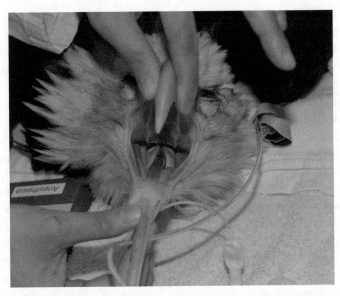

Figure 44.1 Endotracheal intubation in an eagle. Note the obvious airway opening at the base of the tongue. Courtesy of C. Mans.

to the mandible allowing for continued visualization of the mouth and throat during anesthesia [1]. A small syringe or syringe case can be used to prevent the patient biting through the endotracheal tube if they become very light. Figure 44.1 shows intubation in a bald eagle. This is not a typical species seen in general practice, but the photo illustrates the anatomy well.

Q. What kind of breathing circuits are recommended for birds?

A. Most avian patients are small enough to require a non-rebreathing circuit. These systems are lightweight and allow for rapid changes in inspired anesthetic concentrations. As the system does not utilize any kind of carbon dioxide absorbent, a higher oxygen flow rate is required [1]. Recommended flow rate for an Ayre's T-piece is 400 ml/kg/min; recommended flow rate for a Bain system is 200 ml/kg/min [3].

Q. Do I need to worry about ventilating a bird?

A. Yes you do! Birds often do not breathe well under anesthesia. Some of this may be anesthetically induced; premedications and inhalants can depress the respiratory center and cause relaxation of the muscles controlling ventilation [10]. Some of it can be due to positioning; birds lack a diaphragm and when positioned in dorsal recumbency the weight of coelomic viscera further restricts ventilation [1]. Birds have a very efficient respiratory design comprised of lungs and air sacs, with a flow through ventilation system that will not tolerate apnea. Cardiac arrest can occur in a bird after just two minutes of apnea [11]. A spontaneous respiratory rate under anesthesia of 10–25 breaths per min is appropriate for larger birds, 30–40 breaths per min for smaller birds [3]. If manual ventilation is required, a rate of 6–10 breaths per min is sufficient [1]. Avian lungs are rigid and firmly attached to the dorsum. They do not expand well and are susceptible to lung and air sac trauma with overly forceful ventilation. Positive pressure ventilation with a peak inspiratory pressure of 5–15 cm of H_2O will give an adequate breath [3].

Q. How do the air sacs fit into ventilation and gas exchange?

A. The avian respiratory system is designed for flight and it is very different from a mammalian system. Birds have no diaphragm, and large, rigid lungs attached to the body wall. Avian tracheal volume is 4.5 times larger than mammals of equal size. They compensate for the increased dead space of a larger trachea with a lower respiratory rate and higher tidal volume than comparably sized mammals [2]. Most avian species have nine air sacs: paired cervical, cranial thoracic, caudal thoracic, and abdominal air sacs, and a single inter-clavicular air sac. Air sacs are not vascular and do not participate in gas exchange. Birds have unidirectional flow within the respiratory system and air sacs act as a bellows to continually push air through the system. It takes two complete sets of inspiration and expiration to cycle a breath through the entire respiratory system. Again, this illustrates why continuous ventilation is such an important element of avian anesthesia [1].

Q. When would you use an air sac cannula for anesthesia?

A. Air sac cannulas have some similarities to a tracheostomy tube in mammalian patients. The unique design of the avian respiratory system allows air sacs to play a role in ventilation. While air sacs do not engage in gas exchange, anesthetic gas instilled into an air sac will be pushed in a unidirectional fashion through the respiratory system and into the lungs where gas exchange does occur. Air sac cannulas can be used for anesthetic maintenance in birds too small to intubate. They are also indicated in cases of partial or complete upper airway obstruction. Surgical cases involving the head, beak, or upper airway may require air sac cannulation. Air sac cannulas are used to provide additional or long term support for patients with ongoing respiratory distress [1,3,12].

Q. How does one place an air sac cannula?

A. The cannula is generally placed in either the left caudal thoracic air sac or the left abdominal air sac. The right-sided counterparts to those specific air sacs rest near the right liver lobe and should be avoided because of the risk of accidental hepatic trauma. A variety of tubes can be used: red rubber catheters, size 18 gauge or larger intravenous catheters, or standard endotracheal tubes. Cannulas should be shortened to an appropriate length for the air sac. To choose the right size cannula, consider the size tube required for endotracheal intubation and go up at least one size. Placement of the cannula is not a difficult procedure. Using sterile prep and technique, a small incision is made over the desired location and the cannula is fed into the air sac. The tissue is closed around the cannula forming a compete seal [1]. There are few reports

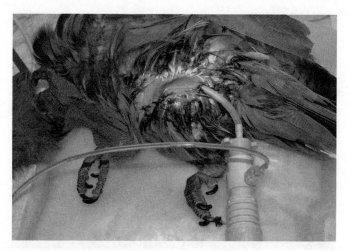

Figure 44.2 Air sac cannulation of the caudal thoracic air sac in an African grey parrot. Courtesy of C Mans.

of complications associated with air sac placement but they include infection at the site, transient subcutaneous emphysema, and blockage of the cannula [1,12]. Capnometry can be used with the air sac cannula, similar to endotracheal intubation. Figure 44.2 shows a parrot anesthetized using a caudal thoracic air sac cannula.

Q. Where are the preferred sites for intravenous catheters?

A. There are three common sites for IV catheter placement: right jugular, ulnar (wing vein), or medial metatarsal vein. Each have pros and cons. The right jugular vein is the largest vessel and catheter placement is not difficult, but may be challenging to maintain. If the patient pulls the IV catheter after anesthesia, they could die from acute blood loss [1]. The wing vein is usually easy to locate and visualize, but is fragile and at an awkward angle. Patients will need to be under general anesthesia for placement of a catheter in the ulnar vein. This location is prone to hematoma formation and pressure should be applied for as long as necessary when removing the catheter. The medial metatarsal vein is an excellent choice in long-legged birds and in some larger parrots. It can typically be maintained post-operatively. It is located on the medial aspect of the leg and can be harder to visualize in heavily feathered or pigmented patients. IV catheter sizes vary based on species but range from 20 to 26 gauge [1,13]. Figure 44.3 shows a medial metatarsal IV catheter in an African Grey parrot.

Q. When would you use an intraosseous catheter?

A. IO catheters are often required for very small patients where intravenous access is unattainable. For critical patients suffering from severe dehydration, shock, or circulatory collapse IO access is often the only option [1].

Q. What is the technique for placing an intraosseous catheter?

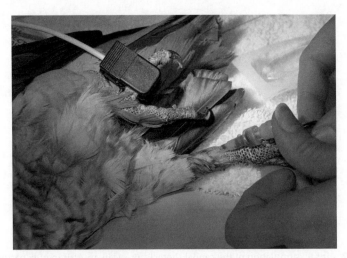

Figure 44.3 IV catheter placement in the medial metatarsal vein in an African grey parrot. Also shows toe placement of a pulse oximeter probe. Courtesy of C. Mans.

A. The technique for placing an IO catheter in birds is the same as in a canine or feline patient. However, when choosing a location, do not use the humerus or femur in avian patients. In most avian species these bones are pneumatized and involved in respiration. Introduction of fluid into these pneumatic bones can drown the patient. Preferred sites of IO placement in birds are the distal ulna and proximal tibiotarsus [3]. IO catheter size will vary based on species but range from 18 to 25 gauge hypodermic needles or 18 to 24 gauge spinal needles [1]. Figure 44.4 shows an IO catheter placed in the proximal tibio-tarsus of an African Grey parrot. A 22 gauge hypodermic needle was used.

Q. What IV fluid rate should I use under anesthesia?

A. Birds have higher fluid requirements than mammals. Standard maintenance fluid rates for birds range from 40–100 ml/kg/day. Under anesthesia, fluid rates range from 10–20 ml/kg/h. In cases of shock or hemorrhage, rates range from 30–80 ml/kg and should be administered over 20 min. Even though the rates seem high, the volumes will be very small. Accuracy is best achieved with a syringe pump, IV fluid pump, or buretrol [11].

Q. What monitoring equipment is used in avian anesthesia?

A. The short answer is to use everything you would on a canine or feline patient. Regardless what equipment is used, nothing replaces hands-on monitoring and a good stethoscope. Limitations for pulse oximetry and capnography are similar to those for other small exotic species.

Q. Can you accurately measure blood pressure in birds?

A. Birds have a "high perfusion" cardiovascular system designed for running, flying, and swimming [4]. An avian heart is both larger and thicker than a mammal of equivalent size. The heart takes up a larger percentage of body weight. To compensate for increased size and weight of the heart, avian blood

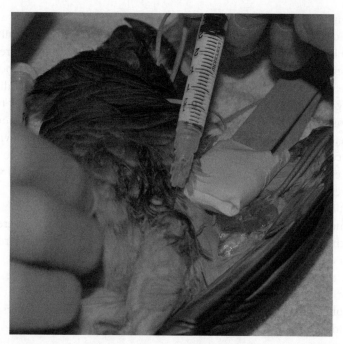

Figure 44.4 Intraosseous catheter placement in the proximal tibiotarsus of an African grey parrot. Also shows placement of the Doppler crystal over the brachial artery. Courtesy of C. Mans.

pressure values are much higher. Mean arterial pressures have been recorded ranging from 100–250 mmHg depending on the species [17]. These anatomic differences often confound traditional oscillometric blood pressure monitors. A study comparing direct arterial pressure to both oscillometric and Doppler blood pressure readings found oscillometric readings to be erroneous more than half the time. However, the Doppler readings were strongly consistent with the invasive mean arterial pressures (MAP) [18]. Extrapolating from studies done on pigeons, MAP should be maintained between 70–100 mmHg under anesthesia [17]. To obtain a pressure reading using a Doppler, the crystal can be placed on the brachial artery, or medial metatarsal artery, with an appropriately sized cuff placed proximal to the crystal. It is not necessary to pluck feathers to place the crystal. In patients too small to obtain blood pressure readings, the Doppler can be used effectively to monitor heart rate and rhythm.

Q. How can I get an ECG to work on a bird?

A. ECG lead placement is the same as in canine and feline patients. Alligator clips can be used with the teeth flattened to prevent tearing of the skin. Alternatively, 25 g needles through the skin with the alligator clip clamped on to the needle will work well in most birds and is often the preferred placement technique [14].

Q. How important is thermal support?

A. The normal temperature of most birds ranges from 102–109 °F. Small patients are at increased risk of hypothermia due to their increased surface area to volume ratio. Patients can drop several degrees within minutes. Hypothermia can result in prolonged elimination of anesthetic drugs, bradycardia, respiratory depression, and increased morbidity and mortality. Monitor temperature using either a flexible rectal thermometer or an esophageal temperature probe. Body temperature should be maintained using warming devices such as circulating water blankets, covered warming pads, or warm air convection devices. Take care that patients are not over-heated with external warming devices [1].

Q. What is defined as bradycardia in birds? How do you treat it?

A. For most species, a heart rate below 200 beats per min warrants treatment. Anticholinergics are the treatment of choice and are effective in birds [1,9].

Q. What emergency drugs should be available?

A. Treat a respiratory or cardiac arrest as you would for any species. Obtain an airway and venous access. Begin chest compressions immediately in the case of cardiac arrest. Atropine, epinephrine, and appropriate reversal agents should be on hand [8]. See Table 44.2 for an emergency chart.

Q. How should I recover a bird?

A. Birds should be extubated once they begin swallowing and coughing. Take care to remove the endotracheal tube before the animal is awake enough to bite through the tube [1]. They should be held wrapped in a towel, without restricting the chest, until all righting reflexes have returned. The bird should be able to stand unsupported and with good balance. Birds that are let go too soon may flail and fracture a wing or leg. Keep patients in a warm, quiet area where they can be monitored closely, but without disturbing the bird. Watch the IV catheter carefully as most birds will chew it out once fully awake [4].

Table 44.2 Emergency drug doses for birds.

Avian ER Drugs	Atropine 0.5 mg/kg IV, IO, IT (0.4 mg/ml)	Flumazenil 0.05 mg/kg IV (0.1 mg/ml)	Naloxone 0.04 mg/kg IV (0.4 mg/ml)	Epinephrine 0.5 mg/kg IV, IO, IT (1:1000)
25 g	0.03 ml	0.01 ml	0.0025 ml	0.013 ml
50 g	0.06 ml	0.03 ml	0.005 ml	0.03 ml
75 g	0.09 ml	0.04 ml	0.01 ml	0.04 ml
100 g	0.13 ml	0.05 ml	0.01 ml	0.05 ml
300 g	0.38 ml	0.15 ml	0.03 ml	0.15 ml
500 g	0.63 ml	0.25 ml	0.05 ml	0.25 ml
750 g	0.94 ml	0.4 ml	0.08 ml	0.4 ml
1000 g	1.25 ml	0.5 ml	0.1 ml	0.5 ml

Q. Do you ever reverse any anesthetic drugs?

A. If the patient still seems "sleepy" or is taking a long time to recover, the midazolam can be reversed with flumazenil at 0.02–0.1 mg/kg. Butorphanol can be reversed, but this does reverse *all* analgesia as well. Naloxone is given at 0.01–0.04 mg/kg IM.

Q. When is it safe to send a bird home after anesthesia?

A. Avian patients are safe to go home once they are able to stand, perch, eat, and drink, and when pain is well managed.

References

1 Hawkins MG, Pascoe PJ. Cage birds. In: West G, Heard D, Caulkett N (eds) *Zoo Animal and Wildlife Immobilization and Anesthesia*, 1st edn. Blackwell Publishing: Ames, 2007: 269–297.

2 Pablo LS. Avian anesthesia. In: Greene SA (ed.) *Veterinary Anesthesia and Pain Management Secrets*, 1st edn. Hanley & Belfus: Philadelphia, 2002:275–282.

3 Gunkel C, Lafortune M. Current techniques in avian anesthesia. *Seminars in Avian and Exotic Pet Medicine* 2005; **14(4)**:263–276.

4 Lierz M, Korbel R. Anesthesia and analgesia in birds. *Journal of Exotic Pet Medicine* 2012; **21(1)**:44–58.

5 Mans C, Guzman DSM, Lahner LL, *et al*. Sedation and physiologic response to manual restraint after intranasal administration of midazolam in Hispaniolan Amazon parrots (Amazona ventralis). *Journal of Avian Medicine and Surgery* 2012; **26(3)**:130–139.

6 Carpenter JW, Marion CJ. *Exotic Animal Formulary*, 4th edn. Elsevier Saunders: St. Louis, 2012.

7 Hawkins MG, Paul-Murphy J. Avian analgesia. *Veterinary Clinics of North America: Exotic Animal Practice* 2011; **14(1)**:62–80.

8 Machin KL. Avian analgesia. *Seminars in Avian and Exotic Pet Medicine* 2005; **14(4)**:236–242.

9 Ludders JW, Matthews NS. Birds. In: *Lumb and Jones' Veterinary Anesthesia and Analgesia*, 4th edn. Blackwell Publishing: Ames, 2007:841–868.

10 Chemonges, S. Effect of intermittent positive pressure ventilation on depth of anesthesia during and after isoflurane anesthesia in Sulphur-Crested cockatoos (Cacatua galerita galerita). *Veterinary Medicine International* 2014;1–7.

11 Muir WW, Hubbel JAE, Bednarski RM, *et al*. Anesthetic procedures in exotic animals. In: *Handbook of Veterinary Anesthesia*, 4th edn. Mosby Elsevier: St. Louis, 2007:438–484.

12 Jaensch SM, Cullen L, Raidal SR. Comparison of endotracheal, caudal thoracic air sac, and clavicular air sac administration of isoflurane in Sulphur-Crested cockatoos (Cacatua galerita). *Journal of Avian Medicine and Surgery* 2001; **15(3)**:170–177.

13 Kramer MH, Harris PJ. Avian blood collection. *Journal of Exotic Pet Medicine* 2010; **19(1)**: 82–86.

14 Nevarez JG. Monitoring during avian and exotic pet anesthesia. *Seminars in Avian and Exotic Pet Medicine* 2005; **14(4)**:277–283.

15 Schmitt PM, Gobel T, Trautvetter E. Evaluation of pulse oximetry as a monitoring method in avian anesthesia. *Journal of Avian Medicine and Surgery* 1998; **12(2)**:91–99.

16 Edling TM, Degernes LA, Flammer K, *et al*. Capnographic monitoring of anesthetized grey parrots receiving intermittent positive pressure ventilation. *Journal of the American Veterinary Medical Association* 2001; **219(12)**:1714–1718.

17 Strunk A, Wilson GH. Avian cardiology. *Veterinary Clinics of North America: Exotic Animal Practice* 2003; **6(1)**:1–28.

18 Zehnder AM, Hawkins MG, Pascoe PJ, *et al.* Evaluation of indirect blood pressure monitoring in awake and anesthetized red-tailed hawks (Buteo jamaicensis): Effects of cuff size, cuff placement, and monitoring equipment. *Veterinary Anesthesia and Analgesia* 2009; **36**: 464–479.

Index

Page numbers in *italics* refer to figures; those in **bold** to tables.

A

abdominal distension, 126, 313, 318
abdominal surgery, 115, 202
abscesses, 202
ACE inhibitors, 3
acepromazine, 3, 33–37, 45, 57–62, 79, 124, 130, 188, 205, 230, 233, 239, 247, 257, **265**, 271, 273, 279, **285**, **286**, 287, 293, 298, 300, 307, 308, 317, 328, 332, 337, **346**
acetaminophen (APAP), 51, 214
acetylcholine (Ach), 53
acetylcholinesterase, 241
acetylcholinesterase inhibitors, 125
acid-base status, 313
acidosis, 97, 264, 265, 277, 278, 284, 313
acromegaly, 289
acupuncture, 217, 310–311
acute respiratory distress syndrome (ARDS), 87, 142
Addison's disease, 77, 297
    see also hypoadrenocorticism
adjunctive therapies, 211
adrenal glands, 294–298
adrenalectomy, 304
Afghan hounds, 328
aggression, 2, 33, 37, 66, 190, **194**, 203–208, 339–340
airway management, 221, 222, 247, 262
airway obstruction, 142, 324
albumin, 65, 68, 269, 269, 270, 272
aldosterone, 296
alfaxalone, 39, 73, 74, 76–77, 80, 87, 90, 91, 103, **104**, 232, 256, 258, 274, 280, **286**, 287, 293, 298, 303, 315, 316, 319, 320, 337
alkalosis, 97, 264, 313
allergies, 2
alpha-1 antagonists, 302
alpha-2 agonists, 33, 36–40, 45, 55, 57, 58, 60, 61, 62, 77, 79, 103, 121, 125, 126, 130, 155, 159, 168, 179, 232, 257, **265**, 271, 273, 279, 286, 287, 291, 293, 296, 298, 300, 317, 338, 339
alveolar collapse, 135
alveolar fluid accumulation, 135
amantadine, 216

amlodipine, 16
amphetamines, 96
amputations, 66, 115, 202
analgesia
    adjunct, 291
    alternative methods of provision, 130
    and alpha-2 agonists, 37–38
    and inhalant anesthetics, 95
    and loco-regional anesthetics, 174, 300, 307
    and orthopedic surgery, 308
    and premedication, 57, 58, 59
    and TIVA, 101, 102, 103, **104**
    by CRI, 163, 164, 166, 167, 169
    definition, 58
    for castrations, 180
    for diabetes mellitus, 300
    for hemoabdomen surgery, 320, 321
    for hyperadrenocorticism, 296
    for hypertension, **127**
    for hyperthyroidism, 293–294
    for IVDD, 318
    for ocular disease, 237
    for pheochromocytoma, 303
    for renal disease, 279
    for urinary tract problems, 283–284, 287–288
    for vomiting patients, 265
    in birds, 357
    in cats, 45, 153, 202, 203, 338
    in herding dogs, 328
    in rabbits and ferrets, 345–346
    in recovery from anesthesia, 188
    local, 309
    multimodal, 211, 212, 217, 306–308, 315
    non-steroidal anti-inflammatory drugs (NSAIDs) for, 51, 58
    opioids for, 47, 60, **62**, 257
    peri-operative, 65, 211, 212, 337
    post-operative, 211–220, 226, 238, 294, 301, 318, 332, 333, 339
    supplemental, 233
    titration, 193
    transdermal, 333–334
analgesic challenge, 205, 208
anaphylactic reactions, 129, 318
anemia, 2, 5, 90, 97, 128, 133, 134, 276, 291, 297, 298, 318

Questions and Answers in Small Animal Anesthesia, First Edition. Edited by Lesley J. Smith.
© 2016 John Wiley & Sons, Inc. Published 2016 by John Wiley & Sons, Inc.